Narrative Intervention Programme

By
Victoria L. Joffe

Illustrations by
Peter Hudspith

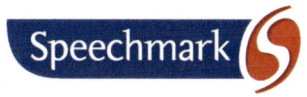
Speechmark

Published by

Speechmark Publishing Ltd, Sunningdale House, 43 Caldecotte Lake Drive, Milton Keynes
MK7 8LF, United Kingdom
Tel: +44 (0)1908 277177   Fax: +44 (0)1908 278297
www.speechmark.net

Reprinted 2012

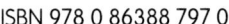**002-5683** /Printed in the United Kingdom by CMP (uk) Limited

British Library Cataloguing in Publication Data
A catalogue record for this book is available from the British Library.

ISBN 978 0 86388 797 0

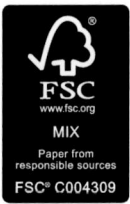

Narrative Intervention Programme

By
Victoria L. Joffe

Speechmark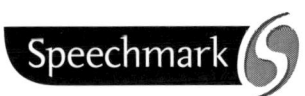

'To be a person is to have
a story to tell.'

Isak Dinesen

Dedication

For my darling mother, Anna Joffe, and in memory of my beloved father, Issy Joffe, and my grandparents Rosa and Barney Kellen and Victoria and Jacob Joffe.

Because of their love and devotion, my own personal narrative is filled with a multitude of happy, inspiring and fulfilling moments and precious memories that will stay with me forever. Thank you.

About the Author

Victoria L. Joffe

Dr Victoria Joffe is a specialist speech and language therapist and Reader in developmental speech, language and communication difficulties in the Department of Language and Communication Science at City University, London. She is programme director of an MSc degree in Joint Professional Practice: Language and Communication, run in conjunction with the Institute of Education, London (www.talklink.org).

Victoria obtained her Honours degree with distinction in Speech and Language Therapy and Audiology in the Department of Speech and Hearing Science, University of the Witwatersrand in South Africa. She obtained her D.Phil degree in the Department of Experimental Psychology, The University of Oxford, UK, exploring the relationship between oral language ability, metalinguistic awareness and literacy in children with speech and language difficulties.

Victoria's expertise is in the area of assessment and intervention of students and young people with developmental speech, language and communication difficulties. She is an experienced teacher and trainer and works with a range of educational and clinical professionals on best practice in enhancing the language, communication and learning of vulnerable students and young people. Victoria runs various workshops for PCT's, LEA's and schools on child speech disorder, evidence based practice in speech and language therapy and collaborative practice in education.

About the Illustrator

Peter Hudspith

Peter Hudspith is an illustrator who produces imaginative, versatile and quick illustrations for a variety of clients, including book publishers, magazines, design groups, advertising agencies and academic establishments across the country. Currently based in Leeds, West Yorkshire, Peter works in both traditional media and digital, to suit the particular job in hand. Peter says about his involvement in the Narrative Intervention Programme: 'I've had enormous fun working with Victoria Joffe on the Narrative Intervention project, which proved to be both challenging and immensely rewarding'. See more of Peter's illustrations by looking at his online gallery at **www.peterhudspith.co.uk.**

Contents

Acknowledgements **1**

Programme background and context **9**

Who are these children with speech, language and communication needs?

Programme overview **13**

Introduction 13

Contextual background to and rationale for the narrative 15
intervention programme

Programme structure 18

Frequently asked questions 22

General strategies that can be used to enhance student
performance and storytelling 29

Session plans **37**

Session 1 . . . . **39**

Teaching notes for Session 1 44

My learning profile 48

Session 2 . . . . **53**

Teaching notes for Session 2 60

Session 3 . . . . **67**

Story train track (no trains) 68

Train carriages 69

Story train track and three carriages 70

Story F1 race track 71

Teaching notes for Session 3 74

Session 4 . . . . **83**

Story football match 88

Story athletics race track 89

Teaching notes for Session 4 90

Session 5 . . . . **93**

Story planner 99

Teaching notes for Session 5 100

Session 6 . . . . **115**

Teaching notes for Session 6 121

Session 7 . . . . **123**

Character word map 130

Teaching notes for Session 7 131

Session 8 . . . . **135**

Character picture cards 142

Teaching notes for Session 8 143

Session 9 . . . . **149**

Session 10 . . . . **157**

    Teaching notes for Session 10 166

    Time word map 171

    Place word map 172

Session 11 . . . . **173**

    Teaching notes for Session 11 180

Session 12 . . . . **193**

    Themed story picture cards 200

    Teaching notes for Session 12 204

Session 13 . . . . **211**

    Teaching notes for Session 13 220

Session 14 . . . . **229**

    Story template form 1 235

    Story template form 2 236

    Teaching notes for Session 14 237

    Range of sequence story cards 242

Session 15 . . . . **245**

    Teaching notes for Session 15 251

Session 16 . . . . **255**

    Teaching notes for Session 16 264

Session 17 . . . . **271**

    Teaching notes for Session 17 276

Session 18 . . . . **299**

    Teaching notes for Session 18 306

Session 19 . . . . **317**

    Teaching notes for Session 19 327

Session 20 . . . . **333**

    My learning profile 340

Session 21 . . . . **347**

    Teaching notes for Session 21 353

References **357**

Appendix 1: Narrative checklist **367**

Appendix 2: An overview of the ELCISS research programme **373**

Acknowledgements

The narrative intervention programme was originally devised by Dr Victoria Joffe from the Department of Language and Communication Science, City University, London as part of a research project funded by the Nuffield Foundation. The research programme was led by Victoria Joffe, the primary investigator, from City University, London. The research team included Nita Madhani, from Redbridge Primary Care Trust, together with Francesca Parker, Emma Dean, Eleni Kotta, Elena Revelas and Clare Lilley from City University, London. The author would like to thank the project team for all their hard work and commitment to the project, as well as the many City University speech and language therapy students and part-time research assistants who were involved in the ELCISS (enhancing language and communication in secondary schools) programme.

The intervention programme was conducted by teaching assistants or learning support assistants[1] in 21 secondary schools in the London boroughs of Redbridge, and Barking and Dagenham. The final intervention programme has been actively shaped by the teaching assistants who participated in the research study and administered the programme to students with speech, language and communication needs (SLCN) in their respective schools. Their comments and involvement has been invaluable and sincerest thanks go to them for their enthusiasm and for showing so clearly the important role that teaching assistants play in the education and support of students with SLCN. The teaching assistants involved were: Amina Ansari; Tanya Bailey; Jean Clarke; Angela Colyer; Denise Day; Jane Dormer; Pat Giles; Hilary Gurden; Doris Guy; Amanda Louise Hahn; Jayne Hart; Tara Low; Anne Marie McDowell; Maggie Millbery; Timea Richards; Jean Roult; Maxine Rowe; Alison Smardina; Tracey Sullivan Sparks; Nicola Stewart; Tricia Turner and Sharon Yates. The passion, commitment and joy that these teaching assistants brought to the programme was truly inspirational.

The author would also like to thank the 21 secondary schools who participated in the study, as well as the school special educational needs coordinators who assisted in the management and delivery of the programme. The schools involved in the project included, from Redbridge: Beal High School; Chadwell Heath Foundation School; Canon Palmer Catholic School; Caterham High School; King Solomon High School; Hainault Forest High School; Loxford School of Science and Technology; Mayfield High School and College; Oaks Park High School; Seven Kings High School; Wanstead High School; Valentines High School; Woodbridge High School, and from Barking and Dagenham: All Saints Catholic School; Barking Abbey School; Dagenham Park Community School; Eastbrook Comprehensive School; Jo Richardson Community High School; Robert Clack School; Sydney Russell School; Warren Comprehensive School.

Valuable support was also provided by the speech and language therapy teams and staff from the local education authorities from Redbridge, and Barking and Dagenham. Particular thanks go to Nita Madhani, Melanie Foster, Annita Cornish, Michelle Meston, Debbie Reith, Karen Powell, Karen

---

[1] The term teaching assistant (TA) will be used throughout the programme.

 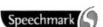

Wright, Glinette Woods and Ann Jones. An advisory team consisting of Mary Hartshorne, Professor Charles Hulme, Elspelh McCartney, Professor Tim Pring, Debbie Reith and Karen Wright gave great support and encouragement throughout the life of this research programme, and their input is greatly appreciated. On the sidelines, Professor Maggie Snowling was a great support and advisor.

The ELCISS programme was funded by the Nuffield Foundation, and many thanks go to them for their continued support and enthusiasm throughout the project. Financial contributions to the programme were also provided by the Redbridge, and Barking and Dagenham Local Education Authorities. A pilot study which shaped the thinking of this research was funded by the Toyne Baby Triathlon and Afasic. Additional funding for the whole school teacher training element of the work was provided by The Communication Trust.

This research and the development of my ideas took place while working in the Department of Language and Communication Science, City University, London. I thank my colleagues for all their support and encouragement and the University for providing me with such a rich and fertile ground in which to develop and prosper.

Many thanks go to my family and friends who had to 'endure' hearing a lot about this programme and kept their interest and support throughout. A special thank you must go to my 'international copyright manager', otherwise known as my dearest uncle, Teddy Kellen, who 'walks with me'.

Final and most important thanks and acknowledgement must go to all the secondary school students who participated in the programme, and to their parents for giving their consent. It has been a joy and privilege to work with them all. Their stories, and the enthusiasm and passion with which they shared them, have enriched all our lives.

Excerpt acknowledgements

I would like to thank the following for permission to reproduce material for this publication:
Excerpts from ANIMAL FARM by George Orwell, copyright 1946 by Harcourt, Inc. and renewed 1974 by Sonia Orwell, reprinted by permission of Houghton Mifflin Harcourt Publishing Company.

Animal Farm by George Orwell (Copyright © George Orwell, 1945) Reprinted by permission of Bill Hamilton as the Literary Executor of the Estate of the Late Sonia Brownell Orwell and Secker & Warburg Ltd.

Excerpts from My Darling, My Hamburger by Paul Zindel, published by Bodley Head. Used by permission of The Random House Group Ltd.

My Darling, My Hamburger by Paul Zindel (1978). COPYRIGHT © 1969 PAUL ZINDEL. Used by permission of HarperCollins Publishers.

The Murder of Roger Ackroyd. by Agatha Christie. Reprinted by permission of HarperCollins Publishers Ltd. © (1993) (Agatha Christie).
Long Walk to Freedom. The Autobiography of Nelson Mandela by Nelson Mandela. Used by permission of Little, Brown Book Group © (1994) Nelson Mandela.

Excerpts from THE NO 1 LADIES' DETECTIVE AGENCY by Alexander McCall Smith, published by Abacus. Reprinted by permission of Random House Inc.

Reprinted with permission of David Higham Associates Ltd:
The No 1 Ladies' Detective Agency by Alexander McCall Smith (2003).

Reprinted with the permission of Atheneum Books for Young Readers, an imprint of Simon & Schuster Children's Publishing Division from ARE YOU THERE GOD? IT'S ME, MARGARET by Judy Blume. Copyright © 1970 Judy Blume.

Approximately 248 words from ARE YOU THERE GOD? IT'S ME, MARGARET by Judy Blume (Hamish Hamilton, 1997) Copyright (c) Judy Blume, 1997. Reproduced by permission of Penguin Books Ltd.

From MATILDA by Roald Dahl, copyright (c) 1988 by Roald Dahl. Used by permission of Puffin Books, A Division of Penguin Young Readers Group, A Member of Penguin Group (USA) Inc., 345 Hudson Street, New York, NY 10014. All rights reserved.

Excerpt from Matilda by Roald Dahl.
Reprinted by permission of David Higham Associates Ltd. © (1988). Roald Dahl.

With thanks to Thomas Howells for use of Ireland. *Blue Guide* by Brain Lalor (1998).

Extract from Pippi Longstocking by Astrid Lindgren translated by Edna Hurup, (OUP, 2002), copyright © Salkraken AB/Astrid Lindgren 1945, translation copyright © Oxford University Press 1954, reprinted by permission of Oxford University Press.

Approximately 279 words from THE DIARY OF A YOUNG GIRL: THE DEFINITIVE EDITION by Anne Frank, edited by Otto H Frank and Mirjam Pressier, translated by Susan Massotty (Viking, 1997) copyright © The Anne Frank-Fonds, Basle, Switzerland, 1991. English translation copyright © Doubleday a division of Bantam Doubleday Dell Publishing Group Inc, 1995.
Reproduced by permission of Penguin Books Ltd.

From THE DIARY OF A YOUNG GIRL: THE DEFINITIVE EDITION by Anne Frank, edited by Otto H Frank and Mirjam Pressier, translated by Susan Massotty, translation copyright © 1995 by Doubleday, a division of Random House, Inc. Used by permission of Doubleday, a division of Random House, Inc.

Excerpts from The Old Man and the Sea by Ernest Hemingway, published by Jonathan Cape.
Reprinted by permission of The Random House Group Ltd.

Reprinted with the permission of Scribner, a Division of Simon & Schuster, Inc., from THE OLD MAN AND THE SEA by Ernest Hemingway. Copyright © 1952 by Ernest Hemingway. Copyright renewed © 1980 by Mary Hemingway. All rights reserved.
Excerpts from TO KILL A MOCKINGBIRD by Harper Lee, published by William Heinemann. Reprinted by permission of The Random House Group Ltd.

Brief quotes from pp.5 (101 words), 6 (63 words) from TO KILL A MOCKINGBIRD by HARPER LEE Copyright (c) 1960 by Harper Lee; renewed (c) 1988 by Harper Lee. Foreward copyright (c) 1993 by Harper Lee.
Reprinted by permission of HarperCollins Publishers

Excerpts from *Charlie and the Chocolate Factory* by Roald Dahl, published by Random House Children's Books.
Reprinted by permission of David Higham Associates Ltd © (2007). Roald Dahl.

From CHARLIE AND THE CHOCOLATE FACTORY by Roald Dahl, text copyright © 1964, renewed 1992 by Roald Dahl Nominee Limited. Used by permission of Alfred A. Knopf, an imprint of Random House Children's Books, a division of Random House, Inc.

Excerpts from *Anne of Green Gables* are reproduced here with the authorization of Heirs of L. M. Montgomery Inc.

Anne of Green Gables and other indicia of "Anne" are trademarks and Canadian official marks of the Anne of Green Gables Licensing Authority Inc.

L.M. Montgomery is a trademark of Heirs of L.M. Montgomery Inc.

Excerpt from Born to Run by Michael Morpurgo, published by HarperCollins Children's Books. Reprinted by permission of David Higham Associates Ltd © (2007).Michael Morpurgo.

Born to Run By Michael Morpurgo
Reprinted by permission of HarperCollins Publishers Ltd
© (2007) (Michael Morpurgo)

Excerpts from Holes by Louis Sachar
Reprinted by permission of Bloomsbury © (2000).Louis Sachar.

Reprinted by permission of Farrar, Straus and Giroux, LLC:
Excerpts from HOLES by Louis Sachar. Copyright © 1998 by Louis Sachar.

Excerpt from The Twits by Roald Dahl, published by Random House Children's Books. Reprinted by permission of David Higham Associates Ltd. © (1980). Roald Dahl.

From THE TWITS by Roald Dahl, text copyright © 1980 by Roald Dahl Nominee Limited. Used by permission of Random House Children's Books, a division of Random House, Inc.

Jonathon Livingston Seagull. A Story by Richard Bach. Reprinted by permission of HarperCollins Publishers Ltd. © (1973) (Richard Bach)

Spells by Aprilynne Pike
Used by permission of HarperCollins Publishers. © (2010) Aprilynne Pike.

Spells by Aprilynne Pike
Used by permission of HarperCollins Publishers Ltd. © (2010) Aprilynne Pike.

Reproduced from **Snatched, by Graham Marks** by permission of Usborne Publishing, 83-85 Saffron Hill, London EC1N 8RT, UK.
Copyright © 2006.Usborne Publishing Ltd.
Excerpt from Buried Alive by Jacqueline Wilson, published by Doubleday.
Reprinted by permission of David Higham Associates Ltd. © (1999). Jacqueline Wilson.

Excerpts from *Buried Alive* by Jacqueline Wilson, published by Doubleday. Reprinted by permission of The Random House Group Ltd.

Excerpts from THE BOY IN THE STRIPED PYJAMAS by John Boyne, published by David Fickling Books. Reprinted by permission of The Random House Group Ltd.

 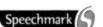

From THE BOY IN THE STRIPED PYJAMAS by John Boyne, copyright © 2006 by John Boyne. Used by permission of David Fickling Books, an imprint of Random House Children's Books, a division of Random House, Inc.

Excerpt from *The Witches* by Roald Dahl.
Reprinted by permission of David Higham Associates Ltd. © (1983). Roald Dahl.

Reprinted by permission of Farrar, Straus and Giroux, LLC:
Excerpt from THE WITCHES by Roald Dahl, illustrations by Quentin Blake. Copyright © 1983 by Roald Dahl.

Excerpts from *James and the Giant Peach* by Roald Dahl, published by Random House Children's Books.
Reprinted by permission of David Higham Associates Ltd. © (1961). Roald Dahl.

From JAMES AND THE GIANT PEACH by Roald Dahl, text copyright © 1961, renewed 1989 by Roald Dahl. Used by permission of Alfred A. Knopf, an imprint of Random House Children's Books, a division of Random House, Inc.

Cards on the Table By Agatha Christie
Reprinted by permission of HarperCollins Publishers Ltd
© (2001) (Agatha Christie)

With thanks to Cartland Promotions for use of *A Castle of Dreams* by Barbara Cartland (2009).

"Matilda, Who Told Lies" by Hilaire Belloc from *Cautionary Tales for Children* (© Hilaire Belloc 1907) is reproduced by permission of PFD (www.pfd.co.uk) on behalf of the Estate of Hilaire Belloc.
"Kidnapped!" from A LIGHT IN THE ATTIC by Shel Silverstein. © 1981 Evil Eye, Music. By permission of Edite Kroll Literary Agency Inc.

"Kidnapped" from A LIGHT IN THE ATTIC by SHEL SILVERSTEIN
COPYRIGHT © 1981 EVIL EYE MUSIC, LLC.
Used by permission of HarperCollins Publishers.

"Walking Away" from The Complete Poems by C Day Lewis published by Sinclair-Stevenson (1992)
Copyright © 1992 in this edition The Estate of C Day Lewis. Reprinted by permission of The Random House Group Ltd.

'Gust Becos I Could Not Spel'
Copyright © 1985 Brian Patten Reproduced by permission of the author c/o Rogers, Coleridge & White Ltd., 20 Powis Mews, London W11 1JN.

With thanks to The Society of Authors as the literary representative of the Estate of Alfred Noyes for use of *The Highwayman* by Alfred Noyes (1996).

'Chocs'. By Carol Ann Duffy, from T*he Nation's Favourite Poems of Childhood* (2000), p. 101.
With thanks to Jenny Joseph for use of the poem 'Warning' (1996).
Reprinted by permission of David Higham Associates Ltd:
'I saw a jolly hunter' by Charles Causley, from *The Nation's Favourite Twentieth Century Poems*.
Edited by Griff Rhys-Jones (1999).

"The Road Not Taken" from The Poetry of Robert Frost edited by Edward Connery Lathem, published by Jonathan Cape. Reprinted by permission of The Random House Group Ltd.

Every effort has been made to trace copyright holders. We would be grateful to hear from any copyright holders not here acknowledged.

 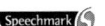

Programme background and context

Who are these children with speech, language and communication needs (SLCN)[2] ?

Children typically acquire and develop language effortlessly without any formal instruction. However, there are some children who experience difficulties learning language without any obvious reasons.

Approximately 7 per cent of primary school children are identified with primary or specific speech, language and communication difficulties (SLCD) (Tomblin *et al*, 1997). This diagnosis is made when the child shows speech, language and/or communication problems which cannot be explained by other reasons, such as an obvious brain injury, environmental or social deprivation or as part of a more global general learning difficulty. Children with other difficulties, including hearing loss, a general learning difficulty, autism, cerebral palsy, Down syndrome or other developmental impairments will also have speech, language and communication needs (SLCN). SLCD are the most prominent special educational needs in primary school children (DfES, 2006). There is far less information available about prevalence rates in secondary schools, but a recent estimate given by Marilyn Nippold is that at least 10 per cent of adolescents have language and communication difficulties severe enough to restrict their ability to express themselves verbally (Nippold, 2010a).

SLCD[3] have been shown to impact adversely on academic and educational performance (Conti-Ramsden *et al*, 2009; Durkin *et al*, 2009; Snowling *et al*, 2001) as well as on broader aspects of development including behaviour (Botting and Conti-Ramsden, 2000; Lindsay and Dockrell, 2000) and social and emotional functioning (Durkin and Conti-Ramsden 2007; Lindsay *et al*, 2008a; Snowling *et al*, 2006; Wadman *et al*, 2011).

Let us consider for a moment what we mean by **language**. Language is a complex system of arbitrary signs which are combined in specific rule-governed ways to form words, phrases and sentences. These signs can take the form of sounds (**speech**), written symbols (text), hand movements (sign language) or raised dots (Braille). The primary role of language is **communication**.

---

[2] For further discussion and information around speech, language and communication, and working with children with SLCN in the classroom, refer to the Primary and Secondary Inclusion Development Programme: Teaching and supporting pupils with speech, language and communication needs. Department for Education: Crown Copyright 2010

[3] SLCD and SLCN are used interchangeably in this resource.

 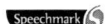

Language is only one of the possible ways for us to communicate. We use systems other than language to relate to and interact with each other and to communicate, for example, body language. By looking at someone with a certain facial expression, one can easily communicate a number of different feelings; anger, disapproval or happiness.

All languages have four main components:

- **sounds** (phonology)
- **grammar** (syntax – the rules)
- **meaning** (semantics – vocabulary)
- **social use of language** (pragmatics).

Effective communication requires an integration of all four of these components. Children with SLCD can experience difficulties with any or all of these four components of language.

Children with SLCD may have difficulties with their speech, including the correct pronunciation of **sounds**, and combining sounds to form syllables and words. They may experience particular problems in pronouncing more complex longer words, for example, multisyllabic words – words with more than two syllables, such as 'hippopotamus' or 'conservation'. Difficulties with the sound system can also lead to problems with literacy when students have to convert the grapheme (letter) into the phoneme (sound) for reading; and the phoneme into the grapheme for writing.

Difficulties with speech may include problems with fluency where speech appears to be hesitant and non-fluent with frequent sound, syllable or word repetitions, or blocks where the child appears unable to get the correct sound or word out.

Children with speech difficulties may also have problems processing sounds in order to understand what is being said.

Problems can also be seen in **grammar**, with difficulties using morphemes (the smallest unit of meaning), for example, to indicate tense – using the incorrect 'catched' for 'caught', as well as problems putting words together to form sentences and build conversations. Children with speech, language and communication needs (SLCN) can struggle particularly with forming more complex sentences, for example, using conjunctions like 'because', 'although', and 'however'.

Problems with **meaning** and semantics involve difficulties in understanding and using words to describe the world around them, finding the correct word and using more complex idiomatic language. Difficulties in semantics may manifest in word finding difficulties, with students struggling to find the target word and overusing general non-specific words like 'thing' and 'stuff' and using conversation fillers such as 'um' and 'er'. Students with semantic difficulties may also show a reduced vocabulary and the words they do have in their repertoire can typically be very literal and limited to very specific items. For example, the word 'sweet' will be used to indicate a tasty snack that one buys from the newsagent, but not be extended to describe the chocolate mousse dessert eaten as the last course of dinner. There will also be less understanding of this word in a more figurative sense, i.e. to indicate the personality of a man, for example, 'the sweet-natured man'. Children with SLCD can also experience problems understanding idiomatic and figurative language and their understanding can be very literal, for example, misunderstanding common idiomatic expressions like 'feeling blue' and being confused by the lack of any blue colouring on the person using this expression. They may also have very rigid understandings of words, for example, understanding the meaning of the word 'jacket' as an item of clothing, but being unable then to accept the term, 'jacket potato' as a food item, or even that people may use the word 'jacket' and 'coat' interchangeably.

Problems with **pragmatics** involve the way children use language. Pragmatic difficulties include problems in interacting with others and/or misunderstanding the rules of communication. This is evident when students use language inappropriately, for example, they may use the same language when talking to their peers and head teacher, not understanding the need to change language depending on the listener. They may also show difficulties maintaining eye contact, either not looking at a person they are talking to at all, or staring in too intense a manner, as well as an inability to start or end a conversation appropriately. Pragmatics also includes choosing the most appropriate words, and the use and interpretation of appropriate non-verbal language (facial expression and body language) to communicate effectively. For example, some children may use incongruent language and facial expressions, such as smiling while talking about a sad event. Difficulties with idiomatic language will also result in problems with pragmatics as children will misunderstand common phrases and are more likely to take the literal interpretation, for example, physically pulling their socks up when told to 'pull your socks up'.

Children with SLCD may show problems in all of these components. All these difficulties can involve the understanding (reception) and expression of language. Students with language problems may also have difficulties with attention, concentration and listening. They also may experience difficulties with memory. All these difficulties can impede learning across all subjects in school and make social interaction more difficult.

Some SLCD are easily identifiable and noticed in the classroom, for example stammering, or a speech problem. However, some are more difficult to identify, for example, difficulties in the understanding of language, and these may go unnoticed or be misdiagnosed. These children can be labelled as naughty, lazy or disruptive.

It is important to remember that children with SLCN are a very heterogeneous group and present with different strengths and areas of need. Rarely will they present with the same pattern of difficulties and strengths. Even when delivering a set programme such as this one, it is important to

 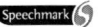

tailor it appropriately to the level of ability of the child. Try asking the child directly what they think their strengths and areas of need are, as this is often helpful in pinpointing more precisely what the focus needs to be.

Programme overview

The narrative intervention programme

Introduction

The focus of this intervention programme is on enhancing the understanding and facilitating the expression of narratives or stories in students with varied SLCN in the later primary years and in secondary schools. It has been piloted on a group of 12–13-year old secondary school students and has been found to be effective in improving the storytelling skills of this age group. The programme was delivered by teaching assistants in groups of between two and six children within the school environment.

Specific aims of the narrative intervention programme are to:

- Introduce the concept of narratives and identify their role and use in language, communication and social interaction.

- Identify different types of narratives and provide examples for each type.

- Explore the behaviours associated with effective active listening and attention.

- Understand and use different means of making story production more interesting through vocal variety, facial expression, body language and print.

- Introduce the structure of narratives using the story planner: beginning (setting), middle (episode/s), end (final outcome).

- Explore characterisation and identify different appearances, feelings and behaviours of characters.

- Set the mood and overall ethos of the story through descriptions of setting, particularly time and place.

- Understand the main components of the middle or body of a story and identify ways of making the story more exciting through choice of plot, themes, climax and resolutions.

- Consider different ways of ending a story through integration of main strands of the story and providing a moral, food for thought, cliffhanger or whetting of the appetite for the next instalment.

- Understand the sequential nature of storytelling with a focus on story sequencing.

- Identify and use a variety of literary devices to enhance storytelling, including rhyme, rhythm,

 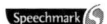

13

repetition, alliteration, personification, double meanings, onomatopoeia and hyperbole.

- Differentiate prose and poetry and explore the narrative poem and limerick in more detail.

- Practise listening and telling stories with a focus on different parts of story structure. This may include the reading and writing of stories where appropriate.

- Evaluate stories produced – own and others'.

- Facilitate and enhance the wonder and enjoyment of storytelling.

- Create an awareness of how storytelling can be used to enhance learning in school; and in social interactions in school and home environments.

- Identify ways of using the story planner to structure homework and essays in all lessons and in exam conditions.

Contextual background to and rationale for the narrative intervention programme

Why narratives?

This programme focuses on enhancing the understanding and expression of narratives or stories. Narrative (storytelling) is an important skill that is an integral part of all our lives. We use stories in our everyday lives to interact with others, form bonds and friendships, explain, excuse, express our innermost feelings, describe, understand and structure our lives. We use stories to help us make sense of the world and to organise our experiences (Meek, 1991). Think for a moment how many times today you have already shared your experiences in some way with others through storytelling. Children typically begin to use stories at a very early age (Applebee, 1978; Peterson, 1990) and are exposed to stories through many different mediums, including books, comics, magazines, children's stories, computer games and imagery, story songs, cinema and television. All cultures use stories to some degree to share experiences and relay familial and cultural history (Meek, 1991).

Stories have a definite structure to them and are sequentially organised into related units (Naremore et al, 1995). A story usually has a clear beginning, middle and end, with a coherent plot, different characters and some type of conflict, problem or main event, climax and resolution. The elements of a story are related to each other temporally and/or causally.

Storytelling can prove challenging to some students as it makes heavy demands on receptive (understanding) and expressive language, requiring more complex syntax (grammar) and semantics (meaning), abstract and imaginative thinking and general knowledge. The art of listening to, understanding and telling stories draws upon a multitude of linguistic and cognitive skills. It draws upon all elements of language and communication (attention, listening, phonology, morphology, syntax, semantics, pragmatics) as well as requiring a general knowledge of events and awareness about the world around us, short and long-term memory and sequencing abilities, an understanding of time and causality, insight into people and typical social interactions, an understanding and insight into feelings and behaviours, and some knowledge of the cultural conventions of storytelling.

Storytelling is a skill required both in the oral and written modalities in school, and its presence is ubiquitous across most subject areas of the educational curriculum in all years of study. Working on storytelling provides students with an opportunity to practise and develop language, communication and language-related skills like attention, listening and memory and social skills, which can enhance and facilitate students' access to the educational curriculum and help improve their social interactions.

Storytelling has been shown to be closely related to educational performance and is a good early predictor of later language ability and educational attainment (Bishop and Adams, 1990; Bishop and Edmundson, 1987; Fazio *et al*, 1996; Stothard *et al*, 1998). Exposure to storytelling in the home and classroom was also found to be an important determinant of literacy development (Wells, 1986).

Narrative ability is not only an important part of educational attainment, but can also play a significant role in the social and emotional development of students. It serves a role in social settings as a means of sharing common experiences, gaining peer group acceptance and forming friendships. Stories can act as a means of linking students to the social life of school and can be used as an opportunity to connect to others and explore relationships (Mello, 2001).

One of the best aspects of working on narratives is that children tend to enjoy the process of telling stories and see it as a FUN activity. They see it as being 'entertaining', 'funny', 'cool' and a help for making information 'interesting' (Mello, 2001).

Considering the complex requirements of storytelling, it is unsurprising that individuals with SLCN have been found to have significant difficulties with telling stories (Liles, 1993; Liles *et al*, 1995; Merritt and Liles, 1987; Van der Lely, 1997). These difficulties are found in the understanding of stories and in telling and writing stories. Students with language difficulties can experience difficulties telling stories that are well structured and coherent. They can also experience difficulties listening and attending to stories, which impacts on their overall understanding.

This intervention programme aims to support and develop SLCN students' understanding and telling of stories.

Why secondary schools?

> **'Many parents reported that services tended to "disappear" over time, especially...on transfer to secondary school. Indeed we found minimal evidence of services for young people at secondary school and beyond.'**
>
> (Bercow, 2008, p37)

Research into typical language development is predominantly focused on early preschool and primary development. However it is well accepted that language continues to develop in complexity and abstractness throughout adolescence and into adulthood (Nippold, 1998, 2007). This focus on early language development mirrors the clinical and educational research activities with limited research on older children and adolescent language and communication impairment. There is also a significant gap in specialist educational and speech and language therapy support for older students in schools with SLCN, with a UK government-led review reporting 'a significant lack of secondary school services' (Bercow, 2008, p105).

It would be misguided to assume from this that children's early SLCN disappear once they reach secondary school. Studies following up primary school children with SLCN show that many of their difficulties are pervasive and long term, and continue into secondary school and adulthood (Beitchman *et al*, 2001; Clegg *et al*, 2005; Johnson *et al*, 2010; Snowling *et al*, 2001; Snowling *et al*, 2006; Stothard *et al*, 1998). The impact of these difficulties is significant and far reaching, not only affecting the young person's language, literacy and academic performance, but can be more widespread with the young person with SLCN at risk of developing problems with poor self-esteem, lack of friendships and social, emotional and behavioural difficulties (Botting and Conti-Ramsden, 2000; Durkin and Conti-Ramsden, 2007; Johnson *et al*, 2010; Lindsay and Dockrell, 2000; Wadman *et al*, 2008; Wadman *et al*, 2011).

A significant proportion of children and young people in secondary school in the UK with special educational needs have SLCN as their primary need (Bercow, 2008). Some children and young people may manage reasonably well in primary education, but experience more difficulties in secondary school as the linguistic demands of secondary school become more complex (Nippold, 2004). Many young people with SLCN are educated in mainstream schools with at least two children in each class having some type of SLCN (Lindsay *et al*, 2008b). Teaching and support staff are, however, given little support on how to meet the needs of these students (Dockrell and Lindsay, 2001). There has been a widespread call both in the UK and worldwide from researchers, practitioners (speech and language therapists and teachers) and government reports to increase the support to secondary school students with SLCN and to the professionals working with them. (Bercow, 2008; Cirrin and Gillam, 2008; Joffe, 2006; Joffe, 2008; Joffe *et al*, 2008; Law *et al*, 2000; Nippold, 2010b; Sievers, 2005; Snow and Powell, 2004).

The paucity of clinical research in this area, the long-term nature of language and communication difficulties and the rigorous demands of secondary school justify increasing specialist and educational support in the older primary and secondary school student. This intervention programme was designed for the older primary and secondary school-aged student with SLCN and therefore fills an important gap in educational and clinical provision. The programme was designed to be delivered by teachers, speech and language therapists, teaching support staff or speech and language therapy assistants with support by a speech and language therapist.

Programme structure

Session details

The narrative programme comprises of 21 sessions of approximately 50–60 minutes in duration. Each session has a detailed session plan which includes aims and activities for the session, the methods used to achieve the aims, and the materials needed to undertake the therapeutic activities. There is also the opportunity at the end of each session plan to record the results of each activity, i.e. details about the students' performance, how the session went and any other comments or observations you may have. It is very important to record results of the session immediately after each session to ensure that we are able to evaluate the programme and the students' progress and responses to the intervention. It is useful to evaluate the performance of the child and the success of the task, as well as your own performance. This triad of evaluation (teaching assistant, teacher, therapist, student and task) ensures an in-depth evaluation of the programme. It is a good idea to read the comments from the previous session before the next session as this will remind you about student progress and what aspects need more or less focus.

There are teaching notes at the end of the session plans which provide further details of the activities and give additional examples of games and activities that can be used to meet the aims of that session. Most of the pictorial materials are included in this resource in the accompanying DVD, but you will need to bring some additional objects, and do some preparation before the session, for example, photocopying some sheets from the teaching notes to use with students during the session, or bringing some examples of different stories. Some activities require the sheets to be cut up into sections which can then be used to play various games with the group. It is advisable to familiarise yourself with the whole programme before it begins, and thereafter to read each session plan the day before the session so you feel prepared and have everything you need to conduct the session successfully.

Each session has a specific structure and all sessions begin and end in the same way. At the start, there is always a review of what was covered in the previous session and what will be covered in the current session. It is a good idea to encourage the students to summarise what was done in the previous session as this helps to jog their memories and direct their attention to the current session. Their recollections of the previous session will also give you an idea of how much information from the previous session has been retained and at what level to begin the current session. All sessions end with a review and summary of what was completed. Again, it is always best to get the students themselves to end the session by summarising the main points that they have learned. If main points are omitted, they can be added by the teacher, therapist or teaching assistant. Each session also includes a 'Mission to Achieve' task to ensure carryover into school and home. This is a homework activity and was termed a 'Mission to Achieve' by the students involved in the programme who preferred this term to that of homework! Time should be given at the beginning of each session to discuss the homework from the previous session and talk about any materials that the students have brought with them to the session.

The original programme consisted of 18 sessions (with 18 session plans) and was delivered three times per week on alternative days (Monday, Wednesday and Friday) over a six-week period, by teaching assistants in groups of two to six children. The programme has been adapted in response to the feedback from the participants and it has been extended to 21 sessions. While the teaching assistants were encouraged to cover all session aims within the duration of each session, and ensure that each session was completed as an entity, they were also encouraged to respond to the groups' needs, which meant that there were times when there was a need to provide more examples and spend more time on some areas. This was appropriate and was encouraged. There are a sufficient number of different examples graded in difficulty to allow for this flexibility and ensure this programme is carried out as instructed while still meeting the individual needs of the students. Please provide as many examples as you feel necessary and go as slowly or as quickly as you feel meets the needs of the majority of the students in your group. Ensure that there is a good understanding of each concept before moving on to the next level.

It is important to make the sessions as fun as possible so that the students want to attend each session. Students should be given a lot of positive reinforcement and encouragement and feel that they are achieving something at each session. Try as much as possible to ignore bad behaviour or lack of participation, and make a fuss of more positive behaviours and good attention and active participation. Your school may have some form of reward system through house points or other forms of reward. If so, it is an excellent idea to encourage participation in the sessions by awarding these points for good group membership and active and positive participation in the session. We want these sessions to help build confidence and rewarding positive behaviour and good performance will greatly facilitate this.

The intervention resource contains most of the materials needed to administer the programme. You will need to provide pens and paper for use by the students. A flipchart or whiteboard is also really useful if you have access to one. Please also photocopy as many of the worksheets as you need for each session.

The resource contains:
- Detailed session plans with teaching notes for 21 sessions.
- A DVD with the following pictures, templates and frameworks:
  - ❑ A variety of cards signifying settings: character, time and place cards
  - ❑ Action picture cards representing various story episodes
  - ❑ Themed story picture cards
  - ❑ A series of sequence stories graded in difficulty
  - ❑ One 4-card sequence story
  - ❑ Two 5-card sequence stories
  - ❑ One 7-card sequence story

- ❑ One 8-card sequence story
- ❑ One 10-card sequence story
- ❑ One 11-card sequence story.
- Story planner
- Story Formula One (F1) race track
- Story football match
- Story athletics race track
- Story train track and train carriages
- Character word map
- Place word map
- Time word map
- Story template form 1
- Story template form 2.

You will also need to provide the following:

- Objects which will be used to facilitate story production. The following seven objects were used effectively in the research programme, but you may like to add your own ideas, and also those of your students.
  - ❑ Plaster
  - ❑ Train ticket
  - ❑ Part of a map (torn)
  - ❑ Lock and key
  - ❑ Whistle
  - ❑ Money
  - ❑ Battery.
- A story pencil or microphone – the person in the group holding the story pencil or microphone is the person who has the floor, i.e. the person who tells the story, continues the story. In the programme we will refer to the story pencil as this is what we used in the original programme. You might like to encourage the children to make their own microphones, or objects which signify that it is their turn to tell parts of or the entire story. This could then develop into an interesting discussion on the importance of turn taking, which is one of the aims of the programme.
- It is a good idea to provide each student with their own folder where they can keep the list of group rules, student learning profile, photocopies, story examples and any other resources from the session.

Some general underlying principles of the programme

- Make explicit the aims and learning objectives of the programme, including reasons for their participation. It is important that students understand why they are involved in this programme, what the aims are and how a greater knowledge of narratives will help their communication and general performance in school and in social settings.

- Discuss with the students the role and impact of language and communication so that they understand how important listening and speaking are to every aspect of their lives.

- Encourage self-generated aims, targets and outcomes. Students should be encouraged to generate their own aims and targets for the programme. These should then be revisited at the end of the programme to assess the outcomes of the programme from the perspective of the student as well as facilitate the planning of future goals. Discuss with students how they will know when they have achieved their targets. This will ensure that the outcomes are meaningful and functional.

- Continually make time for the evaluation of strengths and areas of need, both self (student) and other (their peers). Each session consists of opportunities for self-reflection and self and other evaluation. Evaluation is a key skill and will help students identify the features of active listening, what makes an interesting story and a powerful storyteller.

- Focus at all times on facilitation and elicitation of language. It is important to try at all times to provide an environment where students feel comfortable listening and telling stories and working on their language and communication. Emphasis should be placed on eliciting as much language from the students as possible, rather than taking all the work on you as the facilitator. If the student is experiencing problems with the task, try and break it down or make it easier in some way, for example, using the sequence cards, or giving the student an example. This will help facilitate the student to actively participate in the programme and will help successfully elicit the behaviours you require.

- Always emphasise independent thinking and problem resolution. It is important that students are encouraged to actively participate in all sessions and use the skills and strategies taught to them. At all times, the use of strategies should be explained to students and made explicit, so that they understand why they are helpful and how they can be used in other environments when the trainer is not with them. This is essential for successful carryover into school and home environments and will help the student become an independent learner.

- This programme encourages group interaction skills at all times. Emphasise the importance of working in a group and encourage the group to generate group rules at the start of the programme. These rules should include respect, integrity, acceptance, flexibility and confidentiality. It is interesting to see how much more motivated the students are to keep to the rules when they themselves have generated them.

- Try to always ensure that the examples and tasks you give are relevant and applicable to the student's life. This is the only way to maintain motivation and positive engagement and will support the transfer and generalisation of skills. It is imperative that students are made aware at all times of the relevance of the work you are doing to their lives, both school and home.

 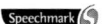

When they can see the relevance and application of what they are doing, their motivation and commitment is ever present. See what happens when you get the students to consider how becoming an effective storyteller will help them in the playground, get a date, get the job they wanted, etc.

- Always emphasise functional outcomes. Ensure that what you include in the sessions, your examples and activities, are functional and based as much as possible on the student's own lives, interests and perspectives. Encourage them to think about how to tell a story that explains why they were late for class, for example.

Frequently asked questions

1 Who can deliver the programme?

The original programme was delivered by teaching assistants supported by speech and language therapists. The TAs were given four-days training in speech, language and communication, in working with children with SLCN and in delivering the two interventions[4] . You will note that the programme consists of detailed session plans and has in-depth teaching notes, as well as a detailed introduction around principles of the programme and recommended strategies to successfully elicit the language and story structures required. It is therefore possible for TAs and speech and language therapy assistants to deliver this programme in schools, supported by teachers, specialist teachers or speech and language therapists. It is important for teaching assistants to read through the programme carefully, including the introduction. It is essential that there is someone available that they can consult about any questions they may have regarding working with children with SLCN.

The programme can also be delivered by teachers, specialist teachers and speech and language therapists, as well as by other professionals working with children with SLCN. Some parents of the children who participated in the original project have asked whether they could use it with their children, as they felt it fitted in well with activities that were taking place in the home environment. The session plans and overall programme are written in sufficient detail to make this possible. It is advisable, however, for parents to consult the professionals working with their children to ensure they receive the necessary support, as well as ensure that all the support structures given to the child are complementary. It is also important to check that the students are happy for their parents to be involved at this level. What frequently occurred in the pilot project was that students took home many of the templates from this programme to help support their homework, for example the story planner and word maps. This is a very good idea and supports the transfer of knowledge and learning into the home and school environments. It is the hope that this intervention programme will be the springboard to a rich and extended programme of narrative development used in schools by a range of professionals to facilitate language and communication, and assist the students in accessing the curriculum.

---

[4] In the ELCISS research the TAs were trained to deliver two interventions, the narrative programme and the vocabulary enrichment programme.

2 Who is this programme suitable for?

The original programme was devised for secondary school-aged students and was delivered to year 8 and year 9 secondary school students with SLCN (ages 11–13 years). The pictures and tasks have been devised particularly for the older child in response to the limited materials available for this age group. The programme would be suitable for all students in secondary school as well as the older primary school years, from around 8 years of age. The content areas are appropriate for children in primary and secondary school, and can be adapted to different levels of ability and age. The content areas have been chosen with a particular relevance to curriculum subjects, and with a strong emphasis on functional communication and facilitation of independent learning. The suitability of this programme will depend on individual ability and interests. It is flexible enough to be used in different ways with different age and ability groups across different countries.

While the programme has been specifically devised for children with SLCN, it is important to remember that the strategies and tasks are based on 'quality first teaching' and the content of the programme covers much of the general content of the educational curriculum. Therefore many of you might find parts of the programme beneficial for use in the classroom when teaching and supporting all students. In this respect, the programme will be adapted more flexibly and it is conceivable that not every session will be used, but the most applicable sessions will be incorporated and used in the general lesson.

3 Does the programme need to be delivered in full to each student?

The programme has been written up as 21 separate intervention sessions which form a coherent programme for narrative development. The sessions are closely related to each other and are progressive in that they build on previous skills and knowledge. It is preferable that it is delivered in full in this format, and in this order, although at the same time, it is important that individual needs of the students are taken into account. Thus it may be the case that students need more than one session to consolidate all the information contained in one of the sessions, and if this is the case, a session can be extended into more than one if appropriate, with further expansion and examples provided. Similarly, if you are working with a more able group who show some knowledge in the area, you may decide to either combine two sessions into one lesson, or to add additional and more difficult examples.

4 How long does the programme take to complete and how frequently should the sessions be given?

The original project consisted of 18 sessions which were conducted over a six-week period with three sessions delivered on alternative days (Monday, Wednesday and Friday) per week. Often the frequency and timing of sessions will depend on the dynamics of the school, classroom and the structure of the school year. While sessions do not have to be delivered three times per week, the teaching assistants did report that they felt this intensity was positive for the child as it kept the work very current and maintained momentum. If at all possible, try and deliver the programme more than once a week. Intervention intensity appears to be emerging as an important component in treatment effectiveness (Gillam *et al*, 2008). Some teaching assistants have settled on using the programme formally with specified groups once or twice a week, but have then ensured that they use the skills and strategies covered in these sessions in the classroom. This is why having teachers or teaching assistants running the programme proves so effective, as they are able to extend the work into the classroom.

As discussed in question 3, the time it takes to complete the programme should depend on the needs and abilities of the students. It may also depend on the number of students in the group, as more students will necessitate longer periods of time. It is important to ensure that the sessions are not rushed and that the students have developed a solid understanding of the concepts covered in each session before moving on to the next session. Some teaching assistants and teachers have reported delivering the programme over a full academic year, expanding each session over a few sessions and adding additional examples and activities. This is fine if appropriate to the needs and levels of the student and if it fits in with the daily structure of the school. Others have successfully completed the 21 sessions within one term, delivering the sessions two or three times per week. The programme is designed to be flexible and to meet the different needs of the students and your own needs too!

5 How many students should be included in the group?

The intervention was delivered in small groups of between two and six students. It is ideal to have more than one student as a great deal of the work is around successfully communicating with others and working effectively in groups. The ideal number of students is four to five as this is quite manageable and allows for sufficient opportunities for discussion and collaboration. However, the programme can be delivered to an individual student as long as they are encouraged to involve others in the homework activities and are encouraged to transfer the new skills into the classroom and home settings. It is also possible to run the programme with groups of six or more students, although this presents challenges of behaviour management, and might need an additional person for support. Again, the word here is flexibility. The programme can be adapted to work with varied numbers. The most important issue is always the needs and abilities of the students. The expertise of the trainer is also important here as someone who is new to the programme may find it easier to run the programme initially with a smaller group.

6 How do I know when to move on to the next session?

Each session has a variety of graded activities and tasks which the students will complete. They will also have brought in work that they did independently as their homework task (Mission to Achieve). Completion, evaluation and discussion of these tasks will provide insight into the understanding of the areas covered. Students are required to explain aspects of what they have learned to other group members, and this too provides a window into their level of understanding. It is important to ensure that the students have a good understanding of the areas covered in each session before moving on, otherwise they will find the sessions get more and more difficult and will fall further and further behind. It is essential that students experience success rather than failure in these sessions, so they should be encouraged to practise the newly acquired skills and use them across different activities and contexts in order to consolidate skills. There will invariably be some students who work more quickly than others. Use them to explain some of the work to other members of the group, or even get them to act as the facilitator, as this will stretch their own abilities while at the same time providing further practice for the rest of the group.

7 How can I help the students generalise the skills from the programme to the classroom?

The very nature of the programme is that it incorporates content and tasks that are functional and relevant to the child's life and are geared to be used in other settings, including the classroom, school and home environment. Each session contains a homework activity or a Mission to Achieve where students are encouraged to trial or test out what has been learned in the session in their own environments. The tasks include discussion with parents, peers and other teachers and suggestions are provided for extending the work to school and home. Students are actively encouraged to bring in examples from school and home, for example, what story they may be covering in their English class that term. This facilitates the link between this programme and their school and home life. Teaching and support staff particularly are in ideal circumstances to extend the work into the classroom, by encouraging students to use the strategies and frameworks to complete school work and homework. Many students on the programme, for example, used the story planner to write and tell stories in the class and for homework. Students also used the story template to structure more difficult or sensitive explanations and discussions they needed to have with teachers or parents or other authority figures. Some TAs used the principles of active listening to encourage listening of all students in the classroom. All of these strategies will assist the student to generalise the skills they learn with you into the classroom, and into their individual familial and social environments.

8 How can I facilitate a cohesive and supportive group?

Group membership and cooperation are key elements of the programme. Many of the students who participated in the intervention commented on how much they enjoyed working in a small group, getting to know the other students better, sharing their experiences and difficulties and realising that they were not the only ones with specific thoughts, problems or difficulties. This is very powerful and group cohesiveness needs to be facilitated from the start. The first session provides an opportunity to meet group members, make introductions, set individual and group aims and targets and establish group rules. It is important that students generate the rules for themselves as this ensures that they are adhered to throughout the programme. It is also much easier to get students back on track when a rule has been broken, as they find it far harder breaking rules that they themselves have not only agreed to but have devised. It is important to encourage self and other reflection and evaluation at all times. A group discussion should take place at the start around what such an evaluation may look like and the difference between constructive and destructive feedback. Behaviour was an issue with some of the groups and some thoughts on behaviour management may be helpful. When students are misbehaving, it is important to remember that they are communicating something, and often the challenge is finding out what that may be. Consider that the work given may be too difficult and think about providing additional examples with more support. Students may also act up in the smaller group, and bring problems they have experienced in other settings to the group as they have developed a feeling of safety and support in the group setting. If this is the case, encourage the students to share what has happened using the various strategies and frameworks for support. If you are aware of a problem that a student is experiencing, it may be effective using this experience within a story and discussing the feelings that are generated by the situation and possible resolutions. In this case it is of course important not to make it identifiable in any way to any one student. We, for example, have had some powerful sharing of experiences when telling 'fictional' stories around bullying in schools.

9 How can I evaluate the success of the programme and measure the students' progress?

It is important to evaluate the success of the programme and measure any improvements made as a result of the intervention. There are numerous ways that one can measure improvement or change in performance and some ideas are provided here which you may like to use. You will come up with your own ideas which may be more appropriate for your particular setting or students.

It is important to differentiate between initial assessment and outcome measures. An initial assessment or diagnostic assessment is an assessment which will be conducted by a teacher, educational psychologist or speech and language therapist and will provide you with a detailed profile of the student's strengths and areas of difficulty. They are routinely used to find out more information about the abilities of the student. This assessment will probably include a variety of standardised language and educational attainment tests.

These standardised tests can also be given at the start and the end of a programme of work in order to assess changes in the student's performance which have arisen as a result of the intervention. This is commonly referred to as outcome measures, i.e. measuring the outcome or changes resulting from the intervention. Standardised tests can be used as outcome measures, to assess change. However, they are not always sensitive enough to pick up the more subtle changes in a student's performance on specific areas that have been targeted during intervention. Many standardised assessments can only be administered by trained professionals, and some are often not accessible to teaching and support staff. It is important therefore to use other outcome measures which can be devised to more accurately reflect what has been covered in the programme. It is also useful to get not only the perspective of the teacher or professionals working with the student, but the student's own perspective of their performance, as well as that of other people working with them in school, and their parents.

You will note that the final session contains a quiz which was originally devised to assess the students' skills informally as a competition at the end of the programme. Some of the teaching assistants have used this quiz successfully as an outcome measure and have shown substantial change in the student's performance as measured before and after the intervention. This can be done quite easily as all that is needed is for the student to be seen individually before and after the programme and tested on this quiz. The quiz covers all aspects of the programme so it is also possible to explore which areas improved and which did not. Ideally, to avoid any tester bias, the person administering the quiz should not be the trainer conducting the intervention, and there should be two different people giving the quiz at the start and end of the programme.

Another suggestion is to use the story planner to assess the complexity of a story produced by the student before and after the intervention. This would entail getting the student to tell a story, using pictures, objects or any other preferred format, and identifying the key parts of the story that the student has included, using the story planner to help you structure your assessment. In this way you will be able to assess the quality of the narrative and ability of the student to use effectively the key aspects of storytelling: beginning, middle; end and all the components within each of these sections. In this way, one could easily chart any changes and developments in storytelling skills that the student showed after the intervention. You could also assess not only the quality of the story with regards to the story elements, but also the language used to tell the story. This may include counting the number of adjectives, adverbs or more complex sentences used, the number of correctly used past tense verbs, the number of coordinators and subordinators and any other language components that you might like to focus on.

In the original pilot project, we also gave each student a narrative checklist which explored their understanding of key narrative terms like 'climax', and their knowledge of what makes up a good story. This narrative checklist was given before and after the intervention, and the students were shown to perform significantly better on this task after the narrative programme. This narrative checklist is reproduced here for you to use as an outcome measure (see Appendix 1).

Remember to try and assess the student's performance not only individually, but if possible in the classroom. You could analyse the student's oral or written story produced in the classroom or for homework, using the story planner as detailed above. Of course you can also use any other school attainment tests that are routinely used in the school which you feel measure narrative skills to some degree. Since the programme also focuses on listening skills, it is useful to assess any changes that might be evident in the student's listening and attention in the classroom. To do this you may decide to talk with the class teacher, or even observe the student's listening skills using some type of rating scale which requires you to rate listening, engagement, participation and any other area that seems relevant to the intervention. Even better, produce this rating scale and get another colleague to rate the student before and after the intervention. If possible, do not tell the colleague what the intervention has focused on, as this will mean she is unaware of what behaviours have been targeted and her responses will be more objective and unbiased. Any changes noted will then be very powerful.

 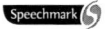

The perspective of the student is also essential. You will recall that at the start of the programme you are encouraged to gather each student's individual aims and targets. It is possible to use this information at the end of the programme to explore how much the student feels has been achieved as a result of the intervention. You may find it useful to carry this out in the group, or individually. Explore with the student the areas they feel they are better at, and what is still difficult. This will give you valuable information about what worked in the programme, and what areas still need further attention.

Remember when looking at outcomes and improvement to look more broadly than at just storytelling, listening and language. Ask the student's teacher and/or parent to tell you in their own words what differences they feel they can see in the student's behaviour and development. Many of our students indentified changes in social skills, making friends, independence and confidence. These are crucial areas that we need to know about, and are often not accessible from more formal assessments.

General strategies that can be used to enhance student performance and storytelling

There are some useful strategies and methods which have been found by researchers and practitioners to be useful in working with students with speech, language and communication difficulties and can be effective in facilitating language and communication. They are listed below. You will not use all of them all the time, but you may find them helpful in enhancing learning. You probably use many of them already in your work with the students. Try and familiarise yourself with them and use them when you feel it is appropriate.

1 Attention. Ensure that you have the students' attention before introducing any new topic. Remind students to look at you, and refocus them through eye contact, use of their names or a change in your voice quality, for example, whispering or raising your voice slightly.

2 Listening. Remind the students of the importance of listening. Good listening should be one of the group rules which will be identified in the first session. If group listening seems to wane, then try changing activities or pace. Simply getting students to stand up and down again is often enough to refocus their attention and enhance listening. The use of the story pencil, microphone or whatever object you decide to use should help group listening as it will cue students in to who is talking and who should be listening. The person holding the story pencil or microphone is the only person in the group telling the story while the other group members should be encouraged to listen and attend.

3 Repetition. Often we need to hear things numerous times before we really understand them. Ensure that new concepts and ideas are repeated within and across sessions. It is important to repeat the information initially using the same vocabulary and sentence structure so that the students can focus on the new information with no distractions. Thereafter it is helpful to repeat the information in different ways using different examples. This is especially important when introducing the story planner, which will be new to the students. Explain each element of the story planner, providing different examples to facilitate understanding. Use the corresponding symbol or picture for each element of the story planner to reinforce understanding.

4 Vary the context of what is being learned. It is important not only to provide many examples of the concepts being covered, but also to vary the contexts in which they are being discussed. For example, when discussing the story component 'setting' within the introduction, provide examples of different settings from classroom texts, stories in magazines and comics, songs and fables. The concept and topic of characterisation is another example of an area that can be explored across many varied contexts. Students can be encouraged to explore the character traits of a specific character in different situations and settings, for example different countries and different circumstances. This leads to enlightening discussions about how people act and behave and how we are influenced by our environments.

 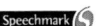

5 Summarising. At different stages in the session, summarise what has been covered before. This provides the students with much-needed repetition as well as giving them an idea of how all the different parts of the session fit together into a coherent whole. Try to get a few students to summarise at the beginning and end of the session to monitor understanding.

6 Monitor your own language and communication. Be aware of the language you use. Ensure that you use language that the students understand, and always check that they understand new vocabulary or concepts that you use. You can always check understanding in a fun way using quizzes and other games. It is just as important not to 'dumb down' your language and underestimate the abilities of the students.

7 Model appropriate language behaviour. Give examples of the language you are teaching and requiring the students to produce. So if you are talking about describing a character using different adjectives, give examples, making up exciting characters for the students. When giving them examples of stories, make sure the stories contain all the elements you are covering and identify explicitly these elements for the students. If you are expecting them to use new words, for example, more adjectives or adverbs, it is important that you model and use them first so the students see how they are used and can copy you. You can not expect them to tell exciting stories, and be boring yourself!

8 Expansion. Always try and take what the student gives as a response, even if you have to change it so that it reflects more of what you are looking for. So, if a student provides an answer which is only half correct, take their answer and expand on it by adding bits so it becomes the correct response. For example, use a more sophisticated or complex word to describe a character while retaining the meaning of the word that the student used initially. Present the student with the new word, phrase, etc as another alternative that they may like to consider using to make their story or sentence even better. So instead of describing the thief as a 'bad' man, suggest the term 'wicked'.

9 Recasting. We can use recasting when students make errors in their language. Instead of bringing attention to these errors in a negative way, and telling them they have said something incorrectly, it can often be better to simply repeat the sentence they have used, but with the correction. So for example, if the student should say, 'We all throwed the ball at camp yesterday', you can simply repeat this by saying, 'Wow, what fun, you all threw the ball at camp yesterday'. You can emphasise the word 'threw' by saying it louder, softer or slower.

10 Cueing. The use of cueing is very helpful when a student is unable to recall the correct response. The adult provides a cue or prompt which helps facilitate recall of the answer. The cue can be phonological (sound based) or semantic (meaning based). For example, if the students are unable to recall that one of the elements of the beginning of a story is 'place', one can use a phonological cue by providing them with the first sound of the word, so you would say, 'it is p___'. You could also provide a semantic cue by saying 'This is where the story or action happens'. You can also use other cues, for example, graphemic cueing by writing down the first letter of the word or concept. It is always a good plan to cue one modality with another. For example, use signs or other visual cues to help recollection of the verbal label. Students may need some prompting to recall and use all the elements of the story planner. Instead of always giving them the story element, try using the visual representations for each story element on the story planner as a cue. For example, if they have omitted information about time and place, show them the picture of the watch and calendar symbolising time on the planner, and the picture of a house and tree signifying place, and this should act as a cue to remind them to add these details. Hopefully, with time and practice, they should be able to cue themselves by thinking either of the story elements or the pictures representing them.

11 Provide a range of different examples. The best way of ensuring understanding of new concepts and newly introduced work is by providing a range of different examples. So, if you are trying to get the students to construct stories with clear beginning, middle and end elements, it is important to provide many different examples of stories that have these elements. Get the students to tell stories using their own experiences and as a group evaluate the story and identify the different elements that are included, as well as those that have been omitted. Encourage group members to provide suggestions on how to improve the stories, make them more exciting and incorporate more of the story elements. Children typically love to hear stories made up by their peers.

12 Reinforce positive behaviour. There will usually be a time when the student is making an excellent effort and showing active and positive participation. It is important at these times to provide praise and positive reinforcement as this will encourage more of this type of behaviour. Try to provide focused praise by explicitly mentioning the specific behaviour that you are reinforcing, for example, 'Excellent, I really liked the way you waited until Jenna finished her story, before asking your question'. Positive reinforcement can be in the form of verbal praise, acknowledging the good behaviour to the group, giving a house point or getting the student to lead the next activity. You will think of more ways to reinforce good behaviour. Behaviour that is ignored and not reinforced usually stops, so try ignoring poor behaviour and lack of participation.

13 Recap and revise. Ensure that you revise and recap at the beginning and end of each session. It is often a good idea to get the students to revise and recap as this gives you a very good idea of what they have understood from the session. It is also a good idea to revise and recap concepts within a session when you are moving from one concept to another.

14 Use a multi-sensory approach. Try using all the senses to reinforce new concepts, vocabulary and ideas. Use visual, auditory, olfactory, tactile and kinesthetic sensations. For example, when introducing a character with a detailed description, get the students to see the character, to visualise all his features, get them to imagine what they sound like, feel like, get them to act out the character so they get a complete sensation of who the character is. This makes the story more exciting for

 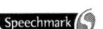

them and brings the elements alive. Ensure that they also then provide all these details when describing their characters. Students like to be active and this programme provides plenty of opportunities for activity. Get students to act out their stories whenever possible. You will find visual cues particularly valuable and the programme includes a DVD with a range of pictures that will support storytelling. The use of sequence pictures will be particularly helpful to support the sequencing of ideas and help structure early storytelling attempts. Use a variety of different modalities and a range of materials to support the work you are covering. Use oral and written language and story songs to reinforce different ways of telling stories; and books, magazines, comics and newspapers will be helpful in reinforcing the concepts included in the programme. I never appreciated the full therapeutic use of *EastEnders* until I used this programme with students who were supported in identifying characters and other elements of a story watching this docu-drama. The students will come up with more ideas than you around the innovative use of objects for role playing and use of different media including computers, iPads, iPods and computer games to generate stories. Go with it…

15 Exaggerate prosodic cues. Use your voice in different ways to emphasise meaning and concepts and provide additional excitement in the sessions. Use more exaggerated intonation patterns, vary loudness levels (whispering is an excellent tool to create tension and get attention), vary the rate of your speech and use slightly higher frequencies and greater pitch variations. This all helps to make the sessions more exciting. Characters and settings can be enhanced through changes in your voice, facial expression and body language. For example, consider the different sounds, facial expressions and hand postures that can be used to describe the setting of a haunted old house on the moors.

16 Facial expression and body language. Ensure that your facial expressions and body language are consistent with what you are saying. So if you are trying to look interested in a story that is being told, ensure that your face and body language are reflecting that interest. Also use the face and body to communicate and teach different concepts and vocabulary. So, for example, if you are talking about a frail old man in your story, use your face to reflect the age and health of the character, and use your body to reflect his frailty. This will bring the story alive for the students, will reinforce meaning and will also encourage them to do the same.

17 Use role play. Students love to act out the characters and stories they hear and tell. Allow them to act out different parts of the story, or to act out different characters. This enhances their understanding and also changes the pace of the session, injecting some much-needed energy and activity, something for which you will all be grateful.

18 Encourage self-monitoring and evaluation. Always try and get the students to self-monitor and evaluate their own work and the input of their peers. Encourage them to look at the positives and also the parts that they can improve on. Ensure that they give constructive criticism and provide suggestions for improvements. Always begin with the positive and then provide suggestions on how their stories can be improved.

19 Ensure new concepts are understood. Check continuously that the students understand what you are covering and that they are at the same stage you are at. It is sometimes hard to gauge this when working in a group, but try and target the level of most of the students in the group. You can provide more simple examples for those who are struggling and also give more complex exercises and tasks to those who appear to be racing ahead of the group. Use their homework tasks to differentiate these different levels, stretching those students who seem to be ready and providing further consolidation for those who appear to be struggling. Use a variety of quizzes and games to check understanding. Getting students to recap, revise and teach each other are excellent ways to check understanding. Use different ways to explain concepts, for example, use the story train track, the story F1 race track, the story athletics race track and the story football match to reinforce the same elements of the story planner.

20 Playing the fool and using verbal absurdity. Once students appear to have mastered a particular concept or idea, it can be helpful to use jokes to reinforce the new learning. So, for example, use the new word incorrectly in a way that is bizarre and clearly funny, or tell a story that obviously lacks correct sequencing. This should be so ridiculous that the students can obviously see the error and usually take great joy in correcting it. When telling a story, for example, omit any details of the main character but refer to 'him' or 'her' throughout the story. Ask the students to evaluate the story and suggest alternatives. Another example is to describe a setting and then have the character act in certain ways that are incongruous with the setting and see if the students are able to identify this. So describe a hot sunny day, and talk about how the character in the story is huddling near an open fire with layers of clothes. Ensure that the character's behaviour is so over the top that this incongruity is obvious.

21 Using negative examples. This is similar to playing the fool, although the incorrect examples here do not have to be funny or ridiculous. It is essential, though, that you only use negative examples when the students have clearly understood the concepts and are able to use them. So, for example, once they understand the concept of story structure and what parts make up a story, then you can give them examples of stories missing one element, so a story missing an ending, for example, or lacking a description of a setting. Then get the students to evaluate the story and identify what is incorrect. Please remember that it is best to do this only once students have a good understanding of the particular concept, otherwise they might not be able to identify or correct the error.

22 Ask focused questions. A very good way to explore and enhance understanding is by asking a range of questions. The answers you get are often only as good as the questions you ask. So when teaching about the different parts of a story, ensure you ask questions about characterisation, setting, plots, motivations of the character/s, morals, etc, as this will encourage students to include all these elements in their stories. After they have listened to a story, ask them specific questions which focus their attention on the different elements of a story. The use of questions will also encourage more active listening. Feel free to make up games and quizzes like '*Who Wants To Be a Millionaire*' and '*The Weakest Link*', which make the use of questions more fun.

23 The use of forced alternatives. Forced alternatives are an excellent means to elicit responses from students. In these types of questions, one includes two options for the student from which to choose: the correct and incorrect options. This is ideal when the students are uncertain of giving an answer without some prompting and hearing the correct item or concept cues them successfully to provide the correct response. For example, when describing a character in a story as malicious, you can ask whether that means the character is spiteful or kind. This allows you to check the student's understanding of malicious and whether they are able to understand that the actions of the character reflect a spiteful rather than kind nature. The choices you provide should depend on the level of understanding of your students: the better the understanding, the closer in meaning the two choices should be to each other.

24 Build on the students' experiences. When introducing new concepts, always try beginning from knowledge and experiences that the students already have, so begin with the familiar and build from that to newer and more complex information. For example, when introducing the story planner, discuss the elements with which they are more familiar (this may be characters) and then move onto the other elements like the plot or theme. When introducing stories, provide examples with which the students are familiar, using their hobbies, favourite activities and topics they have covered in school. This may include talking about *EastEnders*, *Dr Who* or *Harry Potter* and discussing how these are all stories with their own specific characters, settings, episodes and outcomes. Also use football, music and other favourites as themes when constructing stories. Make the stories and themes relevant to the students' daily experiences and passions, so talk about what they have experienced. These may include bullying, making friends, getting jobs, dating, losing homework, coming late for class and other shared common experiences.

25 Make the sessions as functional and real as possible. Always remember that we are trying to arm the students with skills that they will be able to use in the classroom, in the playground, with their peers, at home and in wider social settings. To help with this try and always use examples that they will be able to take and use in their own individual contexts. When constructing stories, or giving them themes around which to tell stories, use functional meaningful examples, for example, telling a story about a young boy having his mobile phone stolen or completing the story about a teenager being the witness to a car accident. These are examples which will possibly help the students deal with similar experiences in their own lives.

26 Upgrade or downgrade tasks. You will need to change the pace of the session and monitor the number and level of examples you give depending on the overall understanding of the group. If you feel the majority of students have not grasped a concept, for example, you will need to go slower and include more examples and explanations, drawing upon more visual cues (use of pictures) and using more simple language. It is fine to play different games with the same aims to ensure a solid understanding. It is best to work at the level of the majority of students in your group. When asking for individual input, you can use more difficult or less difficult questions to reflect more accurately each individual's level of understanding.

27 Emphasise independent learning. It is important to ensure that we give the students the skills and strategies that they can take with them as independent learners. Make explicit what is being taught and explain why and how it will help them. If they have a clear understanding of what they are covering, and the reasons why it is important and how it will help them, they will become more reflective in their learning. Explain to them how knowing about story structure will make them sound more interesting when talking with their friends, and how they can use this knowledge when writing essays in class. This will ensure that the students are aware of the importance of narratives, why they are important and how they can be used to facilitate learning. Provide the students with skills and strategies and encourage them to use these strategies in school and at home independently.

28 Keep the students motivated. Students want to perform and achieve so it is important that we always provide them with the opportunity to get things right. The work should never be too hard but always be at a level that allows them to achieve while at the same time pushes them to a more advanced level. Positive reinforcement should be used at all times to motivate the students. It is important to focus on what they are doing well and acknowledge the effort they are making. The use of rewards can also be very helpful, both intrinsic and extrinsic. Simply completing a task correctly, or winning the game, is an important intrinsic reward, that is the reward is simply about working hard and gaining success at the task. Extrinsic rewards can also be successfully employed. These refer to additional motivators or rewards that students find motivating, and are given to them when they have completed a task successfully, for example, awarding school points, a star or a counter which, when added up, may translate into a more substantial reward. Getting the students involved in each session by asking them to lead certain parts and encouraging them to bring in materials and ideas from home and their school lessons, which reflect the themes of the sessions, will help to motivate them. You might even want to devise some type of achievement chart which encourages group work and individual performance. Try making sure that the students feel they are fortunate to be attending these sessions, and that it is not a punishment. In the first session, ensure you explain to them how these sessions will help them in all their classes in school as well as in their social interactions out of school. This will enhance motivation and ensure regular attendance.

29 And always make sure you are all having FUN. Both you and the students need these sessions to be FUN. The sessions have the potential to be great fun. Storytelling allows for individual flair, role play, use of different materials and examples and experiences from the students' own lives. The best learning takes place in a context of fun, acceptance and security so my hope is that you enjoy the sessions and this enjoyment will quickly pass on to the students. Remember that there is always someone around who can help you problem solve and trouble shoot. Get as much support as you need. Enjoy, enjoy, enjoy. And now after all that, let's go tell a story…

 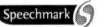

SESSION PLANS

Session 1

Names of students: _____

_____

Facilitator: _____ Date: _____

School: _____

Class: _____

Aims	Method/Activities	Materials
To introduce the members to the programme and provide them with an **overview of the programme** and its main aims and learning objectives.	Introduce yourself to the students if they do not know you already and give them a short overview of the programme and what it entails. Provide information to the students about the programme and explain to them the overall aims, duration of programme, duration of sessions, where it will take place and any other basic pieces of information that will help orient them. It might be useful to explain to them why they have been chosen to attend the group. Elicit their own thoughts and ideas about why they have been chosen and discuss any worries or concerns that may be raised at this early point, for example, missing other lessons. Students will respond very positively if you explain the group as a select group where people are invited to attend and will learn new skills which they will be able to use in the classroom and in their other activities. Discuss with the students how this programme will help them develop some basic and important skills in speaking, listening and storytelling. It might help to use the construction of a building as an analogy, which one of our teaching assistants, Tracey, found to be helpful. She brought in some blocks and asked the students to build a tower or some other building. Once complete, she then took out one	Verbal discussion aided by use of whiteboard and/or flipchart if available and pen and paper. Refer to the aims of the programme in the introductory section on page 13. It is helpful for each student to have a folder in which they can keep all their handouts, group rules, student learning profiles, photocopied notes and homework they have completed. Blocks or bricks may be useful to build a tower or other construction.

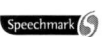

Aims	Method/Activities	Materials
	of the blocks from the bottom of the building, i.e. one of the foundation blocks. The students observed how the whole structure then quickly fell apart. She explained the importance of foundation blocks for a building, and foundation skills for many activities in which the students are involved across school and social settings. It is helpful to explain to students that the aim of the programme is to develop and practise key foundation skills. Without these foundations skills, many tasks, just like the tower or building, fall apart. You might also find it helpful to talk to students about gaps in the building, or weak foundations which make the building very precarious and unsteady. Relate this to gaps in knowledge and discuss how we all have gaps in our knowledge in some way or another. Some of us know much more about some topics than others. But we can plug these gaps and increase our knowledge if we choose to. This is what this programme aims to do, to fill the gaps, strengthen the foundation skills and knowledge around language and communication – crucial skills in our lives. This activity will be in the form of a verbal discussion led by the facilitator. You will find the list of aims in the introduction section on page 13 helpful in summarising for the students the main aims and content of the programme.	
To elicit **group rules** on which all sessions will be based. To ensure that all group members are actively involved in establishing group rules. To **familiarise all group members** with each other and the facilitator.	Brainstorm activity and verbal discussion in which students will be asked to provide suggestions for group rules which will help facilitate the smooth running of the group and ensure it is effective and fun for all participants. The trainer facilitates the suggestions and adds any other important rules that have not been given by the students. See attached teaching notes for suggested rules. Students may come up with additional rules which you may like to add to the list. Divide group into pairs or groups of three if an odd number and group members to exchange three pieces of information about themselves to	Verbal discussion and brainstorm activity using large piece of paper or flipchart or whiteboard if available and coloured pens. The group rules are written on the paper and kept throughout the sessions, revisited if and when needed. Group gelling task through verbal

Aims	Method/Activities	Materials
	a partner. The group come back together and retell their partner's information to the rest of the group. You may also like to use any other group activity that you know which facilitates group cohesion and helps familiarise members with each other.	discussion and sharing of information by dividing into pairs.
To **introduce the students to the importance of narratives or stories** and storytelling in school and in their home and social settings.	Brainstorm activity to elicit what **stories** are and why they are important to learning and to social interaction. Ask students when and where they use narratives or stories in their school and home lives. Emphasise to students how stories are used everywhere. Identify with their help all the situations where one either has to tell a story or listen and understand stories. Identify the use of stories in school; in history for example, when learning about Napoleon, King Henry the Eighth or Hitler and the Second World War; in geography when learning about the animal and plant kingdoms and the solar system; and in English when reading a book written by Charles Dickens or a play by Shakespeare. Discuss how they use stories at home and in making friends, for example, telling people more about themselves, or telling friends what has happened to them at a party. Encourage students to tell you about the stories they have read or watched on television. Explain to them that *Dr Who* and *Coronation Street* are as much stories as more serious stories like *Hamlet*, for example. Generate a list of all the different ways that they use stories in their lives and how being better at listening and storytelling can help them at home, at school and in their social interactions. See the teaching notes that follow for further ideas. Encourage ideas from the students which can be added to the list. The generated list should be retained and revisited where necessary during the course of the programme.	Group discussion using flipchart or whiteboard if available or paper and coloured pens. Teaching notes that follow.

 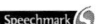

Aims	Method/Activities	Materials
To encourage students to generate their **own individual aims and targets** for the programme using their learning profile.	Once you have discussed the importance and role of stories, it is helpful for students to generate their own targets and individual learning objectives. Use the attached student learning profile to record student aims or get students to make up their own. This activity can work well as a whole group activity, or with students working in pairs. It will help reinforce the aims of the programme, as well as make explicit for the student their own strengths and limitations. They will get the opportunity to devise their own individual targets, as well as how they will measure their own success. This will support more independent and reflective learning.	Pens to record aims and learning objectives using the student learning profile (My Learning Profile) that follows. Start a narrative file or folder for each student where they are able to keep handouts and work from the sessions. Keep these folders somewhere safe where students can easily access them at the beginning of each session.
To sum up and revise contents of the session.	Get volunteers from the group to summarise the main content of the session. Ask other members of the group to help, adding in the parts that may have been omitted.	Flipchart or whiteboard, paper and pen.
Mission to Achieve: Students to go away and think about their favourite stories and what makes them their favourite.	Students will be asked to choose one of their favourite books that they will draw upon and use as an exemplar throughout the programme. These books will be used to provide examples for the students for the different concepts and learning covered. Students should be encouraged to choose any book with which they feel a connection. There is no right or wrong choice.	

Evaluation of session/General comments

Teaching notes for Session 1

Group rules

We encourage students to generate a set of group rules to follow during the sessions. This facilitates the smooth and successful running of the group and ensures that each member is an active participant in the group, has been a part of setting up the group rules and has agreed to follow the rules. It is important to encourage the students to make their own group rules with your support and added suggestions.

The rules should be written on a flipchart or whiteboard or large piece of paper and brought by the facilitator to each session. The facilitator may even decide to photocopy the list for each student to keep in their folder. The rules can then be revisited if and when necessary during the sessions. It is important not only to generate the rules but also to explore the types of behaviour which one might follow or show when upholding the rules, for example, what behaviours would one follow when being supportive of other group members.

Suggested rules that assist in the smooth running of the sessions include:

1   Attendance at all sessions

2   Punctuality

3   Excellent attention and concentration throughout the sessions

4   Active listening to facilitator and each group member

5   Active participation in all tasks and activities

6   Respect for every member of the group

7   Being sensible

8   Being supportive of each member of the group

9   Trying your very best at all times

10 Feeling comfortable enough to say when something is too hard and when you do not understand

11 Asking for help

12 Helping other group members where necessary, for example, providing additional suggestions and giving helpful explanations when other members are experiencing more difficulty understanding

13 Completing homework activities.

Please add other rules which you may think of, and any suggested by the students. Generate a list on paper which can be retained and brought to each subsequent session. The group should be positively reinforced when adhering to the rules they have generated.

Teaching notes for Session 1

The importance of narratives or stories to the student's school, home and social life

Why is it important to learn about narratives?

It is important for the students to understand why they are learning about narratives and how it will be helpful to their learning in school and at home, and with making friends. Try and generate suggestions from the group, but ensure they include the following points which should be raised, extended and explored to form a discussion around why the students are attending the group. These are suggestions to start the discussion, but more ideas should be encouraged and generated.

Learning how to listen and tell stories will enhance performance in the following ways in the following contexts:

In the classroom:
- Improved listening in class will result in better classroom participation.
- Improved and active listening in class will result in greater recall and understanding of the subjects covered.
- Improved listening will result in improved behaviour in the classroom and getting into trouble less frequently at school.
- Better understanding of oral and written stories used in class across all subject areas.
- Enhanced ability to give explanations to teachers, for example, reasons for being late for a lesson or not having done a piece of homework.
- Improved ability to participate in lessons and share with class what has been learned.
- Become a more effective communicator by being more able to listen more effectively and produce sentences and stories that are organised and exciting.
- Provide more descriptive information in the classroom as well as to friends and peers in the playground, school clubs and at after-school activities.
- Improved confidence to participate in the classroom, and in other school activities like school plays, assemblies, etc.
- Being more descriptive about events and using all senses to explain and describe events and experiences.
- Being more communicative and interesting.

In the playground:
- Improved listening to peers and friends.
- Greater understanding of discussions held in the playground.
- Improved ability to recount to friends what has happened and share feelings, thoughts and ideas.
- Ability to solve problems and arguments through discussion and debate rather than physical fights or arguments.
- More active participation in group discussion with improved confidence.

 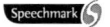

- Sharing information and recounting experiences in a more animated, organised and exciting way which will increase the number of people listening.

At home:
- Better able to listen and understand views of family and friends.
- Greater ability to explain thoughts, wishes and ideas to parents and friends.
- Improved ability to describe and recount what has happened at school.
- Greater understanding of favourite television programmes, books, instructions for putting machinery, furniture, etc together, as well as greater ability to play and understand computer games.
- Improved reading of favourite magazines, newspapers, comics and books.
- Greater ability to explain and describe events in emergency situations, for example, if witness to some robbery, the ability to describe the event to the police in an organised and coherent way is essential.

In social settings:
- Becoming a more popular group member through more active listening and greater ability to share experiences and tell stories.
- Having the opportunity to be the centre of attention at times when everyone is listening to an exciting story or a piece of news that is being shared.
- Greater confidence in speaking to boys and girls and making new friends through a better ability to talk about oneself and share appropriate personal details.
- Be viewed as an exciting and essential guest to have at a party or social event.
- Be a more effective communicator, someone who people enjoy having around and to whom they enjoy listening.
- Making more friends as a result of being a better listener and having an increased ability to share information about yourself and others.
- Having lots of experiences to share and contributing freely and actively to group discussions both with family and friends.
- Understand more about turn taking and giving others more of an opportunity to enter into discussions.

Participating in sports and other hobbies:
- Better understanding of group rules, for example, enhanced ability to follow the trainer's team talk during the football or netball game.
- Improved ability to participate in a team and follow team rules and instructions.
- Taking part in hobbies and events that might previously have been viewed as being too scary, for example, participating in a football club, or doing work experience at a football club or hairdressing salon.

The facilitator can use these suggestions as a beginning point and generate more discussion and ideas through brainstorming.

Encourage students to come up with what they think they can get out of attending the sessions. Get them to make their own aims for the sessions. Explore more specifically what they would like to get out of the programme and what specific aspects they feel they need to improve most on.

You might like to use the learning profile attached, or get the students to make their own learning profile. Use of this learning profile will help make more explicit for the student the aims of the programme, their own individual targets, and their strengths and areas of need around this topic. The profile encourages them to self-reflect and become more reflective and independent learners. It will also help to make them accountable for their own learning.

 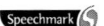

MY LEARNING PROFILE

Name:

Date:

1   The reason that I want to take part in this storytelling/narrative programme is because I…

2   Speaking, listening and storytelling are important in my life in that…

3 The three areas that I am very good at in speaking, listening and storytelling are:

-

-

-

4 I know I am good at these areas because…

5 The three areas which are sometimes difficult for me around speaking, listening and storytelling are:

-

-

-

 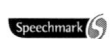

6   I am aware that I have difficulty in these areas because

7   The three main targets that I want to work and improve on by being involved in this programme are:

-

-

-

8   I will know when I have reached these targets because…

I am going to work very hard on this programme and do my very best.

Name:

Signature:

Signature of facilitator:

 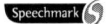

Session 2

2

Names of students: _____

_____

Facilitator: _____ Date: _____

School: _____

Class: _____

Aims	Method/Activities	Materials
To revise and recap themes from previous session, reminding students about the **focus and importance of storytelling**.	Group discussion with students taking turns to give an example of one important thing they learned from the previous session.	Flipchart or whiteboard, paper and pen.
To identify the main features of active **listening**.	Throughout the sessions, students will be encouraged to actively listen to their peers telling stories. **Active listening** is also one of the group rules. In this session, students are to brainstorm what they think active listening is, what behaviours make up active listening and why good listening is so important. Remind students that the human being was born with two eyes, two ears and one mouth! What might this mean? Encourage them to enhance their visual and observational skills, and their listening skills. In this programme, we will use a story pencil, microphone or another object which will denote when a person is talking. The person talking will hold the story pencil and all the other members of the group will listen using their active listening strategies. When it is another person's turn to talk, they have the story pencil, and the other students are the listeners. The students are to be encouraged to generate their own ideas about good listening and can be prompted from the suggestions included in the teaching notes that follow.	Flipchart or whiteboard, paper and pen. Behaviours consistent with good and active listening are included in the teaching notes.

 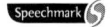

Aims	Method/Activities	Materials
	Explain to students that there are obvious behaviours that we can all adopt to show we are listening, for example, head nodding, body turned to the speaker, looking at the speaker. Similarly, we can behave in certain ways that make it obvious that we are not listening, and in ways that will get us into trouble in the classroom, but also in social situations, as no one wants to talk to someone who does not listen to them. If you look away when I am talking, turn away from me and look bored, fidget and move around, then this signifies to me that you are not listening. Discuss with students how many of them get into trouble because they are not listening. Encourage them to adopt these suggested active listening behaviours not only in these sessions, but at school and at home. Remind students that people like to talk to and spend time with people who listen to them. So let's make sure they are those sorts of people. They can be!	
To identify **favourite stories** of students from homework task. To explore reasons why the stories are their particular favourites.	Group discussion with each group member sharing what their favourite story is and the reasons for this. Students are to be encouraged to give specific reasons for their choices, for example, a favourite fairytale story from their past, a story with an exciting climax, a story with a romantic ending, or a story about their favourite sport. Probe why these stories are their favourites so that they become more skilled at identifying what makes a good story. Use the suggested questions in the teaching notes as a starting point.	Flipchart or whiteboard, paper and pen to record responses of students. Teaching notes for session 2.
To **identify stories that students know or have heard or read or seen**, to include books, comics, television programmes and movies.	Brainstorm all the stories with which the students are familiar. Have a competition to see who generates the most story titles. Stories can be from books, cinema or television and can include famous fairytales, fables, television series and soaps, historical stories and current popular stories like *Harry Potter*. Think of different ways to elicit examples using games and competitions, for example, each member	Flipchart or whiteboard, paper and pen to record responses of students. Teaching notes for session 2.

Aims	Method/Activities	Materials
To discuss the best and worst parts of these stories.	takes turns thinking of a story starting with a different letter of the alphabet. Generate excitement and active discussion about the stories, asking questions about their favourites. See the teaching notes for examples of questions.	
Identify **one favourite book** that each student will use throughout the programme.	Each student will be asked to identify one of their favourite books that they would like to use as an examplar for completing work throughout the duration of the programme. Make a list of all book choices and ask students to provide the reasons for their choice. There is no wrong or right choice here and students should be encouraged to choose the book that is their most favourite. Some students may need some assistance with this, and it is helpful to ask questions and remind them of books they may have read or come across either at home or at school. Some students may choose a book because they have seen the movie. This is a very good way to get some students interested in literature.	Pen and paper to write a list of selected books chosen by the group. This list should be retained in the programme folder and used if necessary to remind students of their choices.
Introduce the three types of stories to students: **fictional, non-fictional and personal.**	Through verbal discussion, explain the three types of stories to students. **Fictional story:** a made-up story which is not based on facts, for example *Harry Potter* or *EastEnders*. **Non-fictional story:** a story that is based on facts. This may include an autobiography of a famous person, i.e. written by that person (for example, the autobiography written by David Beckham) or a biography, a story about the life of a famous person written by another person (for example, other authors have written about David Beckham). Other non-fictional stories include books or television programmes about nature, landing on the moon, the human body, etc.	Flipchart or whiteboard, paper and pen to record the suggestions and discussion.

 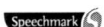

Aims	Method/Activities	Materials
	Personal story: a story told by a person about a specific event that they have personally experienced, for example, going away on holiday, or going to hospital to have one's tonsils removed. This type of story is non-fictional because it is true. Give examples of each type of story and ask students to provide their own examples of the different types of stories. Try and get students to identify when they use or hear different stories, for example, non-fictional stories in geography and history lessons, fictional stories in English classes and personal stories in the playground and at parties.	
Each student to **share a short personal narrative** with the group.	Each student has a turn to share something with the group about themselves. This can include something about their family, their hobbies, their Christmas holiday, etc. The facilitator can begin first by saying something about herself or himself and modelling the personal narrative.	Story pencil or microphone. Introduce the story pencil or microphone to the group. The person who holds the story pencil (or whatever object you are using to denote this) has the floor and talks with the full support and cooperation of all other group members, who are encouraged to show excellent listening and attention skills. Once the person has completed his or her story, they pass the story pencil to the next group member who then has a chance to share their personal narrative. This is an

Aims	Method/Activities	Materials
		important tool to encourage turn taking and active listening skills.
To introduce the concept of **story genres** and generate examples of different types of stories.	Group discussion and brainstorm around the different **types of stories** that exist. Play a guessing game with students taking turns describing the story and other group members guessing the name of the story they are describing. Introduce to the students the idea of the **story genre**. There are many different types of stories and these different story types are called genres. Stories to include: **Fictional stories:** detective/crime, horror, fantasy, mystery, fairytale, fable, romance, science fiction, historical fiction, suspense/adventure, tragedy, action/adventure. **Non-fictional stories**: generate examples of non-fictional stories, for example Neil Armstrong visiting the moon, the story of Anne Frank, Hitler's takeover during the Second World War and other stories from the Education Curriculum. See the teaching notes for further examples. Differentiate for the students between the biography (written by someone else about a person) and autobiography (written by the person about him or herself). Explore students' understanding of the author: the writer of the story. An autobiography will therefore have an author who has written about himself or herself, while a biography will have an author writing about another person. Encourage students to provide examples of each type of story and provide examples for	Flipchart or whiteboard to record responses from students.

 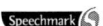

Aims	Method/Activities	Materials
To sum up and revise the contents of the session.	them too – give examples of each type and discuss what makes each story the kind it is, so for example, why 'Lewis' is an example of a detective story. Get volunteers from the group to summarise the main content of the session. Ask other members of the group to help, adding in the parts that may have been omitted.	Flipchart or whiteboard, paper and pen.
Mission to Achieve: Students to bring with them to the next session written examples of two different types of stories. These can be cut out from newspapers, comics, magazines or can come from books or school materials.		

Evaluation of session/General comments

Teaching notes for Session 2

Behaviours of good and active listening

Discuss with students why listening is important, both for school and for home and social settings. Discuss the consequences of poor listening, what it makes the person talking feel when they have not been heard, as well as the impact it has on the listener, i.e. not following what has been said, an inability to carry out the instructions, etc. Encourage them to think about how good it would be for them if they were able to listen more effectively. How much better it would be for them in the classroom, in the playground, making friends and talking in social circles, as well as at home.

Remember: we have two ears and one mouth for a reason

The following are key signs of active listening. Students are to be encouraged to brainstorm what the key behaviours are for good and active listening. These are some suggestions, but encourage students to extend the list further.

You are actively listening when you:

1   Maintain eye contact with the speaker
2   Turn your body to face the speaker
3   Turn your head to face the speaker
4   Focus attention on the speaker
5   DO NOT fidget, fiddle with things or move about
6   DO NOT talk at the same time as the speaker
7   DO NOT daydream or think about other things
8   DO NOT interrupt at inappropriate moments when the speaker is in the middle of talking
9   Ask for further explanation and clarification when you do not understand
10 Nod your head and use other facial expressions (like smiling) at appropriate moments to show your attention
11 Take responsibility when there has been a misunderstanding and help work with the speaker at repairing the communication breakdown
12 Add comments or questions at appropriate times, when the speaker comes to the end of a sentence or paragraph and indicates that this is an appropriate point for additional comments
13 Share your own experiences with the speaker if appropriate, using appropriate turn taking
14 Take short notes if you need to refer to this information at a later point
15 Ask specific questions at the end to show you have heard what has been said
16 Give comments and feedback. Always try and say something positive about what you have heard.

Teaching notes for Session 2

Questions to use to explore the favourite stories of students and the reasons for their choices

The main aim of this session is to allow students to talk about their favourite stories and explore why they like specific stories, and also why they dislike some stories. It is important to try and generate as much excitement as possible around stories and storytelling and every example given by students should be taken and discussed. The following questions might help generate more discussion around each story. Please feel free to add your own as these are only suggestions.

1 What is your very favourite story?
 It can be a story that someone has told you as a child, like a fairytale, or a story that you have read or that someone has read to you. It can be a story that you have heard about in the classroom, maybe in English, geography or history. It can be a real (non-fictional) story or a fictional or make-believe story. It could be a story you have heard about your favourite footballer, or a story that you have seen at the cinema or on television or video. It can also be a story from your favourite comic, magazine or newspaper.

2 What makes this your favourite story? Why do you like this story so much?

3 How does this story make you feel?

4 Can you give us a summary of the story, what is the story about?

5 What kind of story is it, fictional or non-fictional, romantic, fantasy, action or suspense, etc?

6 Where does the story take place – which country, what place, etc?

7 When does the story take place – past, present or future, what year, season, time of day, etc?

8 Who is the story about, who are the main characters?

9 What happens in the story, what is it about, what is the plot of the story?

10 What is the main exciting part of the story, the climax of the story if there is one?

11 How does the story end?

12 Did you like the ending of the story?

13 If you could change one thing about the story, what would it be?

14 What story do you dislike?

15 Why do you think you dislike this story so much?

16 What could you change about this story to make you like it more?

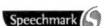

Teaching notes for Session 2

Different types of stories – story genres

There are many different types of stories and these different types are called story genres. A genre is a group or collection of stories or books with a similar theme or style. For example:

- **Mystery:** stories that involve some type of crime or suspense.
- **Romance:** stories that involve deep love and passion.
- **Fantasy:** stories with parts that do not exist in real life, so for example, fairies as characters.
- **Folktales:** stories that have been passed down to us over the years by our grandparents and ancestors. They include fables, myths and fairy tales.
- **Biographies:** stories that tell you all about a person's life or about parts of his/her life. A biography that is written by a person about his/her own life is called an autobiography. These are true and are therefore non-fiction.
- **Poetry:** a piece of writing which expresses thoughts and feelings. They usually consist of short verses and may rhyme. Some poems are narrative poems or story poems in that they tell a story.

Provide examples of the range of different types of stories giving examples for each one and encouraging students to add their own favourites and examples. Here is a list of different stories which you can add to and expand upon.

Non-fictional stories:

Generate examples of non-fictional stories from topics covered in the school curriculum and from experiences of the students and their favourite heroes and stars that they follow and admire. These may include:

1   Historical books on various topics including, for example:

- Neil Armstrong and the landing on the moon – *First Man: The Life of Neil Armstrong* By James Hansen
- The adventures and travels of Christopher Columbus – *A History of the Life and Voyages of Christopher Columbus* By Washington Irving
- The Second World War – *Travels in the Reich, 1933–1945* Edited by Oliver Lubrich
- The Victorian era – *The Victorians* By Jeremy Paxman
- Henry VIII and his six wives – *The Six Wives of Henry VIII* By Alison Weir.

2   Biographies including, for example:

- *Diana: Her True Story* (about Diana, Princess of Wales) By Andrew Morton
- *David Beckham: My Son* By Ted Beckham
- *Tony Blair* By Thomas Collins
- *Posh and Becks* By Andrew Morton
- *Tony Blair: The Making of a World Leader* By Philip Stephens
- *Cheryl Cole: Her Story – an Unauthorized Biography.* By Gerard Sanderson.

3 Autobiographies including, for example:

- *Long Walk to Freedom* By Nelson Mandela
- *The Diary of a Young Girl* By Anne Frank
- *David Beckham: My Side – The Autobiography* By David Beckham
- *The Story of my Life* By Helen Keller
- *Being Jordan: My Autobiography* By Katie Price.
- *Through My Eyes* By Cheryl Cole.

4 Geographical/ecological non-fiction including, for example:

- *Planet Earth: As You've Never Seen It Before* By Alastair Fothergill and David Attenborough
- *Atlas of the World* By Oxford University Press
- *The Living Planet: A Portrait of the Earth* By David Attenborough
- *The Private Life of Plants: A Natural History of Plant Behaviour* By David Attenborough
- *The Life of Birds* By David Attenborough.

5 Home economics, cookery books including, for example:

- *Cook with Jamie: My Guide to Making you a Better Cook* By Jamie Oliver
- *Nigella Express: Good Food Fast* By Nigella Lawson
- *Gordon Ramsay's Just Desserts* By Gordon Ramsay.

6 Self-help books including, for example:

- *I Can Make You Rich* By Paul McKenna
- *Instant Confidence: The Power to go for Anything You Want* By Paul McKenna
- *How to Win Friends and Influence People* By Dale Carnegie.

7 Stories from the Bible including, for example:

- Adam and Eve
- Joseph
- Samson and Delilah.

Students might like to even discuss and debate whether the stories from the Bible are fiction or non-fiction.

Fictional stories:

Here are some different types of fictional stories and some examples of each one. Many stories may fit into more than one story category. Encourage the students to generate examples of their favourite books and try and decide into which category they may fit.

1 Nursery rhymes including, for example:

- 'Humpty Dumpty'
- 'Three Blind Mice'
- 'Jack and Jill'

- 'Baa Baa Black Sheep'
- 'Georgie Porgie Pudding and Pie'.

2 Fairytales, including, for example:

- 'Cinderella'
- 'Little Red Riding Hood'
- 'Hansel and Gretel'
- 'Jack and the Beanstalk'
- 'The Happy Prince and Other Tales' By Oscar Wilde.

3 Fables including, for example:

- 'The Hare and the Tortoise'
- 'The Boy who Cried Wolf'
- 'The Fox and the Grapes'
- 'The Lion and the Mouse'
- 'The Wolf in Sheep's Clothing'.

4 Science fiction including, for example:

- *Dracula* By Bram Stoker
- *The Strange Case of Dr Jekyll and Mr Hyde* By Robert Louis Stevenson
- *Star Wars* By George Lucas
- *The Matrix* By Larry and Andy Wachowski
- *Dr Who* television series
- *Star Trek* television series.

5 Crime/detective stories including, for example:

- *Agatha Christie's Poirot* television series
- *The Bill* television series
- *The Case-Book of Sherlock Holmes* By Sir Arthur Conan Doyle
- *K is for Killer* By Susan Grafton
- *Inspector Morse and Lewis* television series.

6 Fantasy stories including, for example:

- *James and the Giant Peach* by Roald Dahl
- *Alice's Adventures in Wonderland* By Lewis Carroll
- *The Indian in the Cupboard* By Lynne Reid Banks
- *Charlie and the Chocolate Factory* By Roald Dahl
- *The Lion, the Witch and the Wardrobe* By C.S. Lewis.

7 Mystery stories including, for example:

- *Death on the Nile* By Agatha Christie
- *Murder on the Orient Express* By Agatha Christie

- *The Famous Five* series By Enid Blyton (for example, '*Five go to smuggler's top*')
- *Columbo* television series
- *The Haunted House* By Charles Dickens.

8   Modern Realism including, for example:

- *Kiss* By Jacqueline Wilson
- *The Railway Children* By E. Nesbit
- *The Story of Tracey Beaker* By Jacqueline Wilson
- *Blubber* By Judy Blume.

9   Romance stories including, for example:

- *The Boys Next Door* By Jennifer Echols
- *The Princess Diaries* (cinema) By Gina Wendkos
- *The Proud Princess* By Barbara Cartland
- *Wuthering Heights* By Emily Brontë
- *Pride and Prejudice* By Jane Austen.

10   Drama stories including, for example:

- *Casualty* television series
- *Holby City* television series
- *EastEnders* television series
- *Robinson Crusoe* By Daniel Defoe
- *Hollyoaks* television series.

11   Adventure including, for example:

- *The Adventures of Huckleberry Finn* By Mark Twain
- *Treasure Island* By Robert Louis Stevenson
- *Lost* television series
- *White Fang* By Jack London.

12   Adventure/suspense/fantasy including, for example:

- *Harry Potter and the Chamber of Secrets* By J.K. Rowling
- *Harry Potter and the Goblet of Fire* By J.K. Rowling
- *Lord of the Rings* By J.R.R. Tolkien
- *Heroes* television series.

13   Comedy stories including, for example:

- *The Importance of Being Earnest* By Oscar Wilde
- *The Family* television series
- *Little Britain* television series
- *The Catherine Tate Show* television series
- *The Inbetweeners* television series.

14 Tragedy stories including, for example:

- *Salome* By Oscar Wilde
- *Romeo and Juliet* By William Shakespeare
- *Wuthering Heights* By Emily Bronte
- *Tess of the d'Urbervilles* By Thomas Hardy
- *Hamlet* By William Shakespeare.

15 Horror stories including, for example:

- *Carrie* By Stephen King
- *The Shining* By Stephen King
- *Dracula* By Bram Stoker
- *Jaws* (cinema) By Peter Benchley
- *The Texas Chainsaw Massacre* (cinema) By Joseph Stefano.

16 Reality stories/series including, for example:

- *Big Brother* television series
- *I'm a Celebrity, Get me Out of Here* television series
- *The X Factor* television series
- *Pop Idol* television series
- *MasterChef* television series.

17 Poetry – discuss with the students how poems also tell stories, and explore how the use of rhyme and alliteration may help to tell the story. Include, for example:

- 'Dulce Et Decorum Est' By Wilfred Owen
- 'Not Waving But Drowning' By Stevie Smith
- 'The Daffodils' By William Wordsworth
- 'The Owl and the Pussy-Cat' By Edward Lear
- 'The Highwayman' By Alfred Noyes
- 'The Listeners' By Walter De La Mare
- 'On the Ning Nang Nong' By Spike Milligan.

18 Songs – explore with students which songs tell stories and how the music and rhythm helps to tell the story. Include, for example:

- 'Ben' By Michael Jackson
- 'Every Breath You Take' By P. Diddy and Faith Adams
- 'Cat's in the Cradle' By Harry Chapin
- 'A Boy Named Sue' By Johnny Cash
- 'At Seventeen' By Janis Ian
- 'Starmaker' By Fame
- 'The Gambler' By Kenny Rogers
- 'The Windmills of Your Mind' By Noel Harrison
- 'Vincent' By Don McLean
- 'Coat of Many Colours' By Dolly Parton.

Session 3

3

Names of students: _____

_____

Facilitator: _____ Date: _____

School: _____

Class: _____

Aims	Method/Activities	Materials
To revise and recap themes from previous session.	Group discussion with students taking turns to give an example of one important thing they learned from the previous session.	Flipchart or whiteboard, paper and pen.
To introduce the idea that every story has a **story structure** with key elements. To identify the three main parts of a story: beginning, middle and end using train with carriages to pictorially represent the parts of a story.	Show students the train track and separate carriages of the train. Discuss how a story is similar to a train, requiring a front or beginning part or carriage, a middle part and an end or last carriage. Get students to identify the different parts of the train already drawn on the track, making links with the carriages and the three main parts of the story. Some students will prefer to use the story F1 race track to identify the three main elements of a story. The story F1 race track can be used in the same way as the train track, making explicit for students the importance of having a clear beginning, middle and end of a race (and story). Use the students' stories they brought in from last session to identify the three main parts of a story. See teaching notes for examples of stories that can be used in the session with students identifying the different parts of the story. These are examples and you may like to make up your own or bring in favourites from home or school. Discuss how each story has one beginning, middle and end, with the middle being made	Story train track with carriages representing the beginning of the train (story), middle carriages representing the middle of the story and the end carriage representing the end of the story. Story F1 race track with a clear beginning, middle and end. Use written stories that students brought in from last session's homework activity and use these stories to identify the three main parts of a story.

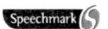

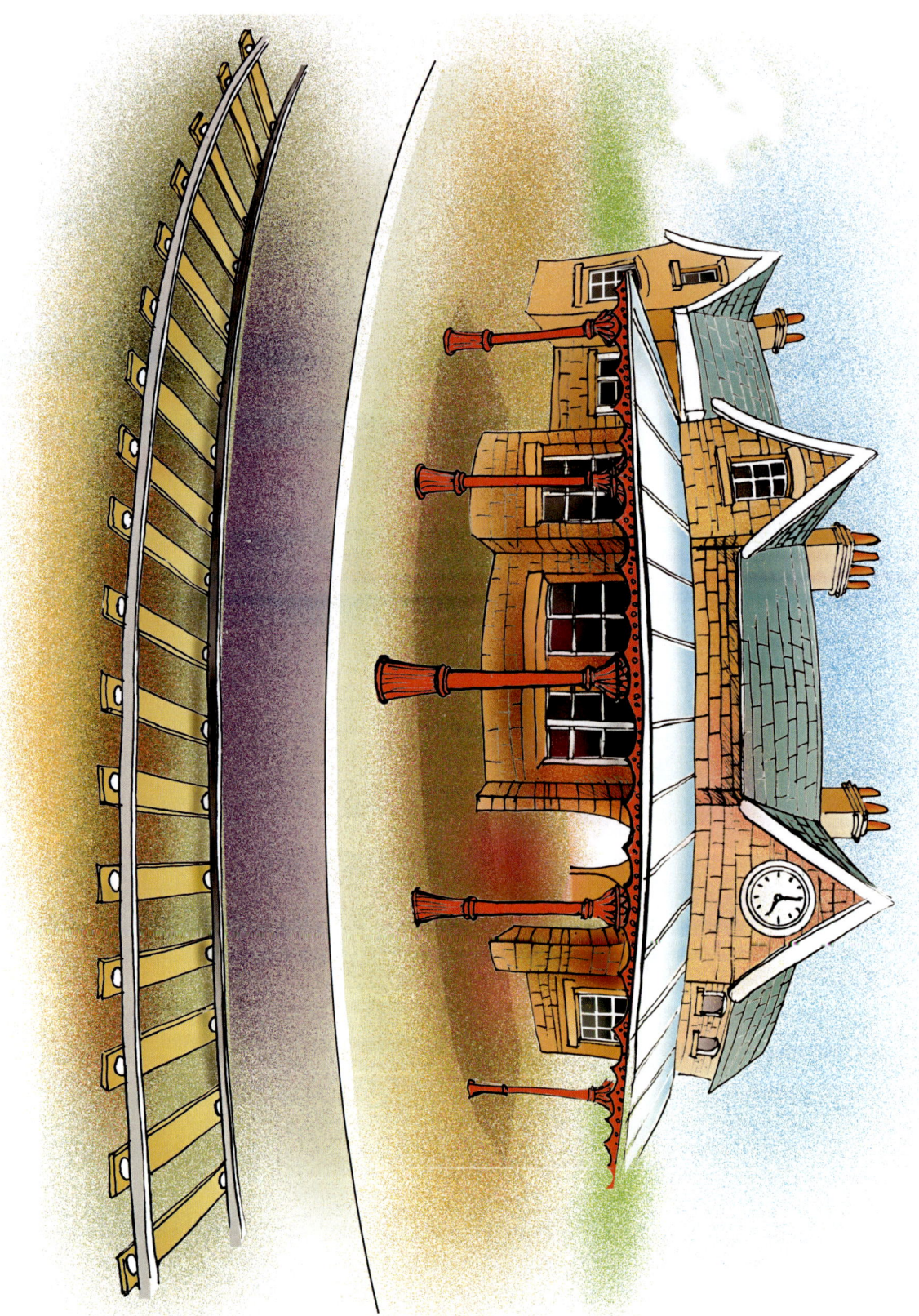

Story train track

Story train track

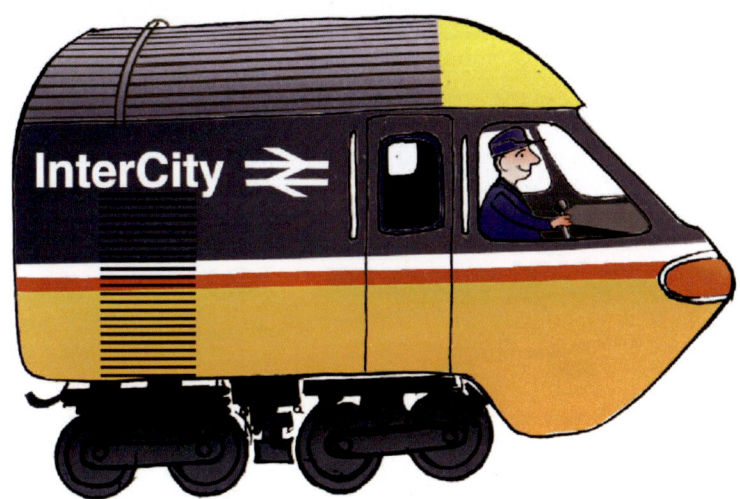

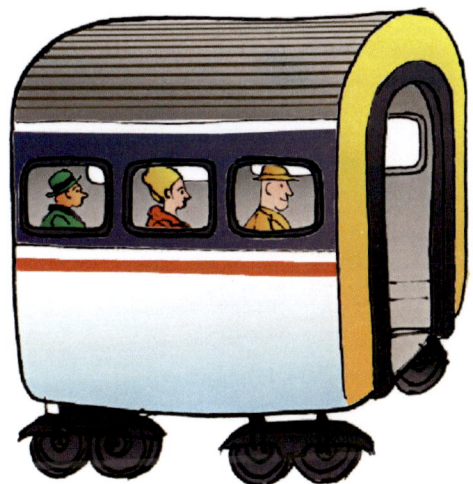

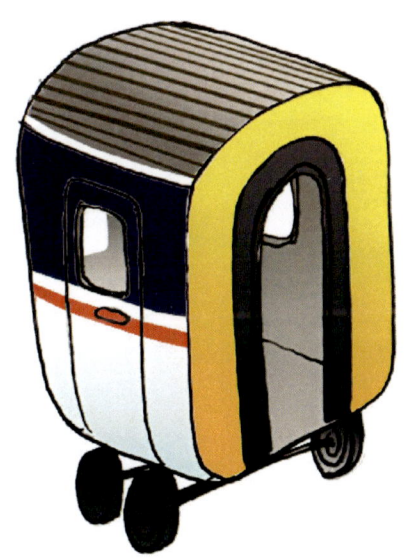

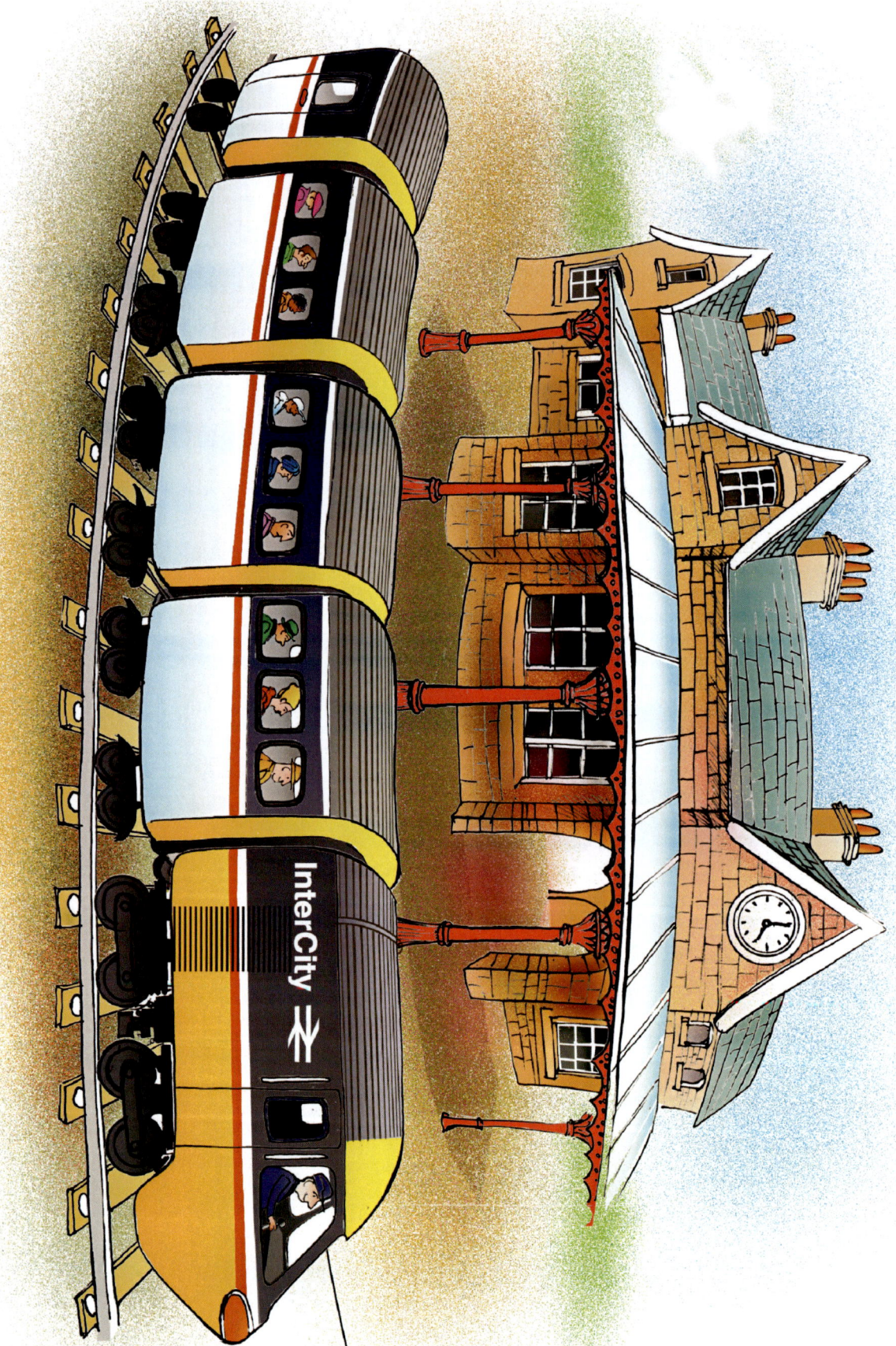

Story train track

Story F1 race track

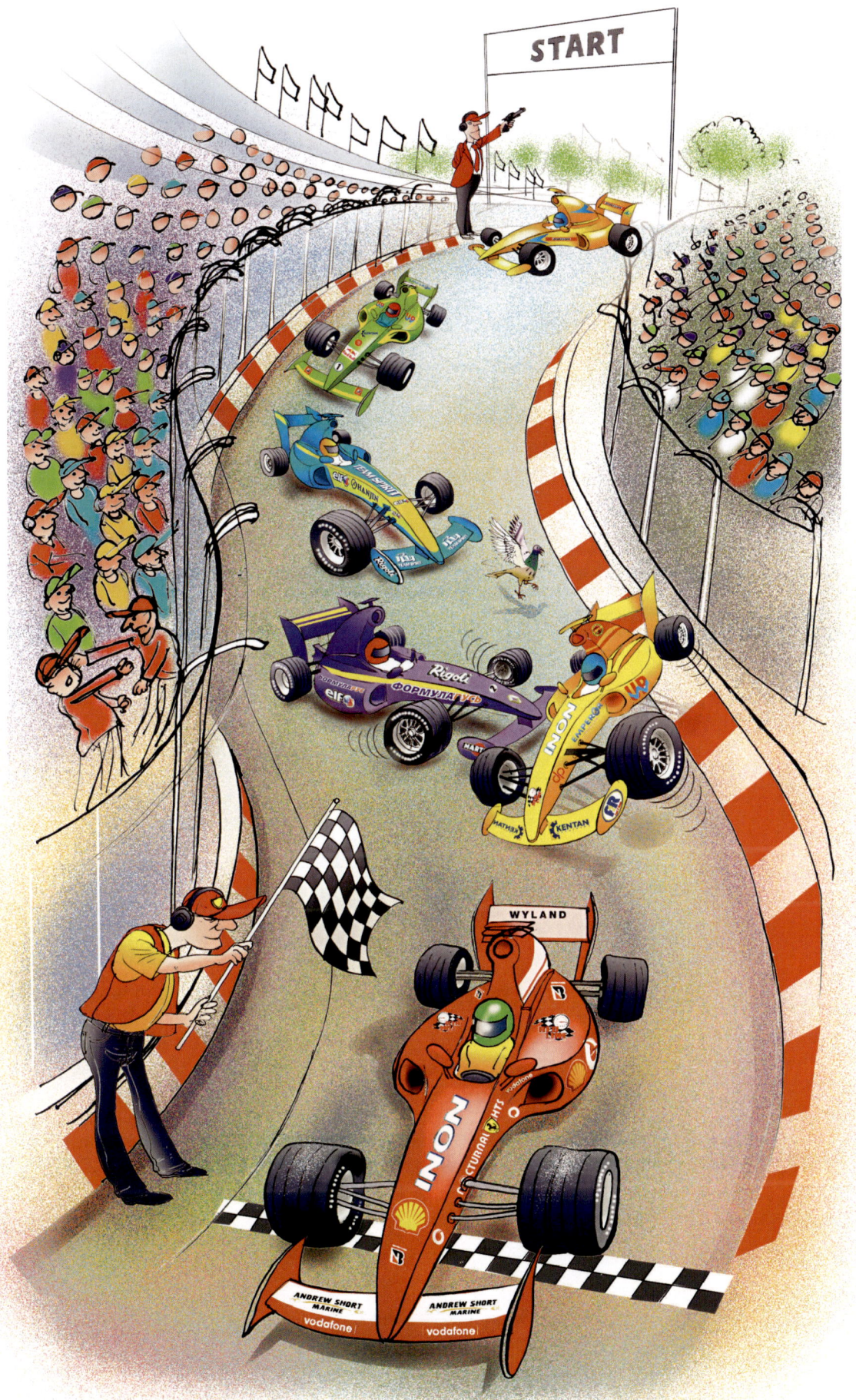

Aims	Method/Activities	Materials
	up of one or more events or episodes, which is why the train can have more than one middle carriage. The story F1 race track has a few events taking place in the middle of the race, for example, a bird flying on the track, two cars smashing into each other and a fight taking place between two people in the stands. Again, this is to emphasise that the middle of a story can be made up of one or many different events.	
To identify what makes a good **beginning, middle** and **end** to a story.	Group brainstorm activity around what makes an exciting beginning, middle and end. Encourage group members to identify for themselves what makes a good beginning, middle and end. See teaching notes for examples and suggestions.	Flipchart or whiteboard, paper and pen.
To produce stories as a group with the three main story elements: beginning, middle and end.	The group sit in a circle and take turns telling parts of a story from a title or beginning and end parts shown or read to them. The story pencil is used to indicate who is telling the story. The story pencil is passed around members of the group, with one member starting the story with a beginning, then passing on the story pencil to the next member who adds a middle, then passes it on to the next student who may add another event for the middle of the story, and then the next student who provides the end of the story. Prompts for these stories can be the story titles and beginnings and ends of stories provided in the teaching notes. You also may like to add your own ideas, or let the students come up with their own story themes.	Story pencil or microphone. Story titles and beginning and end parts of stories from teaching notes. Story train track and carriages. Story F1 race track.
To sum up and revise contents of the session.	Get volunteers from the group to summarise the main content of the session. Ask other members of the group to help, adding in the parts that may have been omitted.	Flipchart or whiteboard, paper and pen.
Mission to Achieve: Each student to make up their own short story with a clear beginning, middle and end to share with the group next session.		

Evaluation of session/General comments

Teaching notes for Session 3

Examples of short stories with clearly identified beginning, middle and end parts

Here are some stories which can be read to the students to help them identify the different parts of the story. Encourage students to identify the different parts of each story.

Discuss how each story usually has:

1   a beginning, which introduces some or all of the main characters of the story and sets the scene for the events that will follow in the middle section;

2   a middle part of the story, which consists of character development, the first, initial or initiating event, and the subsequent actions and reactions that occur which make up the main story theme or plot. The middle section can include one or more separate or related actions, and often contains a problem or conflict which needs to be resolved; and

3   an end, where the outcomes of all actions and events are drawn together and a conclusion is usually provided.

To make this storytelling exercise more interesting, exciting or even challenging for some students, encourage them to add events to the story plot, or even change the beginning and end of the story. For example, perhaps Nathan, the character in the story below, 'The football match', does not find his dad. Get the students to think about what would happen next in their own story. What would he do all alone and lost in London? Many of my Manchester United-devoted students changed the story to Arsenal losing the match!

Story 1
The football match

Beginning: One frosty cold Saturday morning, Nathan woke up early. He was very excited. His dad had promised to take him to watch football. It was Arsenal versus Tottenham Hotspur at the Emirates Stadium in London. He put on a warm coat, a hat and gloves and had a quick breakfast. He was now ready to go.

Middle: Nathan and his dad took the tube to the football stadium. He had never been on the tube before today and felt nervous and excited at the same time. It was packed with football supporters, all singing football songs. They walked the short distance between the station and the stadium. It took them much longer than expected though, as there were thousands of people making the same journey. For a second Nathan panicked as he lost sight of his dad. He looked around him, desperately scanning everyone in front of him. With a huge sigh of relief, he caught sight of the bright scarlet coat which his dad had insisted on wearing.

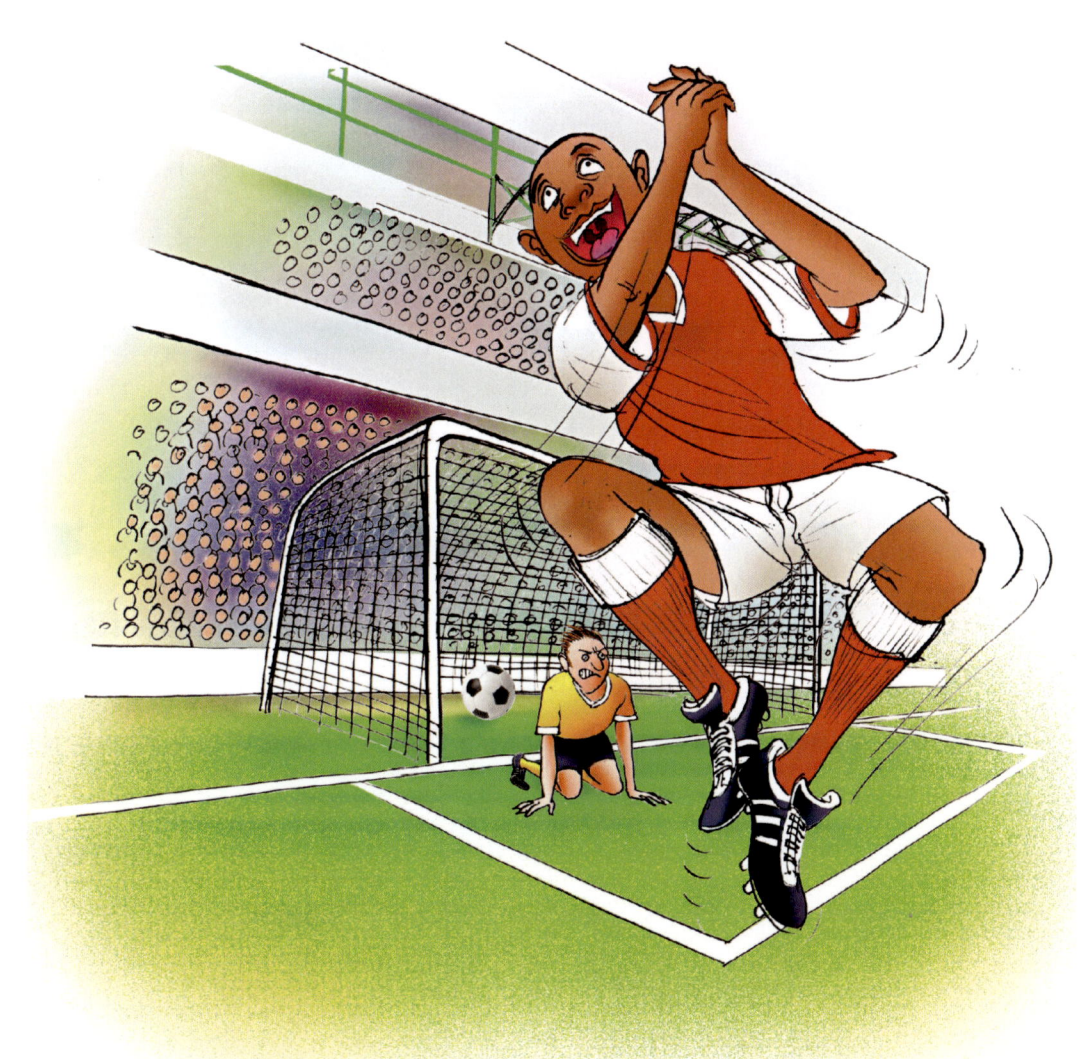

They finally arrived at the football stadium and found their seats. Nathan was delighted when his dad bought him a programme which had been signed by all the players. He knew all his friends at school the next day would be very envious. When the teams and the referee ran onto the pitch everyone cheered. Nathan recognised the Arsenal manager, Arsène Wenger, as he came out on the pitch waving to the fans. The referee blew his whistle and the game started. The game was very exciting but no one had scored. With 10 minutes left to play, Arsenal got the ball. Nathan stood up and shouted 'go on, go on', and he had butterflies in his stomach. Then Gallas got the ball and kicked it into the back of the net. Nathan jumped up and down with excitement and clapped and clapped. The final whistle blew and Arsenal had won – just.

End: Nathan and his dad walked happily back to the tube station. This time there seemed much less people and less of a rush. He felt very excited that his team had won. Nathan thanked his dad for the best day ever. He couldn't wait to share his day with his friends at school on Monday and gleefully looked at his signed programme. He hoped that his dad would take him to another game really soon.

Story 2
A magical Christmas

Beginning: It was still dark and misty outside when Mary woke up and jumped straight out of bed. There was no time to put on her dressing gown. It was Christmas morning and she wanted to go downstairs as quickly as possible and see what surprises awaited her.

Middle: She ran into her mother and father's bedroom to wake them up too. She didn't want to waste a second sleeping on such a perfect day. She was very excited and happy. In fact she was happier now than she had been for a long time. Mary's father had been serving in the army in Iraq and had been away for a very long time. He had just returned home and the family were finally together again. They all went downstairs together happily singing Christmas carols. There under the Christmas tree was a huge brightly wrapped present. It had her name on it. She tore off the wrapping paper to reveal a beautiful pink bicycle. She had never had a bicycle and would now have to teach herself to ride.

End: She gave her mum and dad a big hug and kiss and rushed outside with her new bike. She happily spent the day riding up and down the streets in the neighbourhood. She was so proud of her new bike, but nothing beat the feeling of having her dad home again.

Story 3

The nightmare tube journey

Beginning: It was a hot and sweltering summer's day. Jonah was in a hurry to meet his friends and go to the Arctic Monkeys concert. He was stuck on a packed tube which seemed to be crawling along.

Middle: He looked at his watch in frustration. He never thought he would ever get to the stadium. But finally the tube stopped at his station and he leapt out from the crowds and rushed up the escalator. When reaching the gates at the station, he plunged his hand in his back pocket to get his tube ticket. 'Oh no' he gasped: there was no ticket in his pocket. He looked around him to see if it had fallen on the floor. But he found nothing. People were coming and going and Jonah was looking around randomly, not knowing what to do. He looked at his watch and saw how late it was. He was certain to miss the concert now. He then saw signs about a £10 penalty for not having a tube ticket. Jonah could not afford to pay this amount. He went up to the inspector and explained to him that he had lost his ticket. He promised the inspector that he had in fact bought a return ticket on the way to the concert. The inspector looked at him and told him not to worry. He opened the gates to let him out and told him to enjoy the concert.

End: Jonah could not believe his luck. He had told the truth and the inspector had believed him. The truth is always the best option. Jonah ran out of the station and managed to meet his friends, and get to the stadium just as the band came on stage. Whew, all's well that ends well!

Story 4
The loyal pet

Beginning: Once upon a time there was a little brown and white mongrel dog called Billy. Billy lived in a small terraced house on a council estate with his owner, Jessop. Billy loved Jessop a lot but his owner was often away working and Billy was left alone. He felt lonely and sad.

Middle: Billy would spend most of the day on his own in the garden, in the rain, snow and sunshine. There was no one for him to play with. He would often dream about all the friends he might make if he ran away from home. He often was tempted to do this, but his love for his owner stopped him. He knew that Jessop needed him and couldn't help working so hard. He just wished that he could make friends in the neighbourhood, but he was the only dog in the street. One day as he was snoozing he heard barking in the distance. It sounded like it was getting closer and closer. A large van drew up and a young boy and his dog fell out of it laughing and playing. These must be the people moving into the house next door, thought Billy. The dog was larger than Billy, shaggy and white and she looked very happy and playful. Billy barked loudly and called her over and she came running with her owner. Billy introduced himself and the three of them began playing together. Billy was so happy and excited to meet the new neighbours. He could not believe his luck in having such fun new neighbours to play with.

End: Now Billy would never be alone again. He had his owner Jessop to love and look after, but he also had new friends with whom he could play and have fun. Lucky Billy! He felt like the luckiest dog in the world. Now he would never be alone again.

Story 5
The shiny lost mobile phone

Beginning: Ahmed was walking slowly home from school. It was getting dark and the streetlights were shining brightly, forming sparkling crystals in the large puddles on the pavements. He was tired and fed up after having spent all afternoon in detention. Now he had to go home and face the music! He walked slower and slower the nearer he got to his house.

Middle: 'Hey, what's that in the road', he called out as he passed something vibrating and flashing on the side of the road? He carefully bent down to see what it was. There before his eyes was the most fancy mobile phone he had ever seen. He picked it up and quickly dried off the water. It looked brand new. Ahmed could just imagine what all his friends would say the next day when he brought in 'his new phone'. That would show that irritating boy Oscar who was always showing off his new gadgets! Ahmed looked around him nervously, wondering if anyone had seen him pick up the phone. With relief he saw he was all alone. He could simply put the phone in his pocket and hide it away until school the next day. As he walked home, he thought a little about whom the phone belonged to, and whether they had realised it was lost. He remembered how badly his grandmother had felt when she had lost her purse and how

 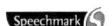

sad she felt that no one had returned it to her. He knew that he could not keep the phone. It was not his to keep, and he would not ever really be able to enjoy it as it belonged to someone else. So, as soon as he got home, he showed it to his parents. They looked at all the phone numbers and managed to find the owner's number. They immediately called her to tell her not to worry as they had her phone. She was so relieved and came over immediately to pick it up. Ahmed's parents told her that it was he who had found it and she thanked him remarking how wonderful it was to meet such an honest person. She insisted on giving him a £20 reward. His parents were so proud of him; so much so that they completely forgot how late he was and that he had got detention. Lucky Ahmed!

End: As Ahmed waved goodbye to the lady, he felt really happy. He knew he had done the right thing by telling his parents about the phone, and now it was back to its rightful owner. Maybe what his grandmother said was true about good deeds leading to more good things. Here he was £20 richer, and had even been forgiven for getting into trouble today at school. A bad day had really ended very well. And now he would start saving to buy one of those fancy phones of his very own.

Teaching notes for Session 3

What makes an exciting and interesting story?

Through discussion with the students, identify what makes a good beginning, middle and end. Encourage students to provide their own views, ideas and beliefs. Here are some examples which can be used to encourage students to come up with their own ideas. Please add your own to this list. These are simply to get the discussion started.

The beginning of a story should:

- Capture the attention of the audience.
- Introduce the main people or characters of the story – the setting (character).
- Describe the characters in enough detail to give the listener a feel for who they are and what they are or were like.
- Describe where the story is taking place, for example, the sun, planets, ocean, sea, what country, house, school or shop – the setting (place).
- Describe when the story is taking place, for example, the past, present or future, morning, afternoon, night, summer or winter – the setting (time).
- Set up what is going to happen in the story, what the problem, plot or theme of the story will be.

The middle of a story should:

- Introduce the main initiating (first) event which begins the story.
- Explore in more detail what the characters are experiencing.
- Describe the thoughts, feelings and actions of the different characters.
- Describe the actions, what happens in the story.
- Introduce the conflicts and problems of the story.
- Detail how the characters deal with the problem/s or events, how they act and react to the situation and what their plans are to deal with the situation.
- Provide the motivations and desires and wishes of the characters.
- Explore how the characters feel about what has happened to them or others in the story.
- Contain the plot of the story, the main part/s of the story, what is happening.
- Be exciting and continue to engage the attention of the audience.
- Include a main exciting part of the story, often called a climax.

The middle of the story may have one or even more events or actions that have happened within the story. These events may be related to each other, or be quite separate. Think of an episode of your favourite soap and all the actions and happenings that take place in the one story episode.

 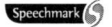

The end of a story should:

- Give the outcome of the story, including the outcomes and results of the actions that have taken place in the middle sections.
- Draw together and integrate all the parts of the story.
- Provide a lesson or moral that has been learned as a result of the story.

The end of the story can either provide the listener with all the outcomes and answers about the story and how the problems were resolved, or leave the listener with unanswered questions so they want to find out more in the next instalment. This is called a cliffhanger and is used to ensure that the audience is curious to know how the story will end, so they come back for the next instalment, or are simply left with lots of unanswered questions.

Include other ways of making a story more exciting. For example, these may include:

- Tell a story with which others can identify, for example, tell a story about current issues that students face in school, when talking to a group of school students, for example, bullying or preparing for exams.
- Use prompts, for example, when describing a tramp as your main character, put on an old coat or a threadbare hat.
- Use role play, so act out as if you were the tramp, with perhaps a limp and shuffle.
- Use direct speech. This means speak as if you were the actual character. So if you were telling a story about a tramp, you might say in a trembling weak voice, 'Excuse me sir, do you have some spare change for a cup of coffee?'
- Use different voices to indicate different characters in the story.
- Make your voice as interesting as you can. Do not speak in one way all the time. Try and vary your voice by changing your loudness levels (loud and soft), the speed at which you talk (fast and slow) and the pitch (high and low).
- Use all the elements of the story: beginning, middle and end, as well as all parts of the story planner which will be introduced in session 4.
- Provide detailed and interesting descriptions which allow the listener to imagine what the characters look like, feel and are experiencing.
- Include humour – humorous stories are fun to listen to.
- Include your own personal experiences when you can. So if you are telling a story about bullying, and you have had some experience of it, then use this experience when telling the story. It will make it seem more real.
- Use interesting and different words, for example, use a variety of different adjectives to describe the characters and/or settings. So, for example, instead of saying 'the small man', you may like to say, 'the tiny gentleman' and instead of saying 'it was summer', you could say, 'it was a warm balmy summer's evening with the humidity clinging to every pore'.

Teaching notes for Session 3

Story titles and beginnings and endings to generate stories

Here are some examples of story titles and beginnings and endings which can be used to get students to provide different and exciting parts of the story in order to complete the story as a group. These are suggestions and you are encouraged to add your own as well.

Story titles

1 The skeleton in the cupboard

2 Sugar and spice and all things nice

3 The haunted aeroplane

4 The magic wheel

5 Walking on Jupiter

6 The evil inventor

7 Things will never be the same again

8 The chef in the cellar

Suggested story beginnings

1   Jason woke up one morning to the sound of rustling in the attic. It was a cold morning and he was all alone in the house.

2   Once upon a time there was an evil wizard who had seven magic wishes that he could use.

3   One sunny morning in August, Lexi went out of her holiday chalet onto the beach. She was horrified at what she saw in the distance.

4   The day had finally dawned for Minnie the mouse. This was the day when her life would finally change.

5   In the beginning, everyone looked calm and collected. There was not a sound to be heard. The crowd waited in anticipation.

6   It was one fine day, in the middle of spring, and Melanie could not hide her excitement. She knew that this was the start of a wonderful adventure.

7   Summertime had finally come and with it the last day of the school year. There was so much to do, and Nita rushed through the school gates with great excitement. How would she manage to sit through her final lessons when all she could think about was the journey they were about to take?

8   Ibrahim walked, behind his parents and sister, into the fancy restaurant. His shoes hurt and his tie was tied tightly around his neck. His eyes caught his sister's and he knew that things were only going to get worse.

 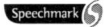

Suggested story endings

1 There were no other options for Jamie. This was the end of the road for him.

2 Charlotte hugged her father closely. She was so relieved that he was OK and felt like she would never let him go again.

3 Johnny looked at the boys in the playground. He finally knew who his friends were. It was a lesson he would never forget.

4 Pushing strongly against the current, Maria finally broke free of his firm grasp. She gasped for air. She was finally free!

5 She would never again walk around while using her mobile phone. She had had a lucky escape and would be more careful in future.

6 Tears flowed down her cheeks. She waved a final goodbye, turned around and limped slowly out of the room. It was the end of her dream.

7 The gargantuan green-eyed monster took one last look at the city he had demolished and stomped off with a bellowing victory cry. He had come to destroy, and destroy he had!

8 Majka held the trophy with trembling hands, and slowly lowered it down until it was resting next to the grave. He had earned it, and it was his to keep, forever more.

Session 4

Names of students: _____

_____

Facilitator: _____ Date: _____

School: _____

Class: _____

Aims	Method/Activities	Materials
To revise and recap themes from previous session.	Group discussion with students taking turns to give an example of one important thing they learned from the previous session. Emphasise story structure and the beginning, middle and end of a story.	Flipchart or whiteboard, paper and pen.
To **share and evaluate the stories** produced as homework.	Students to tell the stories they have produced for homework. Students to identify the beginning, middle and end of each story. Encourage the evaluation of each story with regards to story structure and general interest and excitement. There is a list of suggested questions in the teaching notes for session 15 which can be used to evaluate the stories. Many of the questions will not be suitable at this early point, but some will be appropriate and students should be encouraged at this early stage to begin evaluating their stories and those of their peers.	Stories constructed by students for last session's Mission to Achieve. Use train track and carriages or Story F1 race track to talk about the parts of the story. Questions for evaluation of stories from teaching notes from session 15.
Each student to **produce their own new story** with a clear beginning, middle and end.	Each student holding the story pencil produces a short story using the picture prompts of **story episodes** included in the resource. Students to choose their favourite story episodes from the picture choices provided. Group members to give feedback on each story and critically evaluate how interesting each story is and how the beginning, middle and end parts fit together to form an exciting story.	Story pencil or microphone. Pictures of story episodes included in the resource to be used as prompts. These include: • car crash • footballer scoring a goal

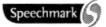

Aims	Method/Activities	Materials
	Other group members can be encouraged to provide a title for the story they hear which reflects the contents of the story.	• boxing match • woman with broken down car • fish under water • lady sunbathing in scorching sun • witch casting a spell • boy getting bullied at school • cat guarding a mouse in a hole • boy drowning. Use train track and carriages and story F1 race track to identify different parts of the story. There is also an option to use the story football match and the story athletics race track, both of which show the main structure of a story and have a clear beginning, middle and end section. These can all be found in the accompanying DVD.
To present a summary of their chosen favourite story and identify the beginning, middle and end elements.	Each student will have already chosen a favourite story that they will be using to work with throughout the programme. The students will be given the opportunity to give a summary of the story, and identify for the group the beginning of the story, the middle parts including the main plot and story theme and the ending of the story. The facilitator should have already written down the students' story choices and have the list in the file as a reminder of the choices made	Story pencil or microphone. Train track and carriages or story F1 race track to facilitate recall of all three story elements.

Aims	Method/Activities	Materials
To produce **middle** and **end** sections of a story to follow the story beginnings provided.	for the duration of the programme. Group members to listen to different story **beginnings** provided in the teaching notes that follow and to provide suitable and exciting **middle** and **end** sections to each story beginning. The student holding the story pencil or microphone is the person with permission to tell the story and he or she can pass the pencil on to another group member whenever they wish for them to continue the story. Group members can be encouraged to rate each story using a 10-point rating scale (1 = poor story and 10 = best story). At the end of the activity, the group can nominate a story star, the person who told the best story. This is a good opportunity to emphasise to the students the importance of having a specific structure to the story, so, for example, the beginning needs to come first to set the scene, and the end needs to come last to tie all the loose ends together. Also raise awareness about the importance of having a structure to anything the students talk about, even when talking with friends, teachers, etc. Encourage them to see the importance of structuring their speaking to ensure their message is relayed as they would like. Their teacher, for example, is going to be less likely to accept or even listen to their reason for coming late to class if their explanation is unstructured and has no clear beginning, middle and end. It is also important to point out to the students the importance of relating the three sections to each other in a coherent way. It is essential for them to see that having the introduction given to them, as in this exercise, constrains them to some degree as they have to make the middle and end parts fit sensibly with the beginning part that was provided. So, for example, if the introduction is set in an airport with pilots, they cannot continue with a plot that centres around elephants in Kenya! Unless of course, that is where the plane is heading…	Story pencil or microphone. Examples of story beginnings provided in the teaching notes.

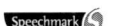

Aims	Method/Activities	Materials
	You might like to have some fun with this and provide your own ridiculous example where the middle and end sections have no relation at all to the beginning, and introduce a completely new set of characters and settings. Ask the students whether the story makes any sense and get them to identify what went wrong and how they could fix it.	
To provide a suitable **title** for their story.	Each group member is to generate an appropriate **title** for their story. Discuss with the group what titles do and what information they provide for the listener and reader. Their title should capture the essence of their stories. Encourage students to explore the importance of a title and how the title provides the listener or reader with information about what the story is going to be about. The title is also important as it can capture the listener's attention even before the story is begun. Get them to think about any titles that may not describe what is happening in a story or some that are more or less interesting.	Flipchart or whiteboard if possible and pen and paper to allow students to write their chosen titles.
To sum up and revise contents of the session.	Get volunteers from the group to summarise the main content of the session. Ask other members of the group to help, adding in the parts that may have been omitted.	Flipchart or whiteboard, paper and pens.
Mission to Achieve: Students to ask two people, one from school and one from home, what their favourite stories are and the reasons for these choices.		

Evaluation of session/General comments

 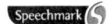

Story football match

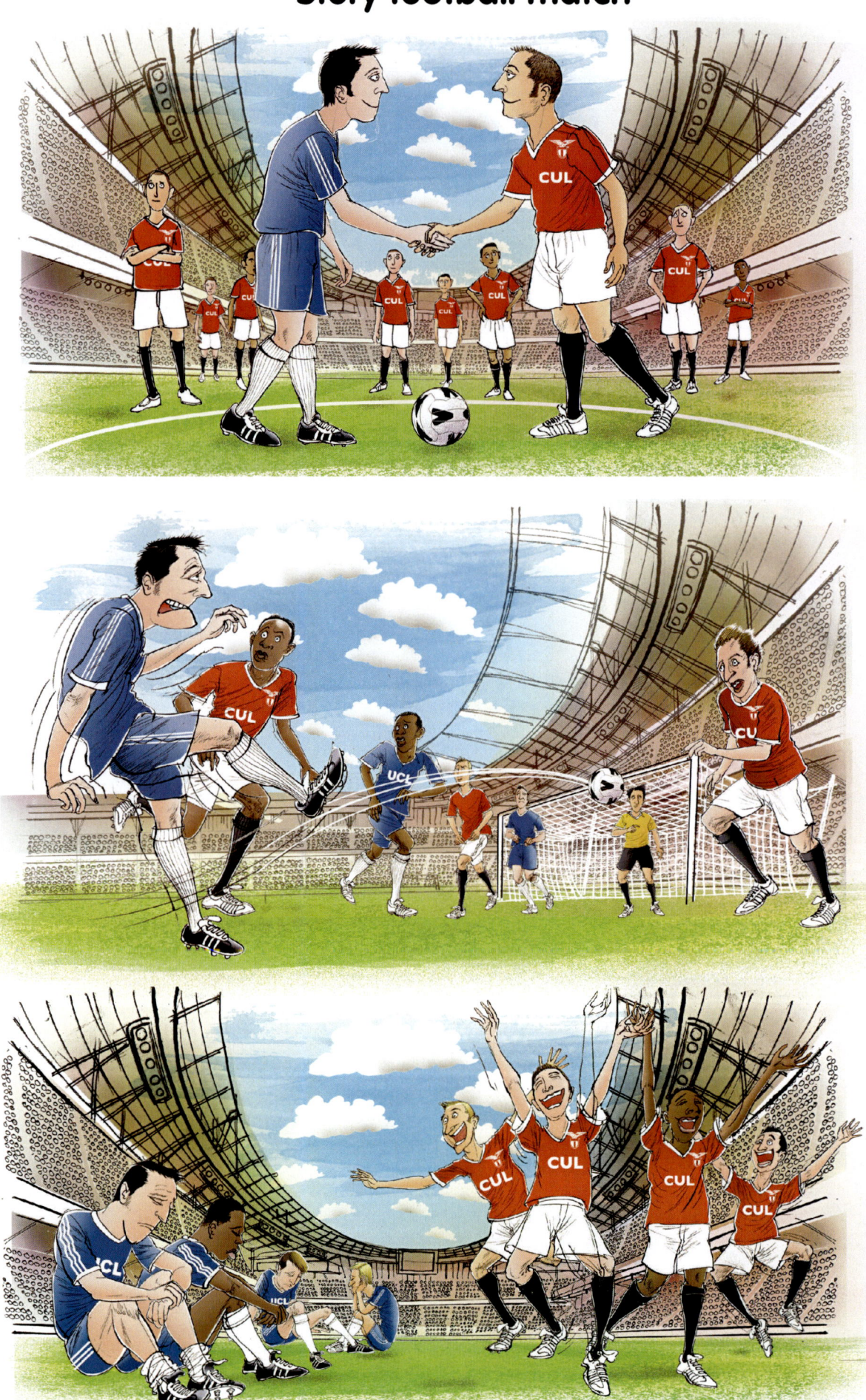

Speechmark

Story athletics race track

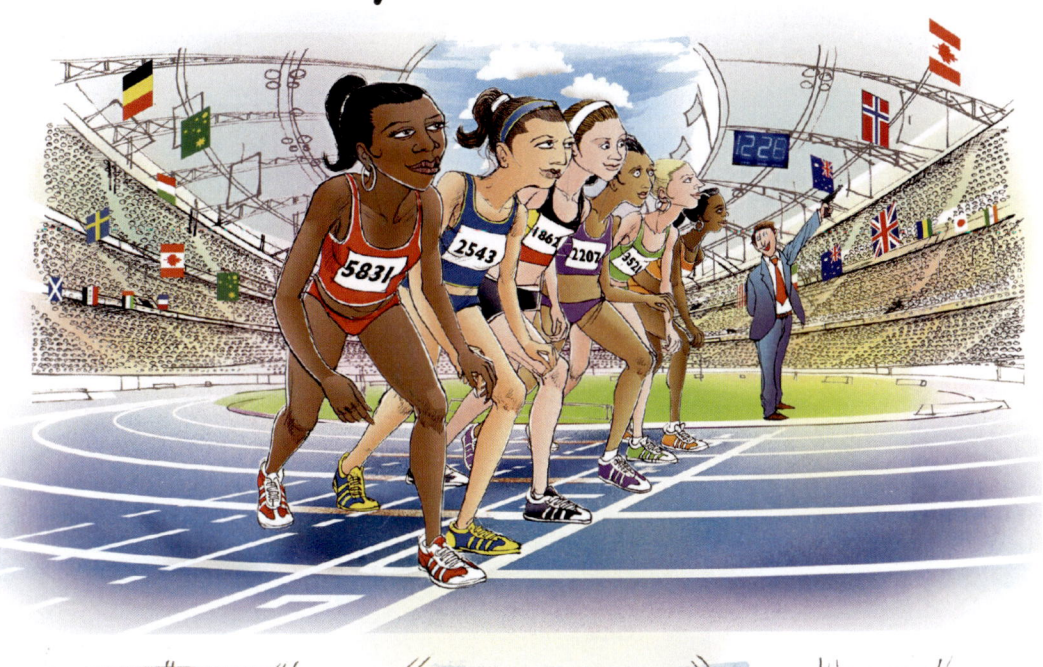

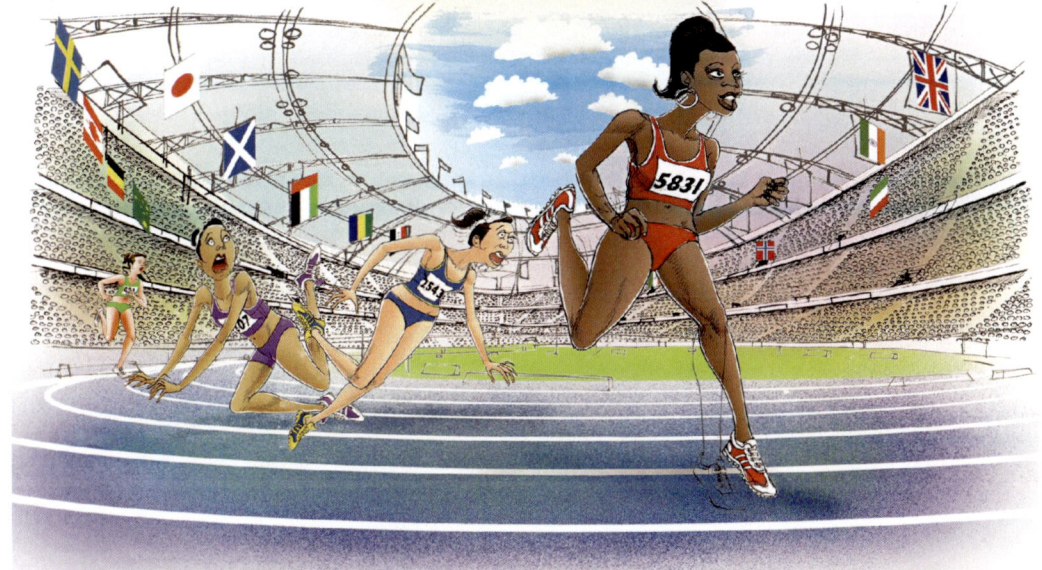

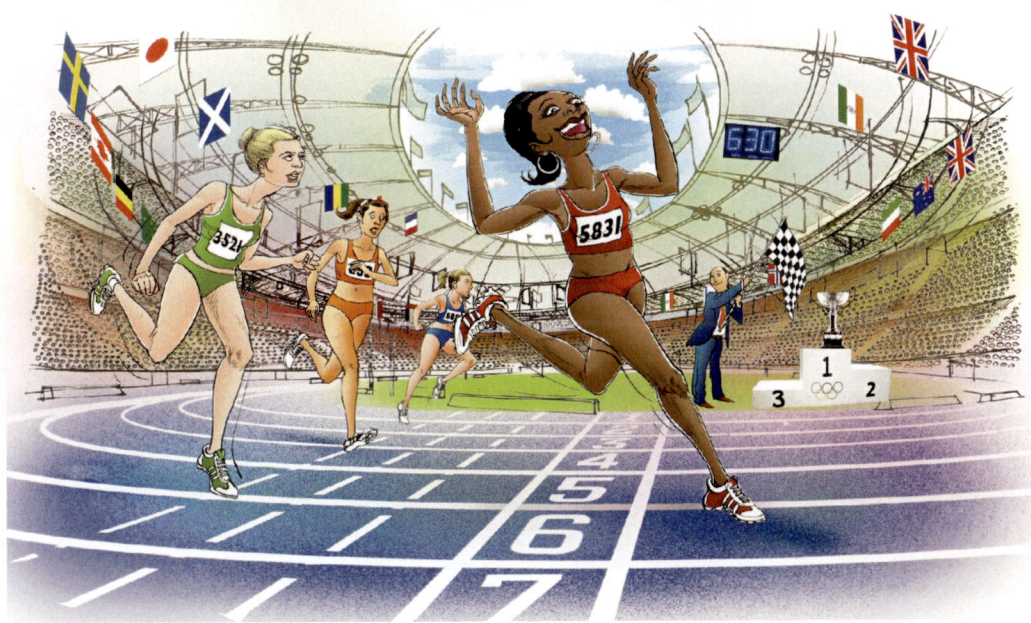

 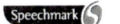

Teaching notes for Session 4

Story beginnings to generate stories

Here are some examples of story beginnings which can be used to get students to provide different and exciting middle and end parts of the story. The facilitator reads out the beginning part and each group member takes turns following on from the story beginning, adding the middle and end sections. The student with the story pencil or microphone is the one who has the floor and tells the story. They can pass the story pencil on to another student whenever they like and the next person then has to continue the story. These are suggestions and you are encouraged to add your own as well.

You will find it useful to use the story train track and carriages and/or the Story F1 race track to indicate the different parts of the story. The programme also includes a story football match for football lovers and a story athletics race track for the girls in the group who specifically asked for something other than football and motor racing! All of these are simply story templates which show the overall structure of any story: beginning, middle and end. Each one of the templates contains a clear start (beginning point), a middle with various actions and an end which brings the event to a conclusion. Some students will just use their favourite one over and over again, while others like to use all at different points. Give them a choice but be sure they are making explicit the different parts to the story. And some will just want to keep using the train and carriages. Let them do so!

Please ensure at various points in the session to emphasise the importance of each story having a structure to it. Explain that the beginning needs to come first, followed by the middle and finally that the story ends with the conclusion. Emphasise the importance of having a structure to whatever is being told, so having a structure to what they say is as important when they are talking to their friends or explaining something to their teachers. Use the following story beginnings as starting points for the students' own stories. Explain any words that may not be understood. Please feel free to come up with your own exciting story beginnings. You may also like to use the story beginnings which were given in the previous session.

Suggested story beginnings

1   Kerry opened the door slowly and with great trepidation. It was heavy and leaned ominously to one side. As it creaked open, Kerry shrieked with shock.

2   After athletics practice, Sally returned home. As she came up the drive, she saw the front door wide open. There was a policeman standing at the door looking at her with a grim expression on his face.

3   Paul took his seat high up in the stadium next to his dad. It was a freezing cold day. Through the thick mist and fog, he could just about make out his favourite players coming on the pitch. The game was about to begin.

4   It was midnight and Raj was fast asleep, warm and snuggled up in bed. Suddenly a flash of light appeared at his window.

5   It was almost Christmas Eve and Marjorie had still not finished her shopping. She arrived at the mall and rushed inside to get her last-minute shopping. The mall was eerily silent.

6   Saturday night had arrived and it was the final of the X Factor competition. Everyone gathered in front of the television, anxiously waiting to see who would be crowned the winner. Suddenly the television went dead.

7   Sebastian and his friends were on the bus one spring morning heading to school. He suddenly heard a piercing scream from the lady in the front row. 'Stop, stop,' she shouted, 'that man has taken my purse. Someone please help me.'

8   Anita had finished playing with her toys and put them all safely in the toy box. As she left the room, she heard voices coming from the toy box. Slowly she approached the box and cautiously lifted the lid.

9   The old wise wizard sat in front of the steaming cauldron mixing the green and blue liquid. He stirred in four frogs' legs and five pine cones. This would do the trick, he thought, and finally put an end to the wicked ways of the witch.

10 The beautiful blonde model walked down the ramp in a ravishing red ball gown. Everyone gasped at her beauty. Suddenly, there was a shout at the back of the room. Everyone fell to their knees and the model cried out in pain.

 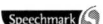

Session 5

Names of students: _____

_____

Facilitator: _____ Date: _____

School: _____

Class: _____

Aims	Method/Activities	Materials
To revise and recap themes from previous session.	Group discussion with students taking turns to give an example of one important thing they learned from the previous session. Emphasise story structure and the beginning, middle and end of a story.	Flipchart or whiteboard, paper and pen.
Encourage students to **share examples of favourite stories** that they had collected from other people for homework.	Discuss with the students their homework task. What favourite examples of stories had they collected and who had they asked. Explore what reasons they got for the chosen favourites and see whether there are some common favourites. Discuss with students some of the classics which people often refer to as their favourite story. These may include *Black Beauty, The Lord of the Rings* or *The Lion, the Witch and the Wardrobe*. Devise a top 20 chart of favourite books and stories from the students' own favourites and those of the people they surveyed. How many members have read these 'top' books and which ones would they choose to read that they have not read already? Get their reasons for their choices. Are there any books on this list that some members would not choose to read, and if so, why?	Flipchart or whiteboard, pen and paper.
To introduce the **story planner**, providing an overview of all parts of a **story**.	Use the **story planner** and introduce the different parts of the story. Explain to the students that the basic **story structure** of **beginning**, **middle** and **end** which have been discussed in previous sessions can be expanded into a more complex story structure	Story planner. Story train track and train carriages. Story F1 race track. Story football match. Story athletics race track.

 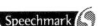

Aims	Method/Activities	Materials
	which allows for the telling of a fuller, more complex and exciting story. Explain how the story planner includes the three main basic story elements of beginning, middle and end and expands on each section. Describe the different components of the story planner using the teaching notes that follow. Draw attention to the corresponding symbols or pictures for each story element on the story planner. For example, the firing shotgun signifying the start or beginning of the story, the film reel representing the middle of the story, and the chequered flag signifying the end of the story. You may need to take some time to explain the use of these visual cues and how they correspond to each story segment. For example: • Firing shotgun or pistol as in a shotgun which is fired to signify the start or beginning of a race. • Film reel – as in a taped movie or DVD and symbolising the main episode/s of a story and its middle element. • Chequered flag – as in the chequered flag used to signify the end of a race. **1 Beginning** • Setting: characters, time, place **2 Middle** • Episode: first event (what happens?), immediate response, action/s, reaction/s **3 End** • Outcome: result, message. Explain to the students how the **beginning** part of the story sets the scene for the whole of the story and describes the different characters that form part of the story, as well as the time and place where the story occurs. The middle part of the story includes the story episode/s which describes the main plot or theme of the story. This will include the initial event, the first event that happens in the story	Make photocopies of both the story planner and story F1 race track or any of the other story structure templates the students choose (football or athletics) for each student.

Aims	Method/Activities	Materials
	which starts the action of the story, followed by the immediate response of the characters to this initial event. This is then followed by the action/s and reaction/s of the characters to resolve the problem or issue that has been encountered in the story. Frequently the episode of a story contains a problem or conflict; however it does not need to do so. It could also describe a happy or joyous event. The end part of the story is the outcome and draws together all the different parts of the story. It describes the result/s of all the actions taken in the story and can also end with a message or moral for the listener or reader which the characters in the story have learned. Use the story train track and train carriages to show how the different components of the story planner map on to the rail track. For example, how the setting matches up with the front of the train, the episode corresponds to the middle carriages and the outcome to the last carriage. Encourage students to first identify the different parts of the train already drawn on the track, making links with the carriages and the different parts of a story from the story planner. Then students can take turns to build the train on the empty track by adding the different carriages and describing what parts of the story they represent. Use the story F1 race track, the story football match and the story athletics race track to show how different parts of a story make up a whole, coherent and exciting story.	
To identify different parts of the story planner: **setting, episode and outcome**.	Use examples provided in the teaching notes to identify different parts of the story using the story planner. Get students to identify the different elements of each story read to them and encourage critical evaluation of each part. Use the story planner and story F1 race track (and story football match or story athletics race track) to discuss the different story components.	Story planner. Story train track and train carriages. Story F1 race track. Story football match. Story athletics race track.

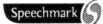

Aims	Method/Activities	Materials
	Associate the start flag at the **beginning** of the race track with the start or beginning of a story, and the chequered flag at the **end** of the race track with the end of the story. The **middle** of the story, the episodes and main content of the story, can be associated with the middle of the race track where various events are occurring, for example, two cars colliding with each other, a car hitting the side of the track and a bird flying on the track.	Examples of stories included in the teaching notes. It is fine to use other examples that you have brought to the session or even examples that the students have brought.
	The same sequence of events can be shown in the story athletics race track with the beginning corresponding to the runners lining up at the start and the firing of the gun representing the start of the race; the middle section corresponding to the actual run (including the action of two runners tripping each other up); and the end with the runners crossing the line at the end of the race, with the chequered flag again signifying the end.	Questions for story evaluation from teaching notes from session 15. Remember only some of these questions will be appropriate at this point.
	Many students will recognise the sequence of events of beginning, middle and end from the story football match where the beginning is clearly signified by the shaking of hands, the middle section contains the actual match with its various trials and tribulations, and the end (outcome) of the match with celebrations and glory for one side.	
	Students will also be able to use these story templates to provide further details of the **setting** of the story, for example, the **place** of the story being an F1 race track (so explore with students where this could be if it was in the UK versus if it was in Italy), a football ground (again this could be any football ground the students choose but this choice will constrain the place where the game (story) takes place, for example, if it is Wembley stadium it will be in the UK, but if it is the Bernabeu Stadium, this must mean that the story (match) takes place in Spain). The same type of discussion can be had with the story athletics race track.	

Aims	Method/Activities	Materials
	In the same way, these story templates can be used to explore **characters** (the players, athletes and drivers as well as the fans in the stands) and also the **time** (present, past or future, day or night, season, etc). For example, what season does football usually take place in, did the race take place in sunshine and so on.	
To sum up and revise contents of the session.	Get volunteers from the group to summarise the main content of the session. Ask other members of the group to help, adding in the parts that may have been omitted.	Flipchart or whiteboard, paper and pen.
Mission to Achieve: Students to watch a favourite television programme and identify the different parts of the story using the story planner.	Students can choose any television programme (for example, *EastEnders* or *Holby City*) and identify each part of the story. They are to record their answers on a copy of the story planner. They are required to record the **characters, time** and **place** of the story, to identify the different episodes of the story and the main parts of the **episode** (ie first event, immediate response, action/s, reaction/s) as well as the **outcome** (including result and message).	Provide students with copies of the story planner which they will use to record details of their favourite television programme.

 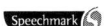

97

Evaluation of session/General comments

Story Planner

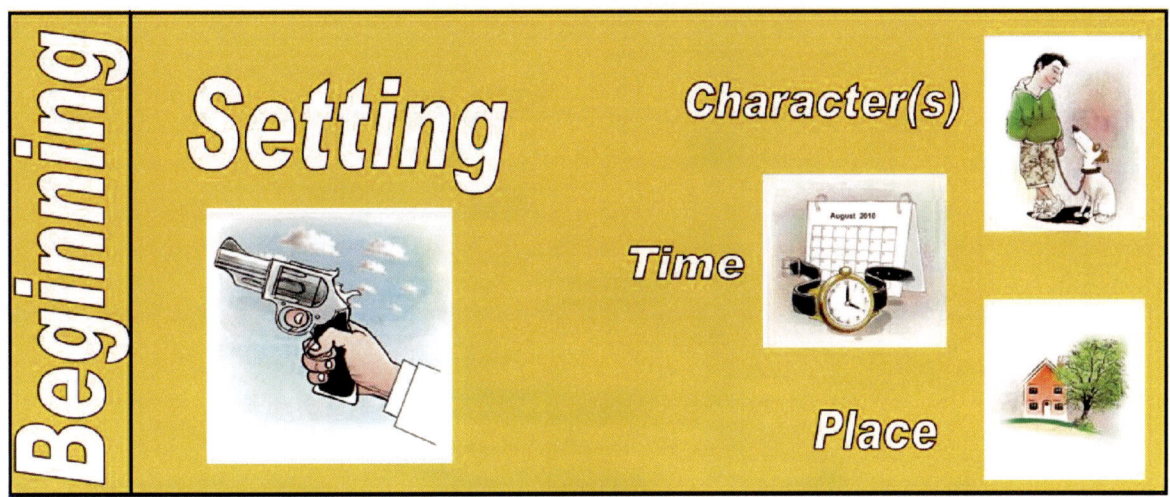

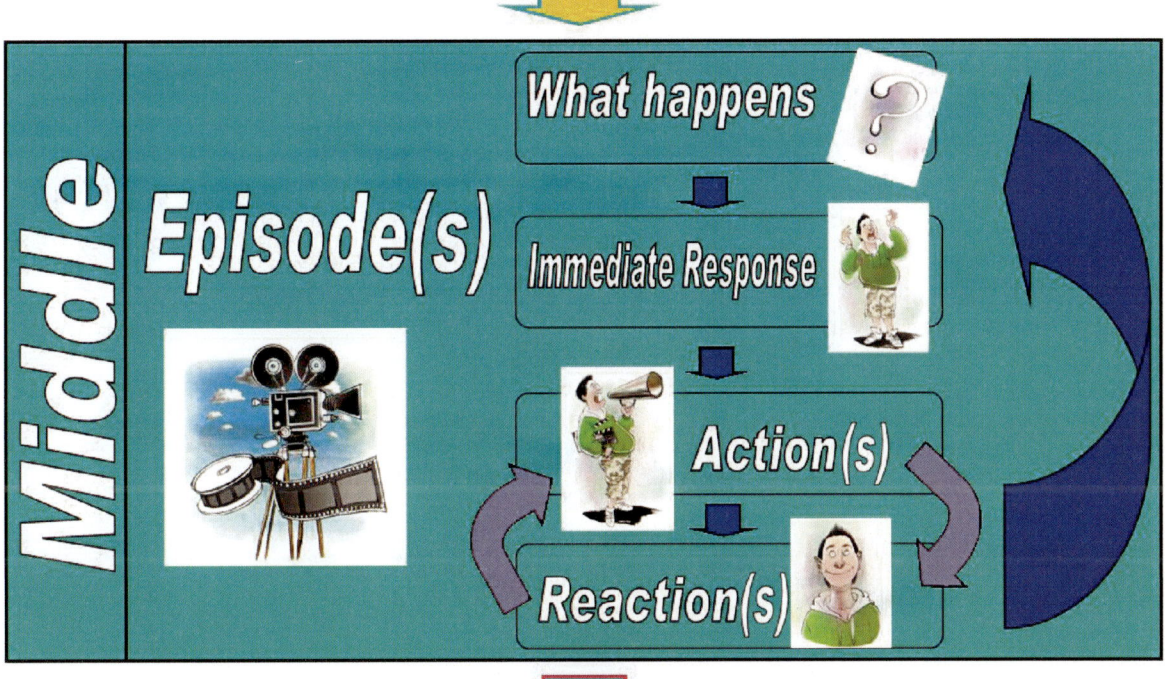

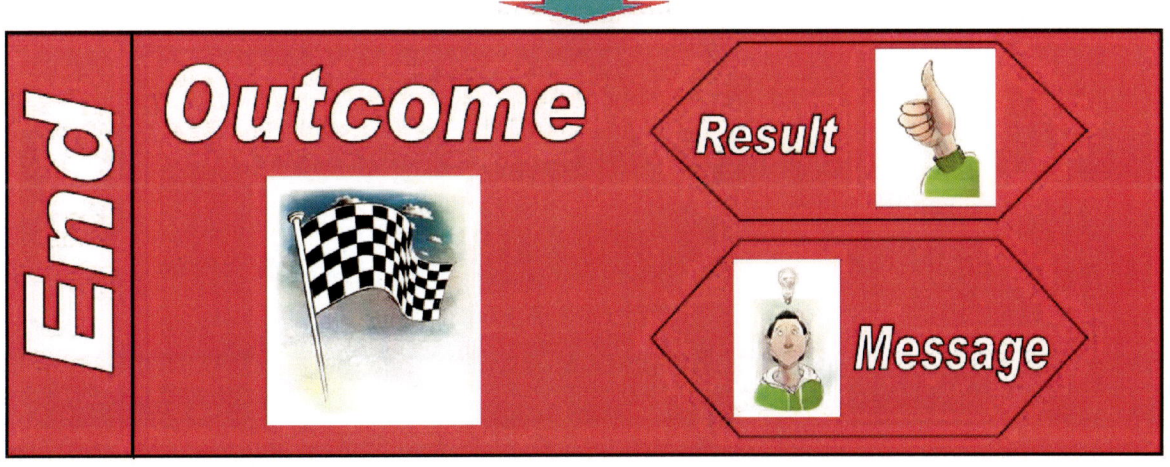

Teaching notes for Session 5

The story planner⁴

In this session, you will provide the students with an overview of the story planner. Photocopy a copy of the story planner for each student. Show them the planner and explain to them how the three basic elements of beginning, middle and end can be expanded into further elements. Talk about each one of these elements providing examples as you go. Explain to the students how their stories will be more interesting if they ensure that they contain each one of the components from the story planner. They should be encouraged to use the story planner as a checklist to ensure that the stories they produce in these sessions contain all the necessary components. Take time to explain the story planner as students may find the concepts quite complex and difficult. Give as many examples as you can and revise and repeat as much as necessary. Encourage the students to explain the story planner in their own words once you have finished explaining it to them. This will give you an idea of how much they understand and what parts need more emphasis and time.

Please note:
It is important to note that there are many different story planners available, all of which categorise story components in different ways, some more complex than others. They all however fit into the main story elements of beginning, middle and end. Usually the main differences occur in the 'middle' section with some planners providing more detailed categories within this section than others. The story planner used in this programme was adapted from Stein and Glenn (1979) and attempts to include a sufficient number of categories to allow students to write and devise complex stories within a structured and coherent framework, while at the same time trying to avoid too much confusion by using too many elements.

Please remember that the story planner is a tool which we want students to use to help structure their stories. The planner will not always successfully categorise all stories. Its use should be flexible and adaptable to different story genres. There will be times when some categories overlap, for example, an initiating event seems to occur in the beginning rather than in the middle of the story, or when the opposite occurs, for example, when the ending does not include an outcome and result. This is fine. Stories will vary and will be different. Remember always that the story planner, like any other tool, template or strategy in the programme, is a means to facilitate and enhance listening, speaking and storytelling. It is merely the vehicle to assist in moving the students forward in their journey to becoming skilled communicators and storytellers.

Explain the components of the story planner in the following way:

1 The **beginning** of a story (symbolised on the story planner with a picture of a firing shotgun) includes the following:

---

⁴ The story planner has been adapted from Stein and Glenn (1979).

Setting: this gives us information about the people in the story, and about where the story takes place. It answers the questions about who, where and when. The setting is therefore made up of:

> ➤ **Characters.** The characters are who the story is about. Characters in a story can be human beings, animals, plants and non-living things like toys or cars. Characters can change as the story is told and things happen to the characters in the story. A good story will provide many details about each character including a physical description, personality traits, likes and dislikes, mood, etc. More and more information is revealed about the character as the story progresses. The actions of the characters throughout the story give us more information about what they are like. Students should be encouraged to explore the actions, thoughts and feelings of the characters. Draw students' attention to the picture cue on the story planner signifying characters, i.e. picture of the boy and dog. Remind them that the characters in stories can be human or non-human.

> ➤ **Time.** This section provides information about when: when does the story take place? The story can be set in the past (for example, the Victorian era), the present or the future. If it is in the present, it provides information about what time, what season, day or night, dusk or dawn, etc. It can include different types of weather, so it may be a windy day, a frosty morning, a boiling evening, etc. A good story will give specific details about the time in which the story takes place. On the story planner, the picture cue for time is a watch and calendar.

> ➤ **Place.** This section provides details about where: where does the story take place? The story can take place anywhere; some stories may not even take place on Earth but will be set on Mars or Jupiter or even on the Sun or Moon. The story can take place in the sea, or in space. It can take place in different countries like England, Thailand or South Africa. It can take place in London or Manchester, or in any other city in the world. A good story will give precise and specific examples of where the story takes place, so not just in London, but in an old haunted house, or a derelict school, or a school playground, football stadium or hotel. The picture of a house and tree on the story planner signifies the 'place' component of the setting of the story.

The beginning of a story sets the scene for the events that will take place in the middle of the story. It provides details of the characters, time and place of the story, but also prepares the listener or reader for the events that will take place in the next section. So the beginning also sets the scene for what will happen and introduces the listener or reader to the beginning of the problem that the character will have to face or the main theme and plot of the story.

Many details about the story setting are given in the beginning part of the story, but more information can be added about the characters, place and time over the course of the story. Some characters may even be added at later points in the story. This has to be planned though and cannot just happen because the characters have been forgotten!

 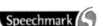

Show the students the story planner and identify where these parts of the beginning of the story fit in as part of the story planner.

2 The **middle** of a story (symbolised on the story planner by a film reel) includes the following:

Episode/s: this gives us the 'meat' of the story, the exciting bits to the story. This is often termed the plot of the story, what happens in the story – the story theme. It tells us **what happens**. It often includes a problem which the characters have to solve, and gives information about what the characters do to try solve the problem/s. A story can have one or more episodes, depending on its length and complexity. Think about an episode of your favourite television programme. This may be *Casualty* or *Dr Who*. Each episode has exciting happenings which occur. An episode often has what is called a climax, a part of the story that is very exciting, and the story usually builds up to that climax, to the most exciting part of the story. Every episode/s can be made up of:

> ➤ ***The initial event: what happens 1?*** This part of the story includes the first event of the story. Sometimes it is called the initiating event, the first event of the story which starts the action. It is the first happening of the story which makes the character/s do things which then lead on to the rest of the story. It can often be the problem or conflict of the story. On the story planner, the question mark signifies this initial event, the 'what happens?' in the story.

For example: 'Johnny sat down in front of the television to watch his favourite programme. He had waited for this the entire day. He put the television on and there was a sudden loud bang.'

> ➤ ***Immediate Response 1.*** This part of the story describes the immediate response or reaction of the character to the initial event. It can include the feelings and thoughts that the characters experience as a result of the first event. This immediate response can be a physical reaction, where there is some physical activity (for example, body shaking), or it can be a cognitive response, where the character shares his thoughts (for example, not believing it is happening), or an emotional response where the character shares his feelings (for example, feeling depressed or worried). Draw students' attention to the picture of the shocked response of the boy, which signifies the 'immediate response' element of the story.

For example: 'Johnny jumped off the sofa in fright giving a short scream as he did so. The television was not working. Oh no, what could he do?'

> ➤ ***Action 1.*** The next part of the episode of a story describes the action or set of actions that the character/s take/s in response to the first initiating event of the story. It explores the action/s that the character/s take/s to resolve the problem, conflict or happening that has taken place. The action part of a story is depicted on the story planner by the picture of a film director shouting 'action' on a film set.

For example: 'Johnny had to get the television working again, and fast. He couldn't miss his favourite programme. That would be terrible! Suddenly he remembered that his neighbour was a television engineer who worked for Sky TV. He didn't know his neighbour at all well. In fact he had never even said hello to him before. He had just noticed that he drove around in a Sky TV van. Could he really ask his neighbour to help him when he had never met him before? He couldn't miss his programme, so he had no choice. He had to go over there and hope his neighbour would help out. He went over to the next door house and introduced himself. He explained to his neighbour what had happened and asked him if he would come over and look at the television. The man did not hesitate. He said he would come immediately. His neighbour brought his toolkit and began fiddling with the television. In five minutes he had the television working again. It was simply a fuse.'

> ***Reaction 1.*** This part of the story contains the subsequent response or reaction to the action that was taken to solve the problem introduced in the first event. So it would describe Johnny's reaction to getting his television fixed. It is the response or reaction of characters to the action that has just been described. It can also include the moods, thoughts and feelings of the characters. This final part of the episode of the story, the reaction to the action, is depicted on the story planner by a boy with a very happy reaction.

For example: 'Johnny was ecstatic. What a relief! He gave his neighbour a huge hug and thanked him profusely. Johnny settled back on the sofa, remote control in one hand and a bag of crisps in the other. The programme had just started.'

Each episode can have multiple parts to it, so may include more than one first event or happening, immediate response, action and reaction. An episode can therefore have more than one happening, response, action and reaction within the same episode which are closely related to each other. For example, something else may have happened to Johnny while he was watching television. Perhaps the television went on the blink again, or maybe he spilt all his coffee on his trousers while he was watching his favourite programme. These initiating events would then lead to further actions and reactions.

> ***What happens 2?***
> ***Immediate response 2***
> ***Action 2***
> ***Reaction 2.***

> ***What happens 3?***
> ***Immediate response 3***
> ***Action 3***
> ***Reaction 3.***

The middle part of a story could also include more than one episode. For example, the story we are using here about Johnny watching television could also include another episode with something else happening to Johnny at a different time and about something completely different. So Johnny could be cooking dinner for his friends after watching his television programme and the second episode of the story could be about him cooking dinner. This new episode would then have a new happening, immediate response, action and reaction which all related to Johnny cooking dinner. If this was a book about the life of Johnny, these different episodes would be separated into different chapters.

Focus first on explaining the components of one episode making up the middle part of the story. You can talk about multiple happenings, actions and reactions making up an episode, and even more than one episode in later sessions.

Show the students the story planner and identify where these parts of the middle of the story fit as part of the story planner.

3   The **end** of a story (depicted on the story planner by a picture of a chequered flag) includes the following:

Outcome: this provides the conclusion to the story. It gives information about how the story ends. It can be used to give a neat finish to the story and tie up all the loose ends from the story. It does not always have to give a neat ending, though. Sometimes it can leave the listener or reader with unanswered questions to ensure that they read or watch the next instalment. It also can provide the listener with an overall message or theme, almost like a lesson. This is not essential but can add a lot to the story and gives the listener or reader something to take away with them. The end is made up of:

> *Result.* This is usually the last few lines of the story, providing the final result of all the happenings and actions that have come before in the story. It gives information about the conclusion of the story, if and how the problem was resolved, how the story ends and what happens to all the characters. It integrates all the different actions and parts of the story. Since the result brings together all the different parts to the story, it is appropriate that the picture used on the story planner to denote the result part of the story is a 'thumbs up' sign. This does not however mean that the result of a story must always be positive.

For example: 'The programme finally came to an end. Johnny took a long and relaxed stretch. It was even better than he had expected. Thank heavens he hadn't missed it.'

> *Message/moral.* The outcome of the story can also include a moral, theme or lesson that the character/s has/have learned as a result of what happened in the story. Sometimes one has to think carefully about what the message of a story is. For this reason, the picture signifying the message part of the story on the story planner is a boy thinking very carefully (about the message or moral of the story!)

For example: 'It was really lucky that his neighbour worked in television. It made Johnny realise how important it is to know your neighbours as you never know when you might need them, or when in fact they might need you!'

Show the students the story planner and identify where these end parts of the story fit as part of the story planner.

It is important to remind students that not every story will fit exactly into this story structure. Some stories, for example, will have an ending where the outcome is not provided or is uncertain. This is often when a cliffhanger is used which leaves an audience or listener in suspense.

 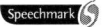

Teaching notes for Session 5

Examples of stories

Use the following examples to identify the different elements of a story from the story planner.

Story example 1

Here is an example of a story that can be read out to students showing the different story elements corresponding to the parts of the story planner. Take time to read this story to the students and discuss how and why each part corresponds to a story element in the story planner.

A fish called Psycho

Beginning

Setting: It was a cold early winter's morning **(time)**. The beach was completely deserted **(place)** except for a lone runner **(character)** who was running along the road. A small turquoise and purple fish called Psycho **(character)** was playing with his friends amongst the coral in the water **(place)**. Psycho was very small, about the size of a 10p coin. His skin was smooth and sleek and he had black piercing eyes **(character)**. He was keeping warm by jumping around. The water in England in winter was always freezing **(place)**.

Middle

Episode: Suddenly, there was a burst and rush of water. All the fish looked up and stopped playing their game. A large vicious fish the size of a tractor came crashing through the waves. He looked very hungry and was on the hunt for breakfast. His large jaws were opening and closing and through them one could see his sharp white teeth **(what happens – initial event)**. Psycho was so scared that every part of his little body was shaking with fear **(immediate response)**. He turned around and swam furiously in the opposite direction to the frightening fish. 'Help me, help me' he yelled with all his might. Luckily his father heard his cries and swam to meet him. Psycho's dad swept him up and took him to the safety of the family home **(actions)**. Psycho almost fainted with relief. He turned to his father and gave him a big hug. 'Thank you so much dad for saving my life.' He went and hugged every member of his family and all of his friends. He felt so happy to be back safe with his family and friends **(reactions)**.

End

Outcome: Everything was quiet again in the sea. Psycho was back safely home with his family and the vicious fish was nowhere to be seen. All Psycho's friends had also managed to escape. Tonight they would have a party to celebrate **(result)**. Psycho had really learned a valuable lesson from today. In future, he would not venture far without his father or another adult **(message)**.

Bring to the students' attention that there can be a main character in the story (Psycho), but that the story can also have many other characters, for example, the runner, Psycho's friends and his father. It is also important for them to see that even though usually the main characters are introduced in the beginning of the story, other characters may be added during the course of the story. So, for example, Psycho's dad is introduced as part of the action of the story, and the vicious fish is introduced to us during the initial event.

Discuss with the students the ways that Psycho tried to resolve his problem, that of the frightening fish. He tried to escape by swimming away as fast as possible in the opposite direction, as well as calling for his dad. These attempts at solving the problem/s presented in a story are usually found in the middle of a story, within the story episode.

Story example 2

The school science project

Beginning

Setting: Nobody likes to do homework and Parminder was no exception (**character**). As she walked wearily home from school (**place**) on a bleak and dark Thursday afternoon (**time**), she felt worried about the school project she had been given (**character**). It was already 5pm (**time**), later than usual, as she had been held up in detention. She trudged home in the dark (**time**), her blazer tightly buttoned around her slim frame, and her oval freckled face and black pigtails at the mercy of the wind (**character**). Finally she reached her house on the outskirts of the town in Essex (**place**).

Middle

Episode: After grabbing a sandwich and drink, Parminder settled down at the table to begin work on the project. She took out everything she needed and put all the materials on the table. Suddenly, to her horror Parminder realised that she could not find her science book. She looked again in her bag, but it was nowhere to be seen. How could this have happened? She could not do the project without her book (**what happens – first event**). Parminder was distraught. She would never be able to complete the project now. 'What a dunce' she thought. She had to stay calm and think what she could do (**immediate response**). Suddenly she had a brainwave. She would invite her friend Louise to come over and work on the project with her. She quickly called Louise who luckily was at home. Louise was working on the same project too and was struggling to finish it. She immediately agreed to come over to Parminder's and work on the project together. Parminder reminded her to bring her science book (**actions**). Louise arrived at Parminder's house with the all-important science book. Parminder rushed to the door and hugged and kissed her friend. The two of them sat at the table and began working on the project together. Parminder was so relieved. Now she would finish the project and not get into any trouble (**reactions**).

 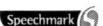

End

Outcome: Parminder and Louise finished the project much quicker than expected. They even had time to watch a bit of television. Their teacher was so happy with their projects and said they were two of the best projects she had seen (**result**). It seems like it is sometimes better to work with others. Two pairs of hands are often a lot better than one pair (**message**).

Story example 3

A surprise visitor

Beginning:

Setting: It was late on a school evening (**time**) and Tony was getting ready for bed (**character** and **place**). It had been a long and arduous day and he had trained hard at football training that day (**time** and **place**). Tony was 12-years old and his favourite sport was football (**character**). He was strong and big-boned. People often thought he was older than his years. He was fit and strong, and was determined to make the football team at school this year. He was very confident that he would be in the school team (**character**). He got into bed and switched off the lights (**place**). His bedroom was on the top floor, in the attic, and was covered in posters of footballers from Chelsea, his favourite football team (**place**).

Middle

Episode: As Tony drifted off to sleep, he began dreaming about how he would score the final all-important goal. In the distance, he heard someone softly call his name. 'Tony, Tony, wake up,' the voice whispered. It was so soft that Tony went back to sleep thinking he was dreaming. A little later he heard the voice again, but this time he felt a slight pat on the shoulder. 'Come on Tony,' the voice said, 'come out to play'. Tony woke with a start and there in front of him was the famous footballer Bobby Moore (**what happens – first event**). Tony couldn't believe it. He worshipped this man. He had been the captain of the team which won the World Cup (**immediate response**). Bobby Moore was beckoning him outside: 'Come on Tony; come play some football with me outside.' Tony leapt out of bed, pulled on a jacket and carefully climbed out of the window following Bobby Moore to the garden. He was shivering with excitement. In the garden, the two of them began to play football. They played and played for most of the night. It was a dream come true for Tony. Bobby Moore showed him some new football moves that he could use during football practice. He coached Tony on how to take penalties and the two of them chatted long into the night. Finally the day dawned and Tony had to say goodbye to his football hero. He shook his hand and waved as the figure of Bobby Moore disappeared as quickly as it had appeared (**actions**). Tony slowly climbed back to his room almost as if he was in a trance. He climbed back into bed and fell asleep, dreaming of his hero and winning the World Cup (**reactions**).

End

Outcome: Tony woke up sharply to the piercing sound of the alarm clock. He couldn't believe what had happened the night before. Surely it had all been a dream. As he slowly got out of bed, he saw something on his bedside table. It was one of the football World Cup medals. Tony took it in his hands as tears streamed down his face (**result**). He knew now that what his grandmother told him was correct – some dreams really do come true (**message**).

Here are a couple more stories which you can read to the students. Identify the key elements of each story as has been done with the previous examples.

Story example 4

The bullies in the playground

It was the last day of the summer school term at Bridgetown Secondary School in London. It was lunchtime and most of the students were outside playing in the playground. The mood was cheery and light. It was almost the start of the summer holidays and the weather was warm and sultry. Jenny was walking out into the playground. Just in front of her walked Penny, another student who was in the same year as Jenny. Penny was small and looked very vulnerable. She had short cropped black hair, a small white face sprinkled with freckles and walked with a distinct limp. She was wearing a jumper and jacket, despite the heat of the midday sun.

Suddenly Jenny heard laughter and sneering. A gang of boys and girls in the same class as Jenny and Penny began teasing Penny and calling her names. They slowly approached her looking mean and menacing. As they got closer, one of the gang, a large gangly boy, leapt out and took Penny's rucksack. He ran off with the bag to sounds of cheering from the rest of the group. Jenny looked around for a teacher, or anyone who could come to Penny's aid. But there was no-one around. She could either watch the group continue to torment Penny or do something herself. Without a second thought Jenny leapt into action and jumped between Penny and the approaching menacing gang of boys and girls. She stood her ground despite the screams and shouts of the crowd approaching her. Jenny was terrified but she knew she had to do something and could not let the bullying continue. In a very loud voice she screamed, trying to sound as menacing as possible, 'Enough, stop'. Her face was stern and serious and she clapped her hands as loudly as possible to get everyone's attention. The gang of students stopped in their tracks. They were afraid that all the loud noise that Jenny was making would draw attention to them and get them into trouble. They turned around and left Penny alone. Jenny picked up her rucksack lying in the corner of the playground and returned it to Penny. Penny was crying with relief. 'Thank you so much,' she said with tears streaming down her face, 'I don't know how I can ever thank you enough'. The two girls embraced warmly in the playground. 'Let's go report this to the year leader,' said Jenny, 'and make sure they never do this again to you or any other student'.

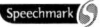

Penny and Jenny became best friends and Penny was never bullied again. Penny became friends with all of Jenny's friends and became part of her social circle. This made her very happy indeed. The bullies were punished by the teacher and the playground is now being monitored much more closely since this event. Jenny knew that sometimes you had to act, no matter how scared you may feel or how outnumbered you are. Bullying is always wrong, no matter what.

Story example 5

The mysterious message in the bottle

It was a cold, dank night in November and the roads were clear for miles ahead in the distance. There was a strange eerie silence that had descended on the town. A silence that was most unusual in this suburb of New York. As the clock struck 12pm, the final lights from the houses were dimmed and the blackness enveloped the town like a thick eiderdown. From the top left window of the smart penthouse, one could make out a small flashing light peeping through the blinds. Chad hated to sleep in the dark and always slept with his torch close by. Of course he could never admit to this, being almost 12 -years old, and a large strapping young man.

Suddenly a ray of multicoloured lights beamed into his bedroom, penetrating through the thick blinds. The lights flickered on and off in a repetitive and hypnotic way. The lights appeared to become more powerful and swirled around the room faster and faster and faster. Chad suddenly felt quite nauseous and hid his head under the duvet. When he thought the lights had faded, he slowly crept out of bed and peeked out of the window. He could see nothing outside except a mangy old fox looking for some shelter. He went to fetch his binoculars and came back to the window, this time looking into the distance to see if he could identify anything out of the ordinary. But everything around him looked calm and peaceful again. Satisfied that there was nothing to see, Chad went back to bed, ensuring that his torch light was on again beneath the covers.

The next morning, Chad checked with the others if they had heard or seen anything strange. No one had seen anything. He walked out of the door carrying his satchel for school, and looking ahead to the bus stop. He completely missed the small bottle lying on the ground with the note inside it. The note had one word on it, spelling HELP. Only Chad was able to see the bottle, and because he missed it, the note went unanswered. There are some mysterious things that happen in life which we can't always explain.

Teaching notes for Session 5

The story F1 race track

The story F1 race track is an excellent tool to use to help students identify and understand the different parts that make up a story. The story race track, like the story train track, is simply another tool to use to help students understand the components of a story and the story structure.

Show the race track to the students and identify what parts of the race track correspond to the main elements of the story on the story planner.

1 The beginning

Draw attention to the start of the race track. There is the START sign and a man with a gun indicating from where the drivers must line up and begin the race. If they do not start from this position, they will be disqualified. It is important that every story has a beginning point from which the story is started. Discuss the setting of the race track. This can include a description of the track, the trees, weather, time of day, etc. There are a number of different racing cars with different drivers. There are also people watching the drivers from the stands. These are the characters; they are all different and have different features and profiles which can be explored, just like the characters that make up a story. The race is happening in the daytime, and it looks like a cloudy day. There are green trees in the background which may indicate the race is taking place sometime in summer or spring. All these details relate to when the race is taking place, to the time of the race. This corresponds to the time of the story. The race track can also give us details of where, the place where the race is happening. We know it is taking place at a race track, and if it is taking place in Britain, then it may be at Silverstone race track. It may of course be taking place at a race track in another country. There are trees in the background, all giving more information about where the race is taking place. All this information tells us where the race is taking place, and corresponds to the place where the story is set.

2 The middle

The middle of the story contains what is happening in the story, the plot and exciting parts of the story. It describes the initial happening or first event in the story, the immediate response of the characters to this first event, and then the action/s that the character takes to solve what has happened, to resolve the problem introduced by that first event. It also contains the reaction/s of the characters as a result of the actions taken. This is where the main part of the story is located. On the story track, there are a number of episodes that are taking place as the race is ongoing. For example, if you look at the race track you will see two cars colliding with each other, another car hitting the barrier, and another car about to go the wrong way. There is also a bird that has flown on to the track. All these events can indicate different episodes which make up the middle part of the story. Each episode will have a different initiating event or happening, some immediate response, an action that the driver takes as a response to this initial happening and then the reaction to the action taken. So, for example, the two cars smash into each other as the initial event or happening, and an immediate response to this will follow, which could be feelings of anger from both drivers. An action or series of actions will usually follow this event and immediate response. This could be the two drivers getting into a fist fight, or getting injured. Then there would be a reaction to the action. This may be the officials ending the race if the two drivers begin fighting with each other. Show the students how the different components of the race track can correspond the different story elements.

3 The end

The race track has a clear end point where the race ends. It is signified by the chequered flag which means 'the end'. All drivers know they have to reach this point to win the race, or at least finish the race. Everything comes together at the end of the race; this is what the whole day has been building up to, what all the drivers have been working hard for, the outcome of the race. It is at the end of the race where we see who has won, we find out the result of the race. The winner of the race will receive a trophy and may even win the championship. There may be a moral to the story, so perhaps the driver with the least experience who worked the hardest wins the race, indicating the importance of hard work. This is the same as the end of the story. Everything that has come before builds up to this ending. The end of the story must be clear to the listener or reader; it must bring the story to an end and provide the final results and outcomes of the story.

The story football match and the story athletics race track have been designed with the same purpose as the F1 racing track, to depict the different story elements. Some students will prefer these story templates, and you can discuss with them the story elements using these templates in the same way that we have used the story F1 race track example above.

The train track and train carriages

It is a good idea to use the train track and train carriages to show the students the overall structure of the story. This helps them see how the different elements of the story included in the story planner fit together in an ordered sequential manner.

Show them how the beginning of the story, the story setting including the characters, time and place, correspond to the first train carriage, the front of the train.

Show them how the middle of the story, the episode/s including the initial happening, immediate response, the action/s and reaction/s, makes up the middle part of the carriage, the middle carriages. The story can have one middle carriage or more depending on its length and complexity. Make them aware how these middle carriages have passengers in them. The middle sections contain the plot, the exciting parts of the story, what is happening in the story.

The train has three middle carriages to indicate to students how stories can be more complex and contain more than one episode.

Show them how the end of the story, the outcome including the result and message corresponds to the end of the train, the last carriage.

Beginning: setting = front carriage of train

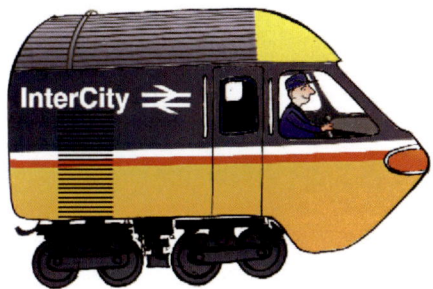

Middle: episode/s = middle carriages of train

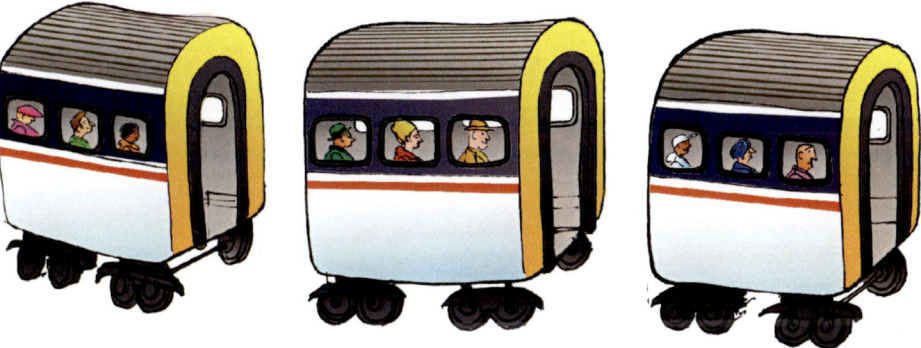

End: outcome = end carriage of the train

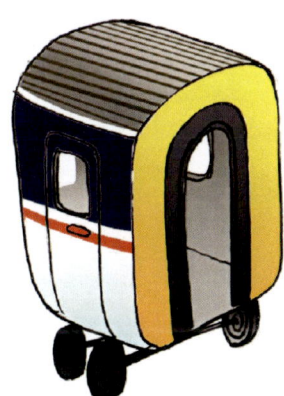

Session 6

Names of students: _____

_____

Facilitator: _____ Date: _____

School: _____

Class: _____

Aims	Method/Activities	Materials
To revise and recap the main elements of the **story planner** discussed in the previous session.	Group discussion with students taking turns to give an example of one important thing they learned from the previous session. Emphasise story structure and the elements of the story planner.	Flipchart or whiteboard, paper and pen. Story planner.
To identify all the elements from the **story planner** of their favourite television programmes.	Students take turns (using the story pencil or microphone) to share their favourite television programmes and identify, using the story planner, each part of the story. Discuss with each student their completed story planner forms that they have filled in as part of last session's Mission to Achieve. Ensure that students have identified the **setting** of the programme including the key characters, the time and place of the programme; the **episode/s** of the programme including what happens (the first initiating event), immediate responses, the actions that followed and the resulting reactions; and finally the **outcome** of the programme, including the result and the message of the story if there is any. Students should provide as many details as possible about the characters of the story, and where and when the story takes place, i.e. the setting of the story. They should also detail the middle section of the story describing the main events and the actions and reactions of the characters. Encourage group participation and discussion around the different stories based on television series and how they map on to the story elements presented by the story planner.	Completed story planner from Mission to Achieve in session 5. Story pencil or microphone. Story train track and train carriages. Story F1 race track. Story football match. Story athletics race track.

 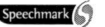

Aims	Method/Activities	Materials
To **evaluate the televised stories** and discuss changes that they would make to improve them.	Students to evaluate the television programmes they have brought in to discuss with the group. They should discuss how interesting the story is, how much detail is provided about the characters, time and place settings, how exciting the main events of the story are, how satisfying the ending of the story is, etc. Discuss with students how realistic the stories were, whether they really believed in the characters and storyline. If so, what made the story so powerful, and if not, how could they have improved it?	Story planner. Examples of stories/television programmes that the students have brought in for their homework.
Students to **practise changing elements of stories** from their favourite television series.	They should be encouraged to critically evaluate the story features AND suggest changes that they would make to enhance the story. This is to encourage flexibility and confidence in story telling. Encourage the students to add in their own characters, change storylines by adding or changing the events of the story, the conflict or story plot, the setting or even the story outcome. Students should be encouraged to provide explanations for their changes.	Use the suggested evaluation questions from teaching notes in session 15. Not all questions will be suitable at this point, but include those that cover content that has been taught thus far.
To identify the main **plot** and **climax** of each story from the television programme.	Students are required to identify the main event, theme or plot as well as the climax from the specific television programme they have brought in to the session to discuss. Explore with the students what the plot and climax of a story are and where they usually occur: The **story plot** is part of the middle of the story and refers to the main theme or topic of the story. The plot is what the story is about. It can also be referred to as the storyline or the sequence of events that happen in the story. One could say that the plot is the most important part of the whole story as it is actually the story itself. A good plot captures the listener's or reader's attention and ensures that they keep listening or reading.	Story planner.

Aims	Method/Activities	Materials
	Take turns to identify the plot of each televised story that the students have chosen. How easily were they able to identify the story plots? Discuss with them how exciting or interesting the plots are, and how relevant they are to their own lives. What is it about the plots in their view that makes so many television series so popular with viewers? Students will provide interesting views on the popularity of such programmes as *EastEnders*, *Coronation Street*, *Hollyoaks*, *Glee* and other popular series. Explore the idea that these programmes have plots and story ideas, with which many people can identify, i.e. they are similar to our own lives, or to which many people aspire. So, for example, we would all like to experience the type of fame in *Glee*. Now begin to discuss the **climax of a story**. The story climax usually occurs in the middle of a story and is the most exciting, intense or important part of the story. It may be where the main problem occurs, or where the danger is at its worst. There is often a slow build-up to this exciting part of the story. Encourage students to see if they can identify the main climax of their chosen television programmes. How successful were these climaxes and did they keep the viewers' attention as would be expected. Explore with students how the climax was built and maintained. What did the writers or authors do to help build the tension and suspense leading up to the climax? Did they leave the end with an uncertain conclusion, or did something bad happen to a favourite character? Encourage students not only to identify the climax in their televised examples, but to analyse how this climax was formed and maintained.	
To identify the **plot and climax** of their chosen favourite story and/or book.	Students are encouraged to think about their favourite book and/or story which they chose in session 2. Encourage them to share with the group what their favourite story is about, the main plot of the story.	Flipchart or whiteboard if available, paper and pen.

 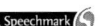

Aims	Method/Activities	Materials
	Then, ask them to identify what the climax of the story is, and share this with the group. Discuss how the climax is built up and maintained. Encourage students to evaluate the plots of the stories, and how successful the climaxes are at building suspense and making the story interesting. We can assume that the students will report the plots of the stories to be very interesting as they have chosen these particular stories as their favourites. Try and get them to reflect on their choices and think about why they are such favourites. Discuss whether their popularity has something to do with the stories having a particularly strong, exciting or relevant plot, or a powerful climax.	Remind students of their story choices by putting up the list of stories gathered in session 2.
To produce their own stories with a clear **story structure, interesting plot and climax**.	Divide the students into pairs or small groups and encourage them to generate their own stories using the story planner as a guide. Their stories should have a clear exciting theme or sequence of events, i.e. a strong plot, together with the three main story elements discussed in the previous session (setting, episode and outcome). Their story should also include an exciting part which can easily be identified as the story climax. Explore with the students how they will choose what their story is about, i.e. what the story plot will be. Explore how their choices will depend on their likes and dislikes, their age, personality, their individual experiences, etc. Discuss with the students ways of making the story, and particularly the climax of the story, more exciting. Explore with students how they can make their voices and faces more exciting when telling their stories. This will be revisited at a later session, but introduce the idea here for students that we can use our faces (different facial expressions), bodies (posture and other physical actions) and voices (loud versus soft, fast versus slow) to make our stories more exciting. This is especially important when telling someone the climax of a story.	Story planner. Story train track and carriages. Story F1 race track. Story football match. Story athletics race track. See teaching notes that follow for suggested story climaxes that can be given to students to incorporate in their self-generated stories.

Aims	Method/Activities	Materials
To sum up and revise contents of the session.	Get volunteers from the group to summarise the main content of the session. Ask other members of the group to help, adding in the parts that may have been omitted.	Flipchart or whiteboard, paper and pen.
Mission to Achieve: Students to think of one exciting character, one specific place and one time around which a story can be constructed.		Story planner.

 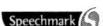

Evaluation of session/General comments

Teaching notes for Session 6

These are some suggestions for a story climax that students can use to build their story around. Encourage them to think about what precedes these climactic events, who the characters might be in the story and where the time and place would be. Explore with the students the events leading up to the climax and the outcomes of the story.

This session should provide students with the opportunity to make up stories using all the components of the story planner. The emphasis should be on making up an exciting story which captures the interests of the listener. Students should be encouraged to think about the middle section of the story, the plot and the climax of their story.

Examples of climactic events which they can draw upon include:

1   Blood spurted from his hands as he tried desperately to stop the bleeding. The man's eyes seemed to roll behind his head. It looked like he was too late.

2   The eagle swooped down with a ferocious force and was about to pick up the small infant.

3   'If you touch that switch,' cackled the evil witch, 'you will be catapulted to the very ends of the earth.'

4   The pilot looked gravely at the air stewardess. There were tears in both their eyes. He nodded slowly and picked up the microphone. There was nothing left they could do. It was time to tell the passengers.

5   Only a few minutes away from the finishing line, and Azaria knew the title and trophy would be his. He kept running, putting one foot in front of the other, completely focused on the finishing line. Then suddenly he heard a snap, followed by a searing pain in his Achilles tendon.

6   'The most important thing you need to remember,' whispered Merlin, 'is never ever ever to breathe any of this to another living soul.'

7   The door swung open, and there before him was Oscar, whimpering and chained to the four-poster bed.

8   The shovel hit something hard and metal. Was this finally going to be the successful end to their long search for the treasure?

 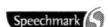

Session 7

7

Names of students: _____

_____

Facilitator: _____ Date: _____

School: _____

Class: _____

Aims	Method/Activities	Materials
To revise and recap the story elements of the **story planner** covered in the previous session.	Group discussion with students taking turns to give an example of one important thing they learned from the previous session. Revise through a group quiz; testing the definitions of each story element of the story planner. Use a popular quiz format such as *Who Wants to be a Millionaire?* or *The Weakest Link* and test the students' recall of the story elements discussed in previous sessions. Students love competitions, so play 'first on the buzzer' games. Allow each student to make up a unique sound and get them to use this as their buzzer and to buzz in when they can answer a question set by the facilitator. Keep a total score and use the format as an excellent reinforcer and motivator. It works!	Flipchart or whiteboard, paper and pen. Story planner.
To explore in more details the **beginning** of the story, the story setting including the character, time and place.	Focus on the first part of a story, i.e. the **story beginning**. Explain the three parts that make up the **setting** of a story, the **characters** that make up a story, the **time** and **place** in which the story takes place. Revisit the teaching notes from session 5 and discuss the features of character, time and place. Remind students to use the story planner and accompanying picture cues to reinforce their understanding. The beginning element of a story (firing shotgun) consists of characters (signified by a picture of a boy and dog), time (signified by a picture of a watch and calendar) and place (signified by a picture of a house and tree).	Story planner. Story F1 race track. Story football match. Story athletics race track – focusing on the beginning of the story.

Aims	Method/Activities	Materials
	Group discussion around the settings of stories. Group members to identify the characters, time and place of their favourite stories (and specifically their one chosen story favourite) and other stories that have been discussed in previous sessions, for example, fairytales, historical stories, stories from the cinema and television.	
To **listen to and evaluate beginnings of stories** from published works.	Provide examples of 'story beginnings' from published stories included in teaching notes. You may also like to bring in favourites of your own, or use examples of stories that the students are covering in the classroom. Get students to evaluate how exciting the beginnings are and encourage them to compare and contrast the different story beginnings. Encourage students to consider the differences in the beginning elements of a 'mystery' versus an 'adventure' versus a 'non-fictional autobiography' versus a 'non-fictional diary' versus a 'travel book'. The varied examples provided in the teaching notes will provide many opportunities for contrasts, comparisons and discussions. Ask students whether the beginning is exciting enough to make them want to read the specific book. Debate which books they would like to read further and which they do not, and encourage them to reflect on their decisions and give reasons for their preferences. This is a good opportunity to emphasise the relevance of this work to their school and home lives. Explore the importance of having one's own point of view and opinion rather than following the crowd. Emphasise how essential it is to make that opinion a reasoned and reflective one, and get students to consider how more influential they will be at school and at home if they are able to offer careful and considered points of view. Encourage them to see how this programme is providing them with practice to do exactly this.	Examples of 'story beginnings' included in teaching notes.

Aims	Method/Activities	Materials
To **identify specific words, phrases or sentences** commonly used to begin stories.	As a group, brainstorm the most frequent words, phrases and sentences that are typically used to begin stories. These can include: • Once upon a time • One fine day • On a cold winter's night • In the beginning • Long ago, in a faraway place • Once there was • This is a story about • The story begins with • It was the night before the wedding and everything looked peaceful. The students take turns to come up with their own ideas and generate sentences using the above phrases.	Flipchart or whiteboard, pen and paper.
To focus more specifically on **characters** and to discuss the importance of characterisation in storytelling.	Group discussion on **characters** and the importance of having interesting characters in a story. It is important to enhance awareness that characters in a story can be non-human and human, and can include people, animals, plants and non-animate objects like football boots. We can see this from example number 11 from this session's teaching notes taken from *Black Beauty* and narrated by the main character in the story, a horse. Example 8 in the teaching notes for the next session (session 8) on characters is all about the character of a dog. In some stories, objects with human traits and voices are characters, for example, the teacup in *Beauty and The Beast*. Think also about the characters in your favourite animated movies like *Toy Story*, *Ice Age*, *Antz* and *The Jungle Book*. Can students give their own favourite animations, and do they know the famous actors behind these characters.	Story planner.
To generate as many potential **characters** as possible for a story.	Stories usually have more than one character. They can have a main character and more minor characters who are less important to the overall plot of the story. The main character in a story is called a **protagonist**. The protagonist is a major character at the centre of the story.	

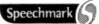

Aims	Method/Activities	Materials
	Group to brainstorm all the possible characters that can appear in any story. Examples may include: girl, ghost, mermaid, rat, pop star, witch, gnome, dragon, dirty ballet shoes, devil, etc.	
	Play a word association game where students take turns at coming up with as many possible characters as they can in one minute. The winner is the person who comes up with the most characters. A variation of this game is for students to give as many different characters as possible beginning with certain letters, so, for example, as many characters as possible beginning with the letter 'd'. Answers here might include: doctor, dentist, detective, dog, dormouse, Diana, Dick, Debbie, etc.	
	Another fun game to play is to award a prize to the person who thinks up the most unique or bizarre character, for example, the eight-legged 40-stone wizard! Then get them to draw this character, or even better, to act it out!	
To identify their favourite characters from stories they have listened to or read.	Group to identify their favourite character/s in any book, television programme or movie that they have seen, for example, Harry Potter, or Nemo (the fish from *Finding Nemo*). Each student to explain why this is their favourite character. Encourage students to describe the character for the group as fully as they can; using all the information the story has provided them with. Group members will try and visualise and understand the characters from this description. This will give students an idea of how well the character was described in the story.	
	Students can also provide details to the group about the characters from their chosen favourite story or book.	
To **enhance character descriptive abilities** by students describing	Students to describe themselves as if they were the main character in a story. Students have the opportunity to draw themselves and identify their main physical traits. In a group they take turns to share their drawings and describe their	Pens, crayons and paper for students to draw themselves.

Aims	Method/Activities	Materials
themselves in as much detail as possible as if they were characters in a story.	characters. Students use the character word map to detail all aspects of their character including physical traits, personality features, moods, likes and dislikes. Other members of group to comment on character descriptions. The character word maps will help students think of as many details as possible about the character in question. Characters will not always be humans; they can be non-humans like animals or plants, or even inanimate objects. Students will not be able to complete all the categories on the character word map with every character description. That is fine. They should complete as many categories as possible and use the character word map to flesh out their characters as much as possible and provide a detailed and interesting character profile. Through the character word map, encourage the students to describe themselves in as much detail as possible, including what they look like, their main physical trait/s, a main distinguishing feature, how they feel, their personality, likes and dislikes, etc. Play a game where students take turns to describe someone in the group using as many details as possible. Members have to then guess who they are describing. This may be a good time to remind students about the group rules and working in a close and supportive collaborative partnership. Character descriptions should be appropriate at all times.	Character word map in DVD to encourage students to describe themselves in as much detail as possible.
To sum up and revise contents of the session.	Get volunteers from the group to summarise the main content of the session. Ask other members of the group to help adding in the parts that may have been omitted.	Flipchart or whiteboard, paper and pens.

 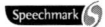

Aims	Method/Activities	Materials
Mission to Achieve: Students to choose their favourite character from a book, comic, television programme or film, and provide a detailed profile of the character using the character word map.	Students are given the character word maps to help them provide as many details as possible about their chosen character, including detailed physical characteristics, personality traits, their likes and dislikes, actions, thoughts, feelings and any other interesting details. They should bring in this character word map with all the details together with their drawing of the specific character.	Photocopy character word maps for students to take home and use to complete the Mission to Achieve.

Evaluation of session/General comments

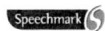

Word Map

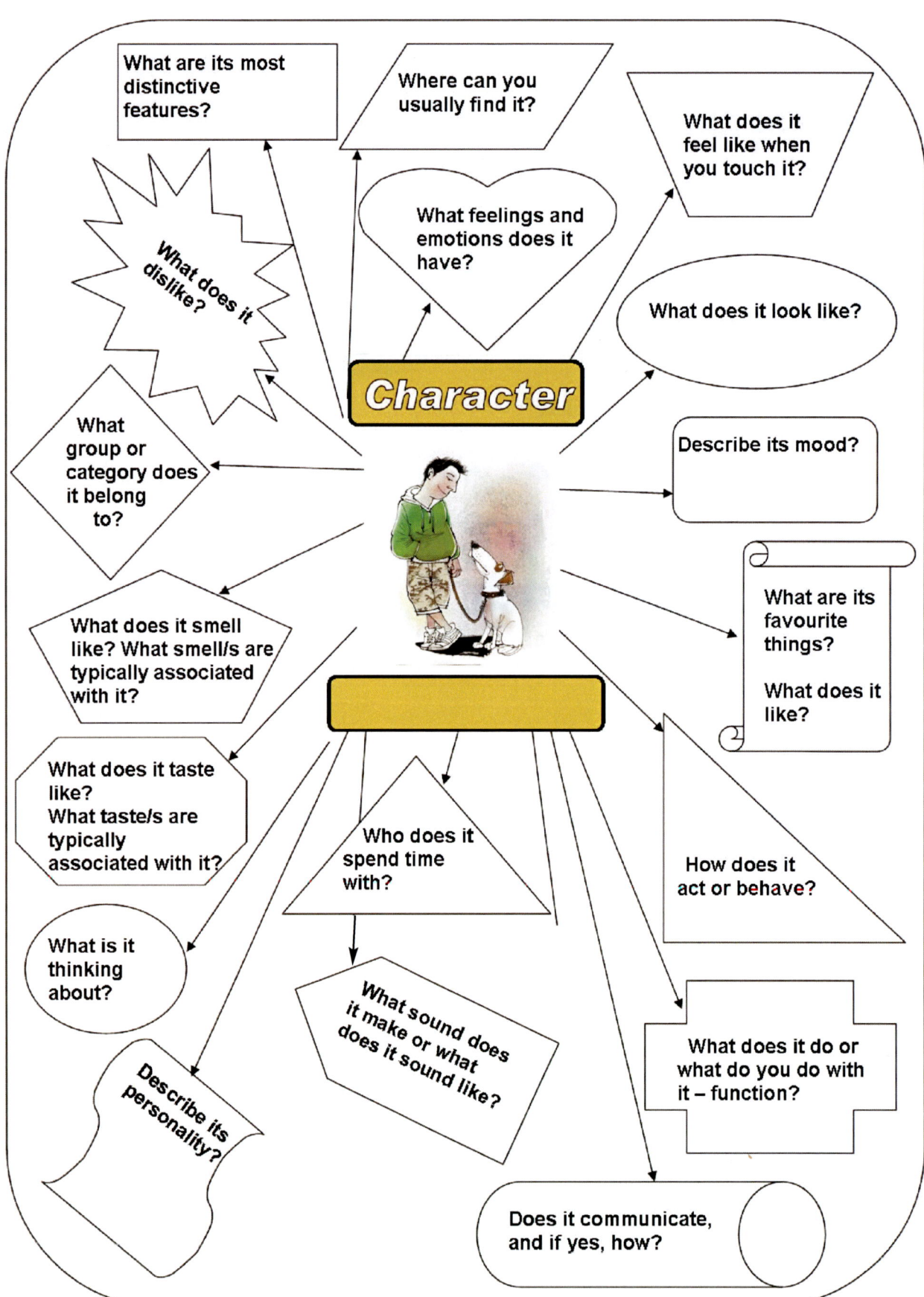

What are its most distinctive features?

Where can you usually find it?

What does it feel like when you touch it?

What does it dislike?

What feelings and emotions does it have?

What does it look like?

Character

What group or category does it belong to?

Describe its mood?

What are its favourite things?

What does it like?

What does it smell like? What smell/s are typically associated with it?

What does it taste like? What taste/s are typically associated with it?

Who does it spend time with?

How does it act or behave?

What is it thinking about?

What sound does it make or what does it sound like?

What does it do or what do you do with it – function?

Describe its personality?

Does it communicate, and if yes, how?

Teaching notes for Session 7

Examples of story beginnings from published works

Here are some examples of the beginning sections which have been taken from a varied selection of published texts. Most if not all of them will be recognisable to the students. Students are to be encouraged at all times to identify their own favourites to share with the group. You may want to read them all out to students, or choose a selected few, or even add your own favourite examples. It is a great idea to find examples from the books with which students are working and reading in the classroom, as well as their own favourite texts.

Read the following beginnings of stories to the students and encourage comments on each one. Discuss how powerful, evocative and interesting each story beginning is. Get the students to compare and contrast each one, comparing, for example the beginning of a mystery, a romance and a travel guide. Ask students whether the beginning part is exciting enough to make them want to read more of the book. If they do find them powerful and evocative, ask them to identify reasons why they think they are so exciting.

Example 1

'Mr Jones, of the Manor Farm, had locked the hen-houses for the night, but was too drunk to remember to shut the pop-holes. With the ring of light from his lantern dancing from side to side he lurched across the yard, kicked off his boots at the back door, drew himself a last glass of beer from the barrel in the scullery, and made his way up to bed, where Mrs Jones was already snoring.

As soon as the light in the bedroom went out there was a stirring and a fluttering all through the farm buildings. Word had gone round during the day that old Major, the prize Middle White boar, had had a strange dream on the previous night and wished to communicate it to the other animals. It had been agreed that they should all meet in the big barn as soon as Mr Jones was safely out of the way.'

Animal Farm. By George Orwell (2003), p1.

Example 2

'"It was Marie Kazinski who asked how to stop a boy if he wants to go all the way," Maggie whispered. Liz dragged her trig book along the wall tiles so it clicked at every crack. "I'll bet she didn't ask it like that," Liz said. "Sexually stimulated" was how she said it, if you must know the sordid details.'

My Darling, My Hamburger. By Paul Zindel (1978), p9.

Example 3

'Mrs Ferrars died on the night of the 16th–17th September – a Thursday. I was sent for at eight o'clock on the morning of Friday the 17th. There was nothing to be done. She had been dead some hours.'

 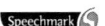

The Murder of Roger Ackroyd. By Agatha Christie (1993), p7.

Example 4

'Apart from life, a strong constitution and an abiding connection to the Thembu Royal House, the only thing my father bestowed upon me at birth was a name, Rolihlahla. In Xhosa, Rolihlahla literally means "pulling the branch of a tree" but its colloquial meaning more accurately would be "troublemaker". I do not believe that names are destiny or that my father somehow divined my future, but in later years, friends and relatives would ascribe to my birth name the many storms I have both caused and weathered. My more familiar English or Christian name was not given to me until my first day of school. But I am getting ahead of myself.

I was born on 18 July 1918 at Mvezo, a tiny village on the banks of the Mbashe River in the district of Umtata, the capital of the Transkei. The year of my birth marked the end of the Great War; the outbreak of an influenza epidemic that killed millions throughout the world; and the visit of a delegation of the African National Congress to the Versailles peace conference to voice the grievances of the African people of South Africa.'

Long Walk to Freedom. The Autobiography of Nelson Mandela. By Nelson Mandela (1994), p3.

Example 5

'Mma Ramotswe had a detective agency in Africa, at the foot of Kgale Hill. These were its assets: a tiny white van, two desks, two chairs, a telephone, and an old typewriter. Then there was a teapot, in which Mma Ramotswe – the only lady private detective in Botswana – brewed redbush tea. And three mugs – one for herself, one for her secretary, and one for the client. What else does a detective agency really need? Detective agencies rely on human intuition and intelligence, both of which Mma Ramotswe had in abundance. No inventory would ever include those, of course.'

The No 1 Ladies' Detective Agency. By Alexander McCall Smith (2003), p1.

Example 6

'Are you there G-D? It's me, Margaret. We're moving today. I'm so scared, G-D. I've never lived anywhere but here. Suppose I hate my new school? Suppose everybody there hates me? Please help me, G-D. Don't let New Jersey be too horrible. Thank you.

We moved on the Tuesday before Labor Day. I knew what the weather was like the second I got up. I knew because I caught my mother sniffing under her arms. She always does that when it's hot and humid to make sure her deodorant's working. I don't use deodorant yet. I don't think people start to smell bad until they're at least twelve. So I've still got a few months to go.'

Are you there, G-D? It's Me, Margaret. By Judy Blume (1980), p1.

Example 7

'I will begin the story of my adventures with a certain morning early in the month of June, the year of grace 1751, when I took the key for the last time out of the door of my father's house. The sun began to shine upon the summit of the hills as I went down the road; and by the time I had come as far as the manse, the blackbirds were whistling in the garden lilacs, and the mist that hung around the valley in the time of the dawn was beginning to arise and die away.'

Kidnapped. By Robert Louis Stevenson (2009), p1.

Example 8

'It's a funny thing about mothers and fathers. Even when their own child is the most disgusting little blister you could ever imagine, they still think that he or she is wonderful.

Some parents go further: They become so blinded by adoration they manage to convince themselves their child has qualities of genius.

Well, there is nothing very wrong with all this. It's the way of the world. It is only when parents begin telling us about the brilliance of their own revolting off-spring, that we start shouting, "Bring us a basin! We're going to be sick!"'

Matilda. By Roald Dahl (2008), p1.

Example 9

'Despite its small size (84.459 sq km), slightly smaller than New York State, about the size of Maine, Ireland presents to the visitor some of the finest unspoilt landscape, dramatic coastline and wilderness areas in Europe, with the attractive prospect of travelling almost anywhere on uncrowded roads in an environment of rain-washed translucent skies while breathing the fresh air of Atlantic breezes.'

Ireland. Blue Guide. By Brain Lalor (1998), p7.

Example 10

'At the end of a little Swedish town lay an old, overgrown orchard. In the orchard was a cottage, and in the cottage lived Pippi Longstocking. She was nine years old, and she lived all alone. She had neither mother nor father, which was really rather nice, for in this way there was no one to tell her to go to bed just when she was having most fun, and no one to make her take cod-liver-oil when she felt like eating peppermints.'

Pippi Longstocking. By Astrid Lindgren (2002), p1.

Example 11

'The first place that I can well remember was a large pleasant meadow with a pond of clear water in it. Some shady trees leaned over it, and rushes and water-lilies grew at the deep end. Over the hedge on one side we looked into a ploughed field, and on the other we looked over a gate at our master's house, which stood by the roadside; at the top of the meadow was a

 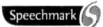

plantation of fir trees, and at the bottom a running brook overhung by a steep bank.

Whilst I was young I lived upon my mother's milk, as I could not eat grass. In the daytime I ran by her side, and at night I lay down close by her. When it was hot, we used to stand by the pond in the shade of the trees, and when it was cold, we had a nice warm shed near the plantation.'

    Black Beauty. By Anna Sewell (2001), p19.

Example 12

'Marley was dead: to begin with. There is no doubt whatever about that. The register of his burial was signed by the clergyman, the clerk, the undertaker, and the chief mourner. Scrooge signed it: and Scrooge's name was good upon 'Change, for anything he chose to put his hand to. Old Marley was as dead as a door-nail.

Mind! I don't mean to say that I know, of my own knowledge, what there is particularly dead about a door-nail. I might have been inclined, myself, to regard a coffin-nail as the deadest piece of ironmongery in the trade. But the wisdom of our ancestors is in the simile; and my unhallowed hands shall not disturb it, or the Country's done for. You will therefore permit me to repeat, emphatically, that Marley was as dead as a door-nail.'

    A Christmas Carol. By Charles Dickens (1979), p3.

Example 13

'12 JUNE 1942

I hope I will be able to confide everything to you, as I have never been able to confide in anyone, and I hope you will be a great source of comfort and support.

COMMENT ADDED BY ANNE ON 28 SEPTEMBER 1942:

So far you truly have been a great source of comfort to me, and so has Kitty, whom I now write to regularly. This way of keeping a diary is much nicer, and now I can hardly wait for those moments when I am able to write in you.
Oh, I'm so glad I brought you along!

SUNDAY, 14 JUNE 1942

I'll begin from the moment I got you, the moment I saw you lying on the table among my other birthday presents. (I went along when you were bought, but that doesn't count.)'

    The Diary of A Young Girl. By Anne Frank (2008), p1.

Session 8

Names of students: _____

_____

Facilitator: _____ Date: _____

School: _____

Class: _____

Aims	Method/Activities	Materials
To revise and recap the story elements of the story planner covered in the previous session with a specific focus on the **beginning** section and the importance of **characterisation.**	Group discussion with students taking turns to give an example of one important thing they learned from the previous session. Revisit the importance of **characterisation** and the details that can be given for each character. Use the character word map as a cue.	Flipchart or whiteboard, paper and pen. Story planner. Character word map.
For students to share their detailed character descriptions of their favourite characters from their homework task.	Students to take turns using the story pencil to share their character maps of their favourite characters from books, television programmes, comics or movies that they have prepared in the previous session's Mission to Achieve. Students to provide the description and show their pictures or drawings of the chosen character WITHOUT divulging the name of the character. The facilitator can write on the board the possible list of books, movies and television programmes that the students are talking about, and they then have to guess which specific character is being described from this list. Group to play a guessing game where rest of group have to guess the character that the student is describing. The better the description the easier it should be to guess correctly. Therefore the winner of the game is the student whose character is identified with the lowest number of guesses.	Flipchart or whiteboard, paper and pen. Story pencil or microphone. Character word maps of favourite characters from students' chosen television programme, comic, book or movie (completed as previous session's homework task).

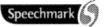

Aims	Method/Activities	Materials
To recognise the importance of characterisation in stories providing a **rich and descriptive character profile**.	Group discussion on the importance of detailed **character descriptions** to enhance the story and ensure that the reader gets drawn into the story and understands and gets to know the character.	Story planner.
	Encourage students to explore all aspects of a character, including (1) what they feel (their feelings); (2) what they do (their actions); (3) what they think (their thoughts) and; (4) what they say (their communication).	Examples of character descriptions from published work included in teaching notes.
	Other areas to describe include the character's personality, physical attributes, mood, his or her likes and dislikes.	Pens and paper for drawing of characters.
To **critically evaluate character descriptions** from published work.	Provide examples of character descriptions from different publications included in the teaching notes that follow. Students to comment on the characterisations, providing a critical evaluation of each character description. The characters include an old man, a knight, young ladies, a smelly boy, a hairy man, a large woman, a dead man, soldiers, a dog and a horse – to name just a few.	Character pictures supplied in the programme.
	Encourage students to visualise the character in their heads from the character descriptions. Discuss whether they are able to do this from the description, and get them to share their visualisations. If they are unable to visualise the characters clearly, what does that say about the details provided?	
	Students can draw the characters if they wish. This can be great fun as students can compare their drawings and see how similar or different they are from the details provided about the characters in the stories. They may find it particularly fun to try to draw Mr Wonka from the description provided in example 7. Discuss with the students this highly descriptive characterisation of Mr Wonka. Explore with them everything they now know about this character from the details provided. Explore why they think he is compared to a squirrel,	

Aims	Method/Activities	Materials
	what features might he share with a squirrel. You might like to extend this discussion further and discuss the use of **simile** here and how the author is making a comparison between two different objects (Mr Wonka and a squirrel). Explain to the students the definition of a **simile**: a figure of speech involving the comparison of two different things which have some similarity. You might like to discuss this figure of speech in more depth and get the students to come up with their own similes to describe themselves and/or their chosen favourite characters. They should explain their simile and make explicit the similarities they are trying to show. Students might like to read through the character description of the headmistress, Miss Trunchbull in example 5 of *Matilda*. Encourage them to visualise Miss Trunchbull and explore whether they are able from the description to get a clear picture of her, both her physical looks as well as her personality. Discuss with the students their perception of Miss Trunchbull and see if they agree with each other. Ask them to provide evidence from the text for their views. For example, if they say she is frightening, ask them to give you evidence from the character description that gives them this information. Ask students to provide a detailed description of their own head teacher and encourage them to compare and contrast their head teacher with the character of Miss Trunchbull. Many of the students may also have seen the film *Matilda* either at the cinema or on television. Ask those who have seen the movie to contrast the picture and image they have of Miss Trunchbull from the written description in the book with the image that they had from seeing Miss Trunchbull in the movie. Discuss with the students their views on seeing movies of books: whether it is best to see the movie first, or read the book first. Another example is *Harry Potter*, as many of the students will have read and seen the *Harry Potter* books and	

 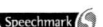

Aims	Method/Activities	Materials
	films. Discuss with students which they did first, saw the movie or read the book, and whether they have a preference. Explore with students the impact of making movies about popular books. Students may even like to debate whether this encourages or discourages the reading of books.	
To describe features of specific **characters** including physical features, personality, likes, dislikes, mood, hobbies, occupations, etc using character word map.	Students to have the opportunity to choose **characters** from a range of character pictures included in the resource and describe the character to the rest of the group. Group to play the game, '**Who am I**?' Each student chooses a character from a range of supplied character pictures and describes the character to the group without divulging who the character is. Group are not to know what character the person is describing and the first person to guess who the character is wins the game. The better the character description, the quicker the group should guess correctly, therefore the person describing the character should aim for the group to guess correctly using as few guesses as possible. Encourage the students to use their five senses when describing a character, so what she or he **looks** like, **sounds** like, **feels** like, **smells** like and in some cases where appropriate, **tastes** like! The character word map should be used to encourage students to use their senses to describe each character. For example, compare the smell of a newborn baby with a crusty old frog. Encourage the group to use new, interesting and descriptive words to describe the characters. Introduce to them the importance of using **adjectives**, which are a special group of words which describe nouns or objects. So, we could say that the witch was bony (physical appearance – visual), crafty (personality), rancid (smell), with creaking bones (sound).	Character pictures include: boy, astronaut, mermaid, dog, footballer, mechanic, wizard, fish, prisoner, old lady, tramp, judge, policeman, pop singer and thief. Continue to use the character word map to encourage students to detail each character as much as possible. A dictionary and thesaurus may also be useful.

Aims	Method/Activities	Materials
	Encourage detailed descriptions with new vocabulary, for example, 'the withered lined old man looked very feeble', rather than simply describing the man as 'old'. It is fine to use the vocabulary that the students know as a starting point, but encourage them to use the knowledge they have to provide as rich descriptions as possible. Extend this knowledge to more descriptive and complex vocabulary where appropriate. Have a dictionary and thesaurus to hand so students can look up word meanings if they need to, as well as different meanings of the same word. Using the thesaurus, for example, get them to look up common adjectives like 'old', 'thin' and 'greedy' and see what other words they can use to make their descriptions more exciting. Students can make up the personalities of their character and build up a whole profile of the character they have chosen from the set of pictures. Their witch, for example, could be kind and generous or mean spirited and cruel. Encourage them to think about how these differences in personality may impact on how they look, what they wear, etc. This can lead on to a fascinating debate about the link between our actions (behaviour) and how we look and feel. So, for example, is there such a thing as a 'kind face'? Would the bad witch look 'cruel' and what does 'cruel' look like? Would the bad witch wear only black and the good witch wear colourful clothes, or is this simply a generalisation? Are appearances in fact deceiving? Students really enjoy such debates, so allow them to have these within the appropriate topic areas. This is how we are preparing students to engage in society and interact with others in a confident and effective way.	
To construct a story with a chosen character.	Students to choose one **character** picture from the range offered and think about how they can construct a story around this character. This task can be undertaken in pairs if appropriate. Students to think about what their chosen	Character cards included in the programme.

 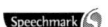

Aims	Method/Activities	Materials
	character is like, what his or her dislikes and likes may be, what motives they may have, etc. Students to take all this information into account when thinking about the story they will construct using this character. Is their character a hero or a villain, for example? Students then to share their stories with the rest of the group.	Story planner.
To sum up and revise contents of the session.	Get volunteers from the group to summarise the main content of the session. Ask other members of the group to help, adding in the parts that may have been omitted.	Flipchart or whiteboard, paper and pen.
Mission to Achieve: Students will identify someone who is their hero and think about how they would characterise that person.	In the next session, students will be asked to tell the story about the hero of their choice. They are therefore given time before the next session to think about who their choice of hero will be, and are asked to find out as many details about this person's character and life as possible. Their choice of hero is their own personal choice and could be someone from their own family, like their grandmother, or a more famous person such as Martin Luther King, Nelson Mandela or David Beckham. Students are encouraged to use the character word map to describe their hero.	Students can use the character word maps to make notes about their hero if they find this helpful.

Evaluation of session/General comments

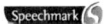

Astronaut	Boy	Businessman	Doctor

Dog	Fish	Fly	Footballer

King (Henry VIII)	Judge	Lion	Mechanic

Mermaid	Old lady	Policeman	Pop singer

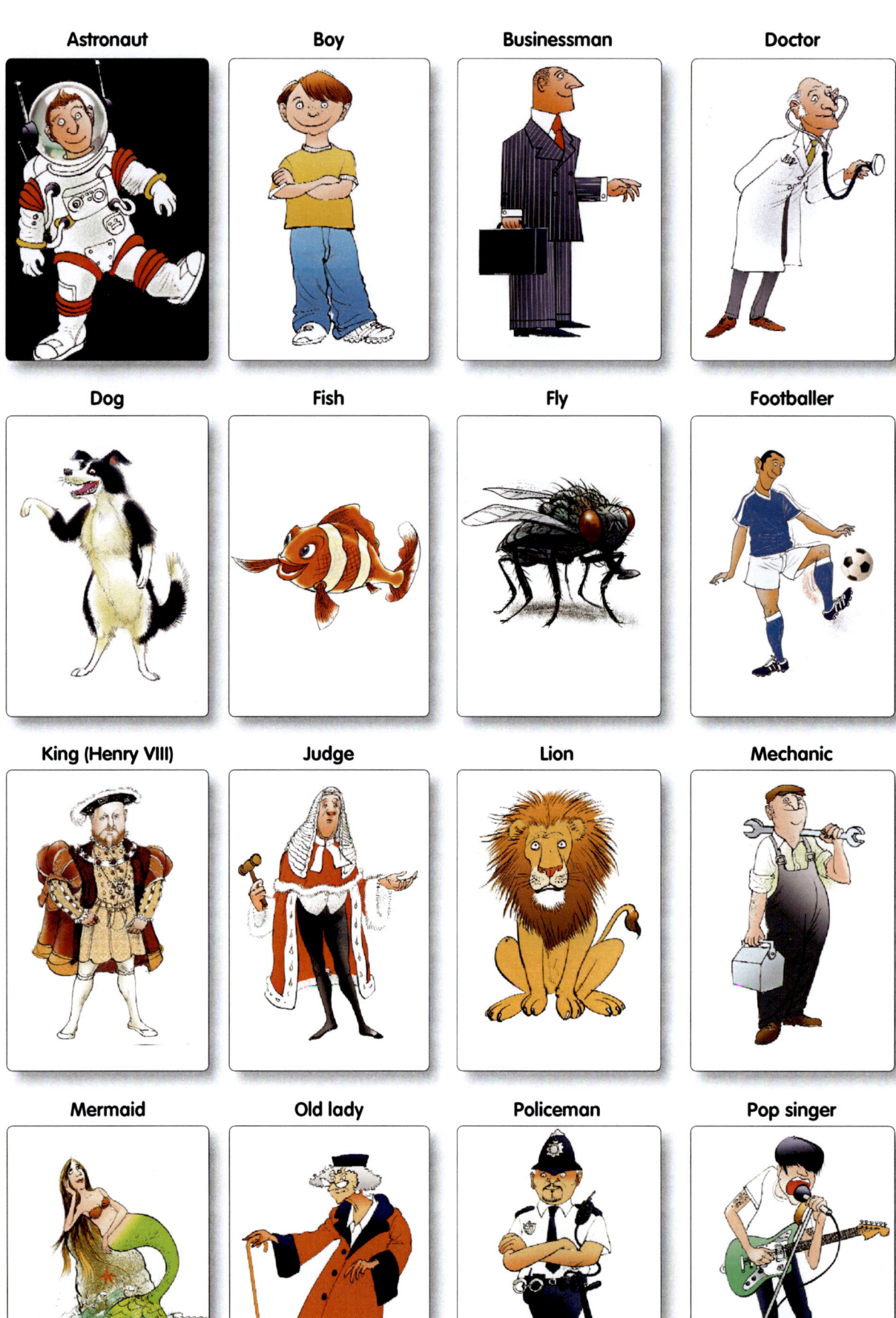

Teaching notes for Session 8

Examples of character descriptions from published works

Here are some character descriptions from a range of publications which you can read to students. You may decide to read them all or select a few and spend longer discussing them in more detail. You may also have your own favourite character descriptions to add to this selection.

Students should be encouraged to critically evaluate each description and comment on how effective and evocative each characterisation is. Members of the group may not always be familiar with or understand some of the new vocabulary or phrases. It is important that as many news words as possible are explained and discussed so that students have a good understanding of the descriptions used.

Students are to be encouraged to see whether they can visualise the character from the descriptions provided and also discuss whether they feel they know the character from the descriptions. Explore with the students what additional details they needed to give them a more in-depth understanding of each character. Students will enjoy drawing the characters from these descriptions and can then compare their drawings with those of other group members.

Example 1

'The old man was thin and gaunt with deep wrinkles in the back of his neck. The brown blotches of the benevolent skin cancer the sun brings from its reflection on the tropic sea were on his cheeks. The blotches ran well down the sides of his face and his hands had the deep-creased scars from handling heavy fish on the cords. But none of these scars were fresh. They were as old as erosions in a fishless desert.'

The Old Man and the Sea By Ernest Hemingway (1978), p5.

Example 2

'Calpurnia was something else again. She was all angles and bones; she was near-sighted; she squinted; her hand was wide as a bed slat and twice as hard. She was always ordering me out of the kitchen, asking me why I couldn't behave as well as Jem when she knew he was older, and calling me home when I wasn't ready to come.'

To Kill a Mockingbird. By Harper Lee (1991), p6.

Example 3

'"Oh, Liz, I thought you were my friend! I wouldn't go anywhere with him. He looks weird." He actually was weird-looking, Maggie thought, studying him closely. How skinny! A face like an undernourished zucchini. She chuckled to herself. And always wearing the same baggy green sweater. He must love that sweater. Any time she ever passed him in the halls, there it was,

 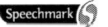

baggy as ever. He wouldn't ask her out, anyway.'
  My Darling, My Hamburger. By Paul Zindel (1978), p11.

Example 4

'Bent double, like old beggars under sacks,
Knock-kneed, coughing like hags, we cursed through sludge,
Till on the haunting flares we turned our backs
And towards our distant rest began to trudge.
Men marched asleep. Many had lost their boots,
But limped on, blood-shod. All went lame; all blind;
Drunk with fatigue; deaf even to the hoots,
Of tired, outstripped Five-Nines that dropped behind'
  From 'Dulce et Decorum Est'. By Wilfred Owen (1996), p20.

Example 5

'Miss Trunchbull, the Headmistress, was something else altogether. She was a gigantic holy terror, a fierce tyrannical monster who frightened the life out of the pupils and teachers alike. There was an aura of menace about her even at a distance, and when she came up close you could almost feel the dangerous heat radiating from her as from a red-hot rod of metal. When she marched – Miss Trunchbull never walked, she always marched like a storm-trooper with long strides and arms aswinging – when she marched along a corridor you could actually hear her snorting as she went, and if a group of children happened to be in her path, she ploughed right on through them like a tank, with small people bouncing off her to left and right.'
  Matilda. By Roald Dahl (2008), p61.

Example 6

'"Now one can breathe more easily," said the Knight, putting back his shaggy hair with both hands, and turning his gentle face and large mild eyes to Alice. She thought she had never seen such a strange-looking soldier in all her life.
He was dressed in a tin armour, which seemed to fit him very badly, and he had a queer-shaped little deal box fastened across his shoulders, upside-down, and with the lid hanging open. Alice looked at it with great curiosity.'
  Through the Looking-Glass. By Lewis Carroll (1994), p115.

Example 7

'Mr Wonka was standing all alone just inside the open gates of the factory. And what an extraordinary little man he was! He had a black top hat on his head. He wore a tail coat made of a beautiful plum-coloured velvet. His trousers were bottle green. His gloves were pearly grey. And in one hand he carried a fine gold-topped walking cane.
Covering his chin, there was a small, neat, pointed black beard – a goatee. And his eyes – his eyes were most marvellously bright. They seemed to be sparkling and twinkling at you all the

time. The whole face, in fact, was alight with fun and laughter.

And oh, how clever he looked! How quick and sharp and full of life! He kept making quick jerky little movements with his head, cocking it this way and that, and taking everything in with those bright twinkling eyes. He was like a squirrel in the quickness of his movements, like a quick clever old squirrel from the park.'

Charlie and the Chocolate Factory. By Roald Dahl (2008), p.80.

Example 8

'Muzzled and caged in the back of a van, I had long hours to think about everything that had happened to me that evening on the park, about how stupid and gullible I had been to allow myself to get caught. And then there were more long, dark hours to remember how happy my life had been before I was so suddenly snatched away from everyone and everything I loved.

In the van there was pitch black all around me. I had no idea whether it was night or day, no idea where I was being taken, only that I was a prisoner, that with every hour that passed I was being driven further and further away from home and from Patrick. I had tried yelping and barking, tried scratching at the door. Now I lay there curled up in my misery, exhausted and dejected, the van shaking and rattling around me. I closed my eyes and tried to think myself home, to blot out the terror I was living through, tried to make myself believe that I was back on the sofa at home with Patrick, that none of this had happened.'

Born to Run. By Michael Morpurgo (2007), pp59–60.

Example 9

'Marilla was a tall, thin woman, with angles and without curves; her dark hair showed some grey streaks and was always twisted up in a hard little knot behind with two wire hairpins stuck aggressively through it. She looked like a woman of narrow experience and rigid conscience, which she was; but there was a saving something about her mouth which, if it had been ever so slightly developed, might have been considered indicative of a sense of humour.'

Anne of Green Gables. By L.M. Montgomery (1994), pp5–6.

Example 10

'It was just then that Miss Minchin entered the room. She was very like her house, Sara felt: tall and dull, and respectable and ugly. She had large, cold, fishy eyes, and a large, cold, fishy smile. It spread itself into a very large smile when she saw Sara and Captain Crewe. She had heard a great many desirable things of the young soldier from the lady who had recommended her school to him. Among other things, she had heard that he was a rich father who was willing to spend a great deal of money on his little daughter.'

A Little Princess. By Frances Hodgson Burnett (2009) pp10–11.

 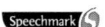

Example 11

'One such young man was Trout Walker. His real name was Charles Walker, but everyone called him Trout because his two feet smelled like a couple of dead fish.

This wasn't entirely Trout's fault. He had an incurable foot fungus. In fact, it was the same foot fungus that a hundred and ten years later would afflict the famous ballplayer Clyde Livingstone. But at least Clyde Livingstone showered every day.'

Holes. By Louis Sachar (2000), p102.

Example 12

'Mr Twit was one of those very hairy-faced men. The whole of his face except for his forehead, his eyes and his nose was covered with thick hair. The stuff even sprouted in revolting tufts out of his nostrils and ear-holes.

Mr Twit felt that his hairiness made him look terrifically wise and grand. But in truth he was neither of these things. Mr Twit was a twit. He was born a twit. And now at the age of sixty, he was a bigger twit than ever.'

The Twits. By Roald Dahl (2008), p2.

Example 13

'Margaret, the eldest of the four, was sixteen, and very pretty, being plump and fair, with large eyes, plenty of soft, brown hair, a sweet mouth, and white hands, of which she was rather vain. Fifteen-year-old Jo was very tall, thin, and brown, and reminded one of a colt; for she never seemed to know what to do with her long limbs, which were very much in her way. She had a decided mouth, a comical nose, and sharp, grey eyes, which appeared to see everything, and were by turns fierce, funny, or thoughtful. Her long, thick hair was her one beauty; but it was usually bundled into a net to be out of her way. Round shoulders had Jo, big hands and feet, a fly-away look to her clothes, and the uncomfortable appearance of a girl who was rapidly shooting up into a woman, and didn't like it. Elizabeth – or Beth, as every one called her – was a rosy, smooth-haired, bright-eyed girl of thirteen, with a shy manner, a timid voice, and a peaceful expression, which was seldom disturbed. Her father called her 'Little Tranquillity', and the name suited her excellently; for she seemed to live in a happy world of her own, only venturing out to meet the few whom she trusted and loved. Amy, though the youngest, was a most important person – in her own opinion at least. A regular snow maiden, with blue eyes, and yellow hair curling on her shoulders; pale and slender, and always carrying herself like a young lady mindful of her manners. What the characters of the four sisters were, we will leave to be found out.'

Little Women. By Louisa May Alcott (2003), p11.

Example 14

'All these details I observed afterwards. At present my attention was centred upon the single, grim, motionless figure which lay stretched upon the boards, with vacant, sightless eyes staring up at the discoloured ceiling. It was that of a man about forty-three or forty-four years of age, middle-sized, broad-shouldered, with crisp curling black hair, and a short, stubbly beard. He was dressed in a heavy broadcloth frock coat and waistcoat, with light-coloured trousers, and immaculate collar and cuffs. A top hat, well brushed and trim, was placed upon the floor beside him. His hands were clenched and his arms thrown abroad, while his lower limbs were interlocked, as though his death struggle had been a grievous one. On his rigid face there stood an expression of horror, and, as it seemed to me, of hatred, such as I have never seen upon human features. This malignant and terrible contortion, combined with the low forehead, blunt nose, and prognathous jaw, gave the dead man a singularly simious and ape-like appearance, which was increased by his writhing unnatural posture. I have seen death in many forms, but never has it appeared to me in a more fearsome aspect than in that dark, grimy apartment, which looked out upon one of the main arteries of suburban London .'

A Study in Scarlet. By Sir Arthur Conan Doyle (2007) pp32–3.

Example 15

'I was now beginning to grow handsome; my coat had grown fine and soft, and was bright black. I had one white foot, and a pretty white star on my forehead. I was thought very handsome; my master would not sell me till I was four years old; he said lads ought not to work like men, and colts ought not to work like horses till they were grown up.'

Black Beauty. By Anna Sewell (2001), p29.

Example 16

'He had changed since his New Haven years. Now he was a sturdy straw-haired man of thirty, with a rather hard mouth and a supercilious manner. Two shining arrogant eyes had established dominance over his face and gave him the appearance of always leaning aggressively forward. Not even the effeminate swank of his riding clothes could hide the enormous power of that body – he seemed to fill those glistening boots until he strained the top lacing, and you could see a great pack of muscle shifting when his shoulder moved under his thin coat. It was a body capable of enormous leverage – a cruel body.'

The Great Gatsby. By F. Scott Fitzgerald (2006), p7.

Example 17

'Everyone thinks I'm showing off when I talk, ridiculous when I'm silent, insolent when I answer, cunning when I have a good idea, lazy when I'm tired, selfish when I eat one bite more than I should, stupid, cowardly, calculating, etc., etc. All day long I hear nothing but what an exasperating child I am, and although I laugh it off and pretend not to mind, I do mind. I wish I could ask G-d to give me another personality, one that doesn't antagonize everyone.
But that's impossible. I'm stuck with the character I was born with, and yet I'm sure I'm not a bad person. I do my best to please everyone, more than they'd ever suspect in a million years. When I'm upstairs, I try to laugh it off because I don't want them to see my troubles. '

The Diary of A Young Girl. By Anne Frank (2008), p81.

 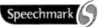

9

Session 9

Names of students: _____

_____

Facilitator: _____ Date: _____

School: _____

Class: _____

Aims	Method/Activities	Materials
To revise and recap the story elements of the story planner covered in the previous session, with a focus on **characters**.	Group discussion with students taking turns to give an example of one important thing they learned from the previous session. Make a list of all the new adjectives that students have learned through their character description tasks from last session. Remind students of the story planner and where characters fit into the planner. Ensure they are mindful of the whole story and have all the story elements in mind during the session.	Flipchart or whiteboard, paper and pen. Story planner.
To **identify their heroes**, giving reasons for their choice.	Group discussion where students share their hero with the group. The facilitator can begin the discussion by stating who her hero is, and providing reasons for her choice. For example, her hero may be Nelson Mandela, and that could be because she lived in South Africa and respected everything he has done for the country and for world peace. She could talk to the students about his bravery, generosity and willingness to forgive and make peace. This is a good example to use as the students will know Nelson Mandela and will be able to provide their own views and participate in the discussion. Each student is then given the opportunity to share their hero with the group. Their heroes can be famous personalities like football stars, movie stars, presidents or prime ministers, Nobel prize winners, scientists, inventors – and	Flipchart or whiteboard, paper and pen.

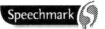

Aims	Method/Activities	Materials
	anyone else who the students admire. They can be alive or dead. Students may identify their mothers, fathers, grandparents or teachers as their heroes. It is important to note that students may disagree on the choices of heroes. This is fine and is a good opportunity to explore appropriate ways of disagreeing with other people which allow the sharing of views from all perspectives in a calm and considered manner. Provide students with the opportunity here to learn that in group debates and discussions, people will often share different points of view and this is healthy and makes for interesting discussion. However, emphasise the importance of respecting everyone's views and allowing each member the time to describe and talk about their hero. Ensure that students provide reasons for their choice. It is not good enough to simply say that David Beckham is their hero, but they need to say why he is their choice. Get them to think about their choices more deeply, so if they chose Beckham because they are football fans, then why Beckham in particularly and not another footballer, for example, Pele? This encourages students to provide rationales for their choices and reflect on the choices and decisions they make. This ability will assist them in all interactions: school, home and wider social settings.	
To **describe their heroes** using the character word map.	Students to use all the information they have learned from previous sessions about detailed and descriptive characterisation, and to provide a description of their chosen hero. The description will include all aspects that have been explored previously, including physical appearance, personality, mood, thoughts, feelings and behaviours. Encourage them to use new words and vocabulary and have the dictionary and thesaurus on hand to facilitate this.	Character word map. Dictionary and thesaurus.

Aims	Method/Activities	Materials
To share the **biographical story** of their hero.	We have already covered the difference between fiction and non-fiction. Revisit this distinction for students:	Flipchart or whiteboard, pen and paper.
	Fiction: stories that are made up and based largely on the imagination and not on facts.	Story planner.
	Non-fiction: stories that are based on facts and are true. They are stories about real events, people and places.	It will be useful to have some general reference books from the school library which students can use during the session to find out more details about their chosen hero.
	Students will share the biographical story of their chosen heroes with the group. The story will be biographical rather than autobiographical as it is someone else telling the story about the person, rather than the person themselves. Revisit for students the difference between biography and autobiography:	
	Biography: a story written about someone else's life. It is about someone else and not written by the person whose life is being described.	
	Autobiography: a biography about you. So it is a story written by the person about himself or herself.	
	Ensure the students understand that the story they will tell about their hero is a biography, as it is told by someone other than the hero in question.	
	Students should share as many details about their hero as they know. They should have looked up some information about their hero as part of their homework task last session.	
	Encourage them to tell their story using the story planner, providing information about the beginning of their hero's life, where they were born (time and place information), what their early life was like, and then going on to describe their life as it is now, or as it was when they became well known to the student.	

 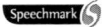

Aims	Method/Activities	Materials
	Students can use the story planner to help structure their stories and provide details of the different episodes of their hero's life. These may include various events, climaxes and outcomes. Many students will talk about messages or morals that they have learned from their hero's activities. Explore this with them and find out why and how these specific people inspire the students. This task can produce some wonderful stories and allows students to share with each other what is important to them and why. Some may share the history and experiences of their grandparents or even great-grandparents, how they fought in the war, fled persecution in another country, and other significant events. This is important as it acknowledges what being a hero is, and what it is not. For example, being a hero is not necessarily about being famous or rich. It can be your next door neighbour or teacher. Other students will share the background and stories of more famous people, who may include Albert Einstein, Walt Disney, Elvis Presley, Michael Jackson, Martin Luther King, Christopher Columbus, Princess Diana, The Queen, Barack Obama, Marie Curie, Bill Gates, Michael Jordan, David Beckham, Madonna, Lady Gaga. This is a great opportunity for students to investigate the lives of people they are interested in and who have achieved great things. The stories of the heroes will inspire the group and provide them with new areas of knowledge and understanding. Students may need to look up some facts and details about their heroes in order to tell a complete story, so make sure you have some reference books available for them to do so.	
To **develop the three questions** that they would most like to ask their hero.	During the pilot study, most students expressed a burning desire to find out more information from their heroes.	Flipchart or whiteboard, paper and pen.

Aims	Method/Activities	Materials
	This was therefore a very popular task. Ask students to think about what they would most like to know about their hero. Get them to develop three questions that would explore these issues and encourage them to think about their choices. Why specifically do they want answers to these questions, how will it change the way they see their heroes, and what answers would they most expect their heroes to give? The latter question is an important one for students as many will pose a question for their heroes with an answer in mind. This is something many of us do in our daily lives. So, for example, if asking David Beckham how he feels before running on to the pitch before an England game, the answer 'petrified' might not be what the student expects or wants to hear. Obviously they will not get answers to their questions, but discuss the possible answers they could get, and whether these may change how they view their hero. So, for example, would knowing that Beckham felt petrified when running onto the pitch change the way they view him?	
To share a **personal narrative** about a difficult time in their life and change the story plot and outcome.	Students are asked to share with the group an incident in their lives which has been difficult for them. This can be a problem, conflict or dilemma they have experienced, for example, a serious disagreement with a best friend, not getting on well with a sibling, continual disagreements with a parent, problems with a step-parent, always getting into trouble in school, not understanding homework, failing exams etc. Students are encouraged to share their personal narrative of this difficult event using the story planner and to ensure that their story is well structured and includes the three main story components. Once the story has been shared, and the outcome of the story given, ask students to evaluate how well they dealt with the problem or conflict or difficulty. Ask them to consider how	Story planner. Flipchart or whiteboard, paper and pen.

 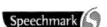

Aims	Method/Activities	Materials
	they think their hero would have handled the same situation. They might like to retell the story, but this time placing their hero as the main character. With everything they have learned and know about their hero, ask them to consider how their hero would address and resolve the issue. Encourage them to explore whether they would have handled it differently in any way, and if so, what these differences may be. Do they feel a different outcome would have been achieved if they had also resolved it in such a way? Explore with the students if there are any lessons they could have learned from their hero about resolving their own issues and if so, what these might be. Explore with students what they have learned from this activity that they might take away and apply when next they have to deal with a problem or difficulty.	
	This activity can be very powerful and provides students with the opportunity to share their own personal narratives and difficulties with the group, and to evaluate how they deal with and overcome their conflicts, and whether they could learn anything from how their hero would deal with similar challenges. Students are often surprised at how similar their problems are to the experiences of other group members and comment on the fact that they had previously thought that no one else would have experienced the same problem as them. They also often come up with excellent ideas for problem solving when thinking about how their heroes would tackle the problem.	
	It is important at the end of this activity to encourage students to explicitly state what they have learned about dealing with problems and difficulties and how they might apply these new skills in their school and home life.	
To provide **biographical portrayals** of other curriculum-based characters.	If there is time in the session, you might also like to take a character from the students' school curriculum, whether it be history, English or geography, and in the same way that students did with their heroes, get them to	Flipchart or whiteboard, paper and pens. Curriculum text. Story planner.

Aims	Method/Activities	Materials
	develop a biographical account of the character under discussion in the classroom lesson. This is a very good way to connect the work covered in this programme to the students' school activity, and will also help to enhance the students' understanding of a specific topic area taught in class. Students should be encouraged to use the story planner and character word map to help them generate the story about the specific character under discussion. Characters may include Macbeth, Anne Frank, Thomas Edison, Alexander Graham Bell, Hitler, Winston Churchill, Henry VIII, to name but a few. Students will be asked to develop this further in their homework activity this session.	Character word map.
To sum up and revise contents of the session.	Get volunteers from the group to summarise the main content of the session. Ask other members of the group to help, adding in the parts that may have been omitted.	Flipchart or whiteboard, paper and pens.
Mission to Achieve: To develop a biographical portrayal of one character that the student is learning about in the classroom.	Students may already have begun this task, but if not, they have the opportunity to do so as their homework task.

Students will choose a main character that they are currently learning about in the classroom. They will explore this character by completing a character word map and providing a rich and descriptive profile of this character. With the knowledge they have from the classroom lessons on the life and times of this character, they will try and generate the biography of this character using the story planner to help structure their biography. | Story planner. Character word map. |

 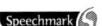

Evaluation of session/General comments

Session 10

Names of students: _____

_____

Facilitator: _____ Date: _____

School: _____

Class: _____

Aims	Method/Activities	Materials
To revise and recap the importance of characterisation in a story. Revisit the three parts that make up the beginning of a story: **Setting = character, time, place.**	Group discussion exploring the beginning element of a story, focusing on character, time and place elements. Revise through a group discussion why detailed and specific characterisation is so important to a story. Test students' recall of all the new characters they have learned about from the previous few sessions.	Flipchart or whiteboard, paper and pen. Story planner.
To share character profile and biographical story on a specific character from a chosen subject of the curriculum.	Students to share homework activity task with group. Provide opportunities for each member to provide character description of character and tell the biography of the person they have chosen. Explore with students what new information they collected that they had not known before about their character in order to tell a complete biography.	Completed character word map on chosen character from curriculum subject. Story planner.
To explore in more detail the beginning of the story, the story setting focusing on **time** and **place** elements.	Focus on the first part of a story, i.e. the story **beginning**. Explain the three parts that make up the **setting** of a story, with this session focusing on the **time** and **place** elements. Revisit the teaching notes from session 7 and discuss the features of time and place. Group discussion around the settings of stories. Group members to identify the possible times and places in which stories can take place. Differentiate for students TIME versus PLACE information. Draw their attention to the different questions one asks to find out more about time and place.	Story planner. Flipchart or whiteboard, paper and pen. Story F1 race track, story football match, story athletics race track – focusing on the beginning of the story, specifically the time and place of a story.

Aims	Method/Activities	Materials
	Where does the story happen? = PLACE **When** does the story happen? = TIME Students to be encouraged to explore all possibilities with regards to time (past, present, future, morning, sunrise, noon, night, dawn, dusk, 3 o'clock, etc) and place (earth, solar system, sea, Mars, America, Australia, house, prison, dungeon, museum, school, prison, etc). Other examples of settings can include: Time (when): present, medieval times, Victorian era, future, e.g. 25th century, tomorrow, yesterday, Second World War, winter, morning. Place (where): alley, bedroom, cupboard, snowstorm, scorching desert, swamp, ark, shopping centre, spaceship, river, different countries.	
To discuss the importance of **time** and **place** settings in storytelling.	Group discussion on **time** and **place** and the importance of having powerful, real and interesting descriptions of the time and place in which stories take place. Group to explore the importance of detailed time and place descriptions to enhance the story and ensure that the reader gets drawn into the story. Students to understand that details about time and place provide a greater understanding of the actions and motives of a character, for example, a tramp living in a box on a cold damp street will act very differently to a billionaire living in a penthouse. Important to enhance awareness that there are many possibilities for time and place settings when constructing stories and students do not have to stick to the present time or the school or home setting. Settings can also change over the course of a story, so a story may start in the morning and conclude later in the day. Similarly, the story can begin in the high street and end in the police station. The place and time word maps that follow will	Story planner. Time word map. Place word map.

Aims	Method/Activities	Materials
	help students think of as many details as possible when describing the time and place of their setting which, together with the characters, make up the beginning section of the story. The time and place of different stories will vary widely. Sometimes, the place may not even be on this earth, but may take place on another planet. Similarly, the time may not always be in the present. A story might be set in the past, or even in the future. The place and time word maps are devised to incorporate all these time and place possibilities. This may mean that students will not be able to complete every category each time on the word maps. That is fine. They should complete as many categories as possible and use the place and time word maps to flesh out the setting details as much as possible and provide a detailed and interesting setting for their story.	
To **identify favourite times and places** and provide reasons for their choice.	Group to identify their favourite time of year and time of day, as well as their favourite places. They should have the opportunity to explain why these times and places are their favourites, for example, a special memory or place where they have the most fun. Students to be encouraged to use the time and place word maps to detail their choices. A fun game to play with time and place is the 'time machine experience'. Students to pretend they are travelling in a time machine and stop the machine at their favourite time and/or place. Students should in turns describe their favourite times and places using the time and place word maps to explore and describe each one in detail. Encourage students to 'observe' their new surroundings carefully and comment on how people dress, act, behave, etc in this new place and time period.	Time and place word maps.
To critically evaluate **setting descriptions** (time and place) from published works.	Provide examples of **setting** (time and place) descriptions from different publications included in teaching notes. Students to	Story planner. Examples of time and place descriptions from

 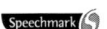

159

Aims	Method/Activities	Materials
	comment on these descriptions providing a critical evaluation of each description. Encourage students to visualise the settings and describe them verbally. Discuss how powerful each description is. Students may enjoy trying to draw each setting from the description provided. Drawings can then be compared and similarities and differences noted. Students will find interesting how different their drawings are, and how much interpretations of the same descriptions can vary.	published works included in teaching notes.
To describe features and characteristics of specific time and place settings from different setting pictures.	Students to have the opportunity to choose time and place settings from a range of setting pictures included in the programme and describe the setting to the rest of the group. Group to play the game, 'Where am I?' Each student chooses a setting from a range of setting pictures and describes the setting to the group without divulging where it is. Group are not to know any details about the time or place of the chosen picture that the student is describing and the first person to guess the setting wins the game. The better the description, the quicker the group should guess correctly, therefore the person describing the setting should aim for the group to guess correctly using as few guesses as possible. The time and place word maps should be used to encourage students to describe each setting in as much detail as possible, using all senses, for example, describing the sound, sight, smell and touch of the place. They can describe the setting of a dungeon, for example, using all their senses: 'dark, dense, damp, putrid, with jagged pointy edges and filled with ghostly sounds and a musty stale smell'. Students to consider how settings will impact on feelings and behaviour of characters, so consider how a little boy will feel and act differently in a dungeon compared to a bedroom. Consider also the difference with the everyday activities of the same boy living in a palace versus a flat in town.	Setting pictures supplied in the programme. Setting pictures include: lounge, aeroplane, cinema, daytime, galaxy, ocean, night time, rainy day and snow. Continue to use the time and place word maps to encourage students to detail each picture as much as possible.

Aims	Method/Activities	Materials
	This topic allows you to discuss many issues relevant to group members. The group, for example, may like to explore the places where they are from, and where their ancestors have come from. In this case, encourage discussion on the differences in places, and how these differences may impact on the way we live. Many of the students will have heard their grandparents perhaps talking about Britain many years ago, and some will have grandparents and even parents from different countries. Get them to talk about these experiences and share details about these different places. Ensure all students are involved in some way in this discussion. Invite students to talk about their favourite holiday destinations and all the places they have visited. Encourage students to explore the differences and similarities between these places and how these differences impact on the way people live. So, for example, how do they think the difference in weather impacts on how people live in Britain and in Australia? And what about Iceland? What impact does this have on the clothes we wear, on our personalities, on the food we eat (so, for example, salads versus stews, and certain fruits available in certain climates). You can explore with students the different wildlife and animals we find in different places, and in different times and eras; so what did we use as transport before the motor car? You can also discuss the difference living in a country at peace versus one at war. You will of course not necessarily have time for all such discussions, but choose the ones that are most relevant for the members of the group. Use the story F1 race track, story football match and story athletics race track if appropriate to explore details of the setting. Encourage students to comment on the setting of the race track, the football match and athletics race, the	Story F1 race track. Use of story F1 race track to explore details of the setting. Encourage students to comment on the setting of the race track, the characters in the cars, the audience watching the race, the time and place where the race is taking place. Story football match. Story athletics race track.

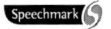

Aims	Method/Activities	Materials
	characters in the cars, on the football pitch and the runners, the audience watching the races and match, the time and place where the races and match are taking place. Draw their attention, for example, to the time of day, the trees, ground, sky, etc around the car track, football stadium and athletics stadium.	
To construct a story with a chosen character, time and place setting.	Students to choose one **setting** picture from the range offered and think about how they can construct a story around this specific setting. This task can be undertaken in pairs if appropriate. Students to construct a story using a **character** chosen from the character pictures, and place that character in the **time** and **place** settings chosen from the picture cards available. Students should be encouraged to think about how the time and place elements they have chosen impact on the character and vice versa and think about what details the beginning of their story will contain. Students to take all information about the three elements of setting (character, time and place) into account when thinking about the story they will construct. Students to share their story with the group, ensuring their beginning elements are sufficiently detailed with regards to time, place and character. Students holding the story pencil or microphone hold the floor and tell their story.	Story planner. Story pencil or microphone. Time, place and character picture cards included in the programme.
For students to change their stories by mixing and matching different **character, place** and **time** picture cards.	Students to mix and match different characters and time and place settings from the setting and character pictures provided and consider how different setting combinations change the story. Students, for example, swap one card with another member of the group. This could be a character, place or time card. They then have to incorporate this new information into their story and change their story accordingly. So, for example, students to explore the difference in	Character, time and place picture cards included in the programme.

Aims	Method/Activities	Materials
	telling a story about a boy fighting with another boy in the playground or classroom, versus a story about a boy fighting with another boy in a prison. This helps create an awareness of the importance of time, place and character in storytelling and how these factors impact on behaviour, events and story outcomes.	
To **produce well structured stories from varied combinations of character, time and place** cards.	This is a fun activity with students required to make up well structured and coherent stories using strange combinations of character, time and place cards given to them by the facilitator or other group members. The combinations are meant here to be as strange and incongruous as possible. Students are encouraged to combine completely opposing characters and pictures, for example, an old lady windsurfing on the ocean at midnight. The challenge is for them to construct exciting, well structured and coherent stories using this information. Their stories should not be too silly, and they need to try and make some sense of the combination of cards they have received. Other combinations might include the Queen in Thailand on Christmas day or David Beckham at a ballet class in Russia. The group to evaluate each story told and discuss how well fellow members managed to integrate the different parts of the setting. The picture cards from the programme will be a starting point, but students should be encouraged to think up other strange character, place and time details to further challenge their imaginations and storytelling skills!	Story planner. Character, place and time picture cards.
To sum up and revise contents of the session.	Get volunteers from the group to summarise the main content of the session. Ask other members of the group to help, adding in the parts that may have been omitted.	Flipchart or whiteboard, paper and pen.
Mission to Achieve: Students to choose one place or time period that they have	Students are required to choose one time period or place that they have learned about in lessons. This may be a different country they have learned about in geography or history,	Time and place word map.

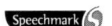

Aims	Method/Activities	Materials
learned about in school and describe it using the place or time word map.	such as Germany or America; it may be somewhere in space that they are learning about, for example, Mars or Saturn or the Sun; or it may be a piece of agricultural land. They could also choose a time period, for example, the period of the First World War, the Victorian era, the Roman or Tudor period. They might even choose the time when dinosaurs roamed the earth. The choice is theirs, and they are to use the place or time maps to provide detailed descriptions. Students should be encouraged to ask their teachers or other helpers for more information and also refer to school texts or library books where they will find additional helpful information.	

Evaluation of session/General comments

 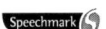

Teaching notes for Session 10

Examples of setting descriptions, specifically time and place descriptions from published works

Here are some time and place descriptions from a range of publications which can be read to the students. You might decide to read them all, or to choose some of your favourites and go into them in more detail. Feel free to add any of your own suggestions too.

Students should be encouraged to critically evaluate each description and comment on how effective and evocative each description is. Students should try and see whether they can visualise the setting and place and time from the description provided and also discuss whether they feel that it is so detailed and evocative that it is as if they are there themselves. Many of these settings, but not all, can be found at the beginning of the book. It is important to emphasise that detailed setting descriptions of time, place and character can be provided throughout the story where appropriate.

Example 1

'It was the sweetest, most mysterious-looking place anyone could imagine. The high walls which shut it in were covered with the leafless stems of climbing roses which were so thick that they were matted together. Mary Lennox knew they were roses because she had seen a great many roses in India. All the ground was covered with grass of a wintry brown and out of it grew clumps of bushes which were surely rose bushes if they were alive. There were numbers of standard roses which had so spread their branches that they were like little trees. There were other trees in the garden, and one of the things which made the place look strangest and loveliest was that climbing roses had run all over them and swung down long tendrils which made light swaying curtains, and here and there they had caught at each other or at a far-reaching branch and had crept from one tree to another and made lovely bridges of themselves. There were neither leaves nor roses on them now and Mary did not know whether they were dead or alive, but their thin gray or brown branches and sprays looked like a sort of hazy mantle spreading over everything, walls, and trees, and even brown grass, where they had fallen from their fastenings and run along the ground. It was this hazy tangle from tree to tree which made it all look so mysterious. Mary had thought it must be different from other gardens which had not been left all by themselves so long; and indeed it was different from any other place she had ever seen in her life.'

The Secret Garden. By Frances Hodgson Burnett (2002), pp107–8.

Example 2

'I had a new suit and a small velvet hat. My mother said everyone wears new clothes for the Jewish holidays. It was hot for October and my father said he remembered it was always hot on the Jewish holidays when he was a kid. I had to wear white gloves. They made my hands sweat. By the time I got to New York the gloves were pretty dirty so I took them off and stuffed them into my pocketbook. Grandma met me at our usual spot in the bus terminal and took me in a taxi to her temple.

We got there at ten-thirty. Grandma had to show a card to an usher and then he led us to our seats which were in the fifth row in the middle.'

Are you There, G-D? It's Me, Margaret. By Judy Blume (1980), p60.

Example 3

'He could see the green of the shore now but only the tops of the blue hills that showed white as though they were snow-capped and the clouds that looked like high snow mountains above them. The sea was very dark and the light made prisms in the water.'

The Old Man and the Sea. By Ernest Hemingway (1978), p28.

Example 4

'It was morning and the new sun sparkled gold across the ripples of a gentle sea. A mile from shore a fishing boat chummed the water, and the word for Breakfast Flock flashed through the air, till a crowd of a thousand seagulls came to dodge and fight for bits of food. It was another busy day beginning.'

Jonathon Livingston Seagull. A Story. By Richard Bach (1973), p13.

Example 5

'Maycomb was an old town, but it was a tired old town when I first knew it. In rainy weather the streets turned to red slop; grass grew on the sidewalks, the courthouse sagged in the square. Somehow, it was hotter then; a black dog suffered on a summer's day; bony mules hitched to Hoover carts flicked flies in the sweltering shade of the live oak on the square. Men's stiff collars wilted by nine in the morning. Ladies bathed before noon, after their three o'clock naps, and by nightfall were like soft teacakes with frostings of sweat and sweet talcum.'

To Kill a Mockingbird. By Harper Lee (1991), p5.

Example 6

'I wander'd lonely as a cloud
That floats on high o'er vales and hills,
When all at once I saw a crowd,
A host of golden daffodils,

 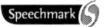

Beside the lake, beneath the trees
Fluttering and dancing in the breeze.

Continuous as the stars that shine
And twinkle on the Milky Way,
They stretch'd in never-ending line
Along the margin of a bay:
Ten thousand saw I at a glance
Tossing their heads in sprightly dance.'
        'From The Daffodils'. By William Wordsworth (1996), p17.

Example 7

'But there was also the view, which again could appear on no inventory. How could any such list describe what one saw when one looked out from Mma Ramotswe's door? To the front, an acacia tree, the thorn tree which dots the wide edges of the Kalahari; the great white thorns, a warning; the olive-grey leaves, by contrast, so delicate. In its branches, in the late afternoon, or in the cool of the early morning, one might see a Go-Away Bird, or hear it, rather. And beyond the acacia, over the dusty road, the roofs of the town under a cover of trees and scrub bush; on the horizon, in a blue shimmer of heat, the hills, like improbable, overgrown termite-mounds.'

The No. 1 Ladies' Detective Agency. By Alexander McCall Smith (2003), pp1–2.

Example 8

'Matilda saw a narrow dirt-path leading to a tiny red-brick cottage. The cottage was so small it looked more like a doll's house than a human dwelling. The bricks it was built of were old and crumbly and very pale red. It had a grey slate roof and one small chimney, and there were two little windows at the front. Each window was no larger than a sheet of tabloid newspaper and there was clearly no upstairs to the place. On either side of the path there was a wilderness of nettles and blackberry thorns and long brown grass. An enormous oak tree stood overshadowing the cottage. Its massive spreading branches seemed to be enfolding and embracing the tiny building, and perhaps hiding it as well from the rest of the world.'

Matilda. By Roald Dahl (2008), p178.

Example 9

'They both jerked as the door to the chemistry lab flew open, smacking loudly against the wall beside it. The earsplitting clang of the room's smoke detector filled the hall as blue smoke billowed out of the doorway and several students emerged from the cloud, coughing. "Out, out!" Ms Pehrson's voice sounded above the din as she shooed a bunch of sophomores from

Speechmark

the classroom. The blue haze spread down the hallway and somebody pulled the fire alarm, setting off the entire building's cacophonous alert system.'

Spells. By Aprilynne Pike (2010), p194.

Example 10

'The night's storm was over, as quick and angry as a torrential late-summer downpour can sometimes be. It had left the air cooler and smelling like a wet dog, the ground waterlogged. The ragged encampment slowly came back to life, caravan doors opening, spilling out flickering lamplight and tired voices; no one in Hubble's Circus had slept well, the hammering rain, the lightning and the thunder that sounded like the world was coming to an end had seen to that.'

Snatched. By Graham Marks (2006), p7.

Example 11

'There is no lake at Camp Green Lake. There once was a very large lake here, the largest lake in Texas. That was over a hundred years ago. Now it is just a dry, flat wasteland.

There used to be a town of Green Lake as well. The town shrivelled and dried up along with the lake, and the people who lived there.

During the summer the daytime temperature hovers around ninety-five degrees in the shade – if you can find any shade. There's not much shade in a big dry lake.

The only trees are two old oaks on the eastern edge of the "lake". A hammock is stretched between the two trees, and a log cabin stands behind that.

The campers are forbidden to lie in the hammock. It belongs to the Warden. The Warden owns the shade.'

Holes. By Louis Sachar (2000), p3.

Example 12

'It was one January morning, very early – a pinching, frosty morning – the cove all grey with hoar frost, the ripple lapping softly on the stones, the sun still low and only touching the hilltops and shining far to seaward.'

Treasure Island. By Robert Louis Stevenson (2008), p8.

 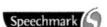

Example 13

'Scrooge took his melancholy dinner in his usual melancholy tavern; and having read all the newspapers, and beguiled the rest of the evening with his banker's-book, went home to bed. He lived in chambers which had once belonged to his deceased partner. They were a gloomy suite of rooms, in a lowering pile of building up a yard, where it had so little business to be, that one could scarcely help fancying it must have run there when it was a young house, playing at hide-and-seek with other houses, and have forgotten the way out again. It was old enough now, and dreary enough, for nobody lived in it but Scrooge, the other rooms being all let out as offices. The yard was so dark that even Scrooge, who knew its every stone, was fain to grope with his hands. The fog and frost so hung about the old gateway of the house, that it seemed as if the Genius of the Weather sat in mournful meditation on the threshold.'

A Christmas Carol. By Charles Dickens. (1979), pp18–19.

Example 14

'The apartment was on the top floor – a small living-room, a small dining-room, a small bedroom, and a bath. The living-room was crowded to the doors with a set of tapestried furniture entirely too large for it, so that to move about was to stumble continually over scenes of ladies swinging in the gardens of Versailles. The only picture was an over-enlarged photograph, apparently a hen sitting on a blurred rock. Looked at from a distance, however, the hen resolved itself into a bonnet, and the countenance of a stout old lady beamed down into the room.'

The Great Gatsby. By F. Scott Fitzgerald (2006), p29.

Example 15

'The rainstorm had ended and the gray mist and clouds had been swept away in the night by the wind. The wind itself had ceased and a brilliant, deep blue sky arched high over the moorland. Never, never had Mary dreamed of a sky so blue. In India skies were hot and blazing; this was of a deep cool blue which almost seemed to sparkle like the waters of some lovely bottomless lake, and here and there, high, high in the arched blueness floated small clouds of snow-white fleece. The far-reaching world of the moor itself looked softly blue instead of gloomy purple-black or awful dreary gray.'

The Secret Garden. By Frances Hodgson Burnett (2002), p85.

Time Word Map

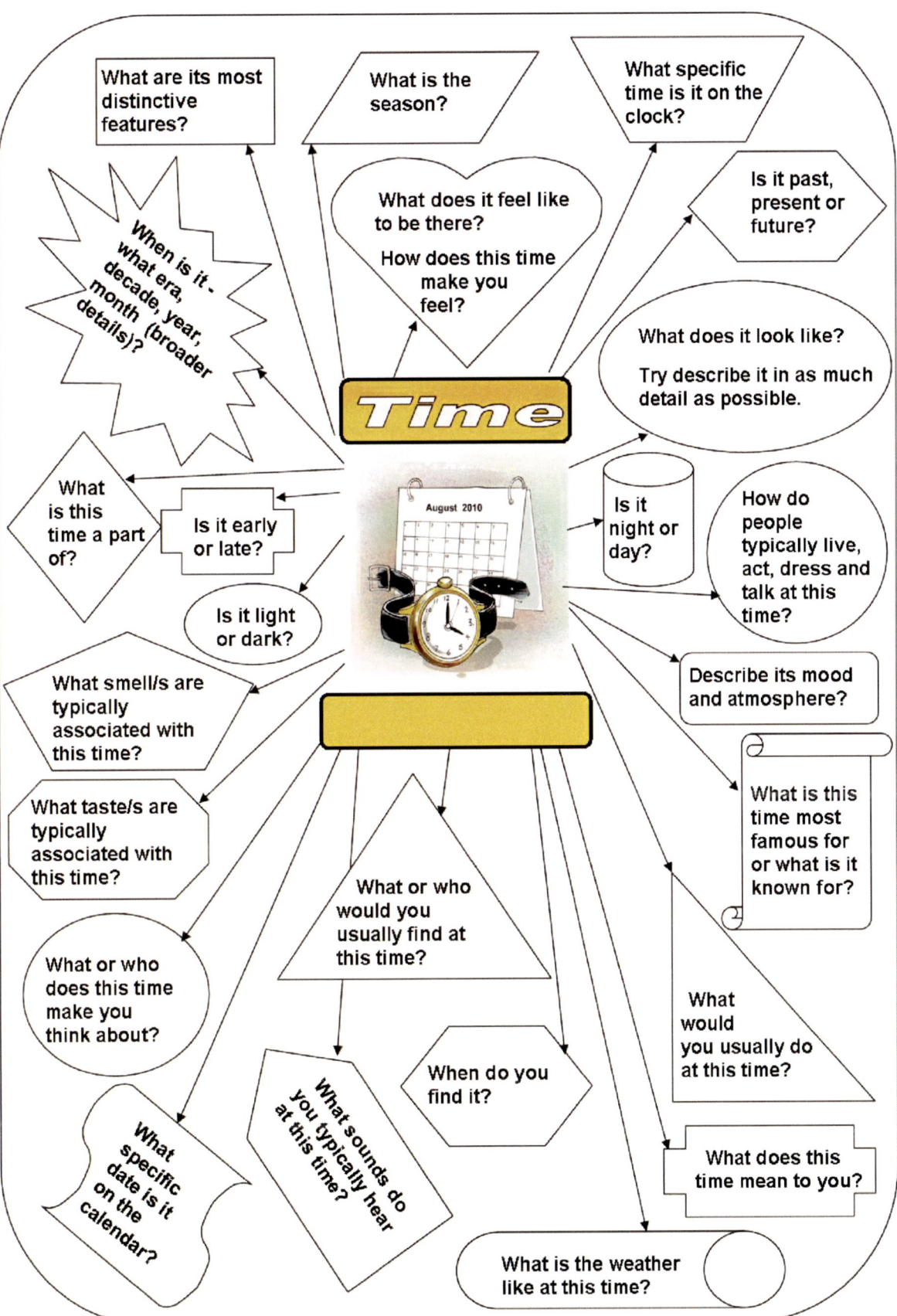

What are its most distinctive features?

What is the season?

What specific time is it on the clock?

What does it feel like to be there?

How does this time make you feel?

Is it past, present or future?

When is it - what era, decade, year, month (broader details)?

What does it look like?

Try describe it in as much detail as possible.

Time

What is this time a part of?

Is it early or late?

Is it night or day?

How do people typically live, act, dress and talk at this time?

Is it light or dark?

What smell/s are typically associated with this time?

Describe its mood and atmosphere?

What taste/s are typically associated with this time?

What is this time most famous for or what is it known for?

What or who does this time make you think about?

What or who would you usually find at this time?

What would you usually do at this time?

What specific date is it on the calendar?

What sounds do you typically hear at this time?

When do you find it?

What does this time mean to you?

What is the weather like at this time?

Place Word Map

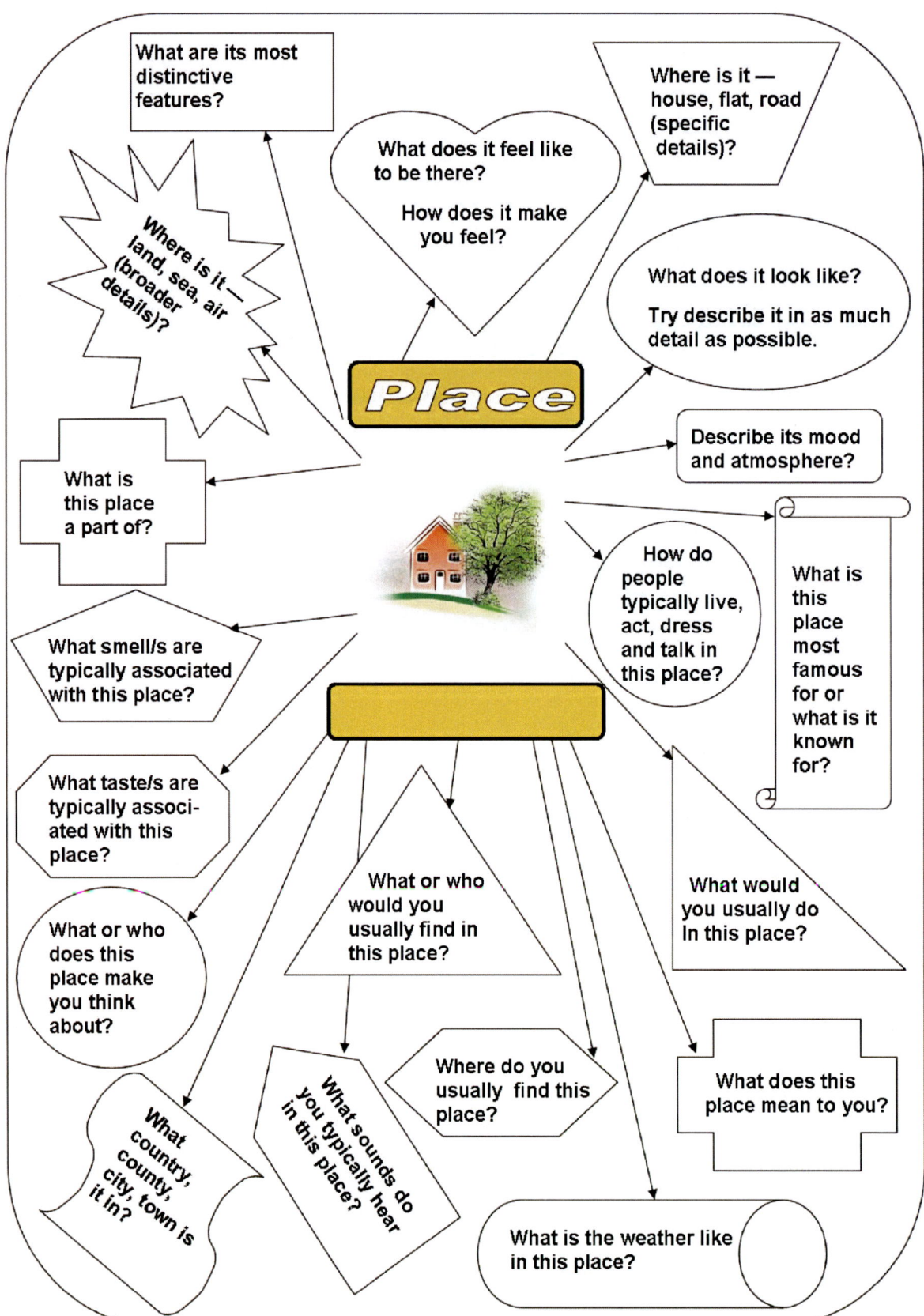

What are its most distinctive features?

What does it feel like to be there?

How does it make you feel?

Where is it — house, flat, road (specific details)?

Where is it — land, sea, air (broader details)?

What does it look like?

Try describe it in as much detail as possible.

Place

Describe its mood and atmosphere?

What is this place a part of?

What smell/s are typically associated with this place?

How do people typically live, act, dress and talk in this place?

What is this place most famous for or what is it known for?

What taste/s are typically associated with this place?

What or who does this place make you think about?

What or who would you usually find in this place?

What would you usually do In this place?

What country, county, city, town is it in?

What sounds do you typically hear in this place?

Where do you usually find this place?

What does this place mean to you?

What is the weather like in this place?

Session 11

Names of students: _____

_____

Facilitator: _____ Date: _____

School: _____

Class: _____

Aims	Method/Activities	Materials
To revise and recap concepts from the previous sessions, i.e. the beginning element of the story planner. **Setting = character, time, place.**	Group discussion recapping the main ideas from the previous session on the beginning of the story from the story planner.	Flipchart or whiteboard, paper and pen. Story planner.
To **review place and time settings** prepared by students around a curriculum topic area.	Provide the opportunity for students to share details about their chosen time and/or place from their homework activity. Discuss their completed word maps and their reasons for choosing the specific settings. Assist students to understand that a greater knowledge about the time and place of a topic covered in class will facilitate their understanding of the entire topic and will help make the subject more interesting and relevant for them. Explore with them their examples brought to the session and the links between the settings they describe and behaviour or dress. You may, for example, consider the typical dress code for ladies in the Victorian era and how this impacts on their physical movement.	Completed time and place word maps.
To focus on the **middle** element of a story, providing insight into what the middle part of the story consists of.	The students have now developed a good understanding of the first element of a story, the beginning, with detailed information on characters, time and place settings. The group discussion now moves on to the main part of the story, the middle of the story. Draw students'	Flipchart or whiteboard, pen and paper. Story planner focusing on the

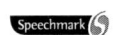

Aims	Method/Activities	Materials
To introduce concept of **middle** of the story and the concept of a **story episode**.	attention to the picture of a film reel on the story planner which depicts the middle element of a story. This incorporates the story plot, i.e. what happens in the story. Explain to students that the middle of the story is where the exciting 'bits' occur; this is where one describes what happens in the story. The middle section is often referred to as the plot where the events of the story take place and are described. In the story planner, the plot or events are referred to as an **episode**. This is where the problem, conflict or main action/s or happening/s of the story occurs. These events drive the character/s and lead to their actions and reactions. Every middle section of a story has an episode. Stories can also have more than one episode or a main event. Give the example of episodes of *EastEnders* or *Hollyoaks* to help students identify with the meaning of an episode. Revisit the teaching notes from session 5 and provide students with the examples of the middle section of stories.	middle section of the story. Train track and carriages. Story F1 race track – draw students' attention to the different events happening on the race track (cars colliding, bird on track, etc). Use the story football match and the story athletics race track in the same way, describing all the different actions that take place in the middle section, during the football match and race. Teaching notes from session 5 giving examples of the elements contained in the middle section of the story.
For students to identify favourite episodes of stories and provide a rationale for their choices.	Group discussion where students talk about their favourite **events, plots, episodes** from their favourite stories. Encourage discussion about the most exciting episodes or events from television programmes like *Dr Who*, *One Tree Hill*, *The OC*; from favourite movies, for example, *The Matrix*, *Spider-Man*, *Titanic*, *Grease*, *Mean Girls*; and from favourite books, for example, the *Harry Potter* series, *Lord of the Rings*, *Twilight*. Students to share their favourite episodes or events and explain why these are their favourites.	Story pencil or microphone. Story planner. Compiled list of favourite stories chosen by students in previous session.

Aims	Method/Activities	Materials
	Students also to share the most exciting story plot and theme that they have ever read, heard or seen. Encourage them to explain their reasons for this choice, and describe what made it such an exciting plot. Students can also be given the opportunity to identify the plot and main episodes of their chosen favourite story. Encourage them to identify the main conflicts or problems that the characters faced, and allow them to describe for the group the main actions taken by the characters to resolve the conflicts.	

To explore in more depth the elements of an episode: **initial event – what happens, immediate response, action, reaction = episode**.	Group discussion to explore the four main elements making up an episode of a story:
	
	Middle
	• Episode:
	
	   ➤ **First event:** what happens? – the first initiating event which drives the plot or theme of the story (symbolised by a question mark on story planner).
	   ➤ **Immediate response:** describes the immediate response or reaction of the character to the initial event. It includes the initial feelings or thoughts of the character (symbolised by picture of boy with shocked response on story planner).
	   ➤ **Action/s:** the actions that take place after the initiating event, usually in an attempt to resolve the story problem or conflict (symbolised by picture of film director shouting 'action' on story planner).
	   ➤ **Reaction/s:** further reactions or responses by the characters to the subsequent actions (symbolised by picture on story planner of boy with happy reaction).
	
	Use the story train track and train carriages with the middle carriages representing the episode/s of a story. There are different people
		Story planner. Train track and middle three carriages indicating different episodes of a story.
		
		Story F1 race track with happenings on the track representing different episodes in a story.
		
		Some students may prefer using the story football match or story athletics race track. All the templates can be used to show how the middle section of a story has different events happening, and reflect the story episodes.
		
		Teaching notes from session 5.

Aims	Method/Activities	Materials
	in the middle carriages, indicating that the middle parts are where the main action, the exciting part, occurs. Use the F1 race track to show different events/happenings occurring along the race track between the beginning and end of the track, representing the episodes of a story, for example, the cars colliding with each other, colliding with the barrier, bird on track, fighting in the stands. Use the story football match and story athletics race track in the same way. Revisit the teaching notes from session 5 for detailed examples of the elements of the middle section of stories. Also see the teaching notes that follow for this session on episodes and read examples to students.	Teaching notes for session 11.
Students to listen to and evaluate middle sections of story plots from published works.	The facilitator reads out the examples of different short extracts from a range of published stories in the teaching notes. Students are encouraged to listen to each example, and evaluate how interesting, captivating and exciting the story episodes are. Explain to students that they will only be hearing a small part of the story, so they will not be able to judge the entire story. However from the piece that is read out to them, they should be able to identify certain themes and the main plot of the story, particularly if they know the book from where the extracts have been taken. They should also be able to identify some of the actions that the characters have taken in response to the conflict or problems presented in the story, as well as some of the reactions by the characters. Encourage students to evaluate the parts of the story they hear, and explore whether they now want to read the book to find out more. Consider with the students why some of the stories appeal more to some students than	Examples of story plots from published works from teaching notes for session 11.

Aims	Method/Activities	Materials
	others. Discuss personal preferences, as well as the power of the story to draw the reader in. Discuss with the students how exciting the parts of the story are: does the theme or plot appeal to them, does it make them want to read more and find out what happens? Is there an exciting build-up of events, a climax, is the plot or storyline exciting and relevant to them, does it interest them, and if not, why not? Ask them to consider where possible the actions that the characters have taken and the appropriateness and success of such actions. What would they have done in similar circumstances to resolve the situation?	
	Students will not be able to answer all these questions with the short extracts provided, but these should give them a feeling for different story plots and events that take place and are part of the essence of stories. This is what the middle part of stories are all about, and these extracts will provide students with opportunities to hear some different examples. Emphasise to students that stories are not about a sequence of unrelated events, but exciting actions and responses and subsequent actions of various characters to meet an aim or respond in some way to a problem or conflict faced by the character/s.	
	You might also like to draw students' attention to the use of direct speech (the actual words of the characters spoken), descriptive words and other literary devices like onomatopoeia (the word used mimics the sound of the action or object it describes) which have been used and the effect this has on the overall level of excitement and involvement in the story. Some further points to consider are included in the teaching notes. Take the time to read the extracts to students and allow them to really feel and analyse what has been written. You may even choose to read each extract more than once.	

 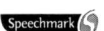

Aims	Method/Activities	Materials
To sum up and revise contents of the session.	Get volunteers from the group to summarise the main content of the session. Ask other members of the group to help, adding in the parts that may have been omitted.	Flipchart or whiteboard, paper and pen. Story planner.
Mission to Achieve: Students to begin to produce the autobiography of their lives detailing two major events that have occurred thus far.	Students have already had the opportunity in previous sessions to profile themselves using the character word map. They will now be encouraged to produce their own autobiography, i.e. story based on their own life. Remind students that an autobiography is the biography or true story of that person's life. They are to begin thinking about the story of their own life and consider the following questions: • Who are the characters in their autobiography (besides themselves as the main character, who are the other important characters in their life)? • Where does their story take place, for example, where were they born, where do they live? Ask students to think about two main episodes or events that have taken place in their lives. They are to think about these events using the story planner and prepare an autobiographical story to share with the group next session about one of these events.	It might be helpful for students to have the story planner to help them with their autobiographies.

Evaluation of session/General comments

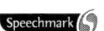

Teaching notes for Session 11

The story planner: middle

In this session we are discussing the middle section of the story. This can be difficult for some students. Read through the detailed explanations which will assist you in explaining the middle components to students. Remember that what is most important is that they learn that stories have a definite structure to them, and that the middle section describes a sequential course of actions which result from an initiating event. Avoid getting bogged down with trying to identify every initiating event, action or response in all future stories. This is a tool to support exciting, complex and structured storytelling, and I encourage you to use it with appropriate flexibility and adaptation where necessary.

The middle section of the story planner consists of one or more episodes.

Episode/s

An episode corresponds with the main part of the story, what happens in the story, the plot or main events. It can revolve around a problem that the character has to overcome, for example, losing a passport at an airport. This is the **first initiating event** which starts the sequence of events of the story. One can then describe the **immediate response** or reaction of the character/s to this event. This, for example, may be the feeling of desperation at possibly missing an important flight. Following this immediate response to the initial event come the **action/s** that the character/s takes to resolve this problem, so the things they do, for example, to try and find the passport in time for the flight. There may then be further **reaction/s** or responses to the actions taken to resolve the problem. The reaction, for example, may be the character bursting into tears after finding the passport, or hugging the person who kept the plane waiting for them.

The episode can also involve what is referred to as a climax, the most exciting part of a story. Events in each episode can build up to the main climax of the story.

A story episode consists of four main parts:

Initial event – what happens?

This refers to the first happening in the episode, the event which initiates or begins the events and actions of the story. It is the trigger for the rest of the story, and is what causes the characters to act in certain ways. This initial event typically causes a problem, conflict or issue that the character/s needs to resolve or work on.

Immediate response

This refers to the immediate response/s of the characters after experiencing the initial event. It may describe a feeling, a thought, or even a physical reaction like being sick or trembling.

Actions

This part of the story details what the character/s does or do in response to this first initiating event. It describes the actions taken by the character/s to solve the problem, conflict or issue that has arisen from the first event.

Reactions

This final part of an episode of a story details what happens as a result of the main action/s taken by the character/s. It could be a further action, a feeling or a thought that the character experiences as a result of the action taken.

Within the one episode, it is possible to have subsequent actions and reactions, all of which are set into motion as a result of the first initial event. This can all take place within one episode. This is why, in the story planner, there are arrows running between elements in the middle component of the story. Think about an episode of *EastEnders* or *Coronation Street*, and how many different problems, crises and events take place in each episode.

A complex story can also have more than one episode. The events or episodes can be about the same characters, and take place in the same setting, which is why they still make up one story, but they describe a different event or crisis which is not directly linked with the previous one. This is why we can refer to this as being a separate episode. Again, using the example of *EastEnders*, you can see how there is a different episode every second night. The episodes are all about the same characters and in the same settings, but the initiating events and actions are different and take place within separate episodes. Different episodes are usually separated in books as chapters.

The following story is an example of how a simple story can consist of more than one episode, and how one episode can have two (or even more) initial events, immediate responses, action/s and reaction/s. Read this example to the students and discuss the different parts with them.

Do not let them get confused by the different labels. There are many different ways of categorising the middle section of stories. However, the most important thing for them to understand is that the middle part of a story contains one or more episodes, and that this is where the main part of the story takes place, where the events and actions and main happenings of the story are described. What is most important is for them to understand that each episode has different parts, i.e. an initial happening or first event, an immediate response, an action and a reaction. This will ensure that when they tell stories, their middle sections are full of depth and excitement. Here is an example of the different parts of the middle section from the story planner:

Johnny's eventful day at school

Episode 1

Initial event – What happens? 1:
Johnny overslept and is very late for school.

Immediate response 1:
He is worried that he will get a detention.

Action 1:
He decides to run as fast as he can to the school gates. As he runs so fast, he does not see the hole in the road and falls headlong on to the kerb. Johnny gets up very slowly. There is blood oozing from his knee where he has grazed himself really badly.

Reaction 1:
He tries to be brave but feels the tears seeping through his eyes. He limps slowly to school. Johnny got to school late. He was very nervous as he had been late before and knew how much trouble he was in.

(Note: there is no second initiating event as all subsequent actions result from the first initiating event.)

Action 2:
As Johnny tries to slip into the classroom without being seen, his teacher calls out his name sharply, 'Johnny, you are late, come here now!' As he limps to the front of the classroom, she notices the blood congealing by his knee. 'Oh dear, Johnny, you have hurt yourself, you must go to the first aid room. The nurse will want to have a look at that knee.'

Reaction 2:
'What a relief,' thought Johnny. He would not get into trouble if the teacher thought he had actually hurt himself. Result!

Action 3:
Johnny made his way to the first aid room where the nurse was sitting. She had a kind round face and he felt really relieved to see her and get out of trouble. 'Poor Johnny,' she crooned, 'you have been in the wars. Never mind, let's fix you up and send you back to class.' The nurse put some disinfectant on the knee and bandaged it up. 'There you are, all sorted. Now you can go back to class.'

Reaction 3:
Johnny felt so much better. His leg had stopped throbbing and he was no longer scared about getting into trouble. He thanked the nurse and went back to the classroom to rejoin his class for his first lesson of the day, science.

Episode 2

Initial event – What happens? 1:
At the end of the day, Johnny walked home with a couple of friends. It had been a very good day after all and they were kidding and messing around. Suddenly some boys from the neighbouring school started shouting at them and throwing firecrackers in their direction.

Immediate response 1:
Alarmed, Johnny's friends ran in opposite directions to avoid the approaching firecrackers. Johnny was unable to run with his injured knee. What will I do? he thought.

Action 1:
Quick as lightening he slipped between two parked cars and managed to avoid all the firecrackers. When his friends came to look for him, he was sitting safely between the parked cars.

Reaction 1:
They were so relieved to see that he was OK. They continued on their journey home. 'I managed to get a good look at those boys,' said Johnny; they were from the school down the road. 'First thing tomorrow we will report this to Mr Pearson, the head teacher,' promised Johnny, 'but for now, after such an eventful day, all I want to do is go home!'

And the story about Johnny can go on and on and one can add more and more episodes to this story.

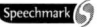

Teaching notes for Session 11

Here are some extracts of story episodes and story events from published books. Read them to the students and facilitate a discussion around the story plots, the main themes, the presenting problem or conflict and the various actions and reactions of characters. These extracts are not long enough to give students a complete idea of the story plot; however, they should provide students with opportunities to listen to various different types of exciting and interesting events and episodes that make up the 'meat' of a story and are found sandwiched between the beginning and end of a story. Encourage students to listen out for the story climax, the actions of different characters to resolve their problems and the reactions of the characters to the actions taken. Provide opportunities for discussion and evaluation about what they feel works well, what appeals to them, what makes them want to read the book immediately and find out more, and what leaves them cold. Encourage them to provide reasons for their answers. Facilitators can use all or a selection of these examples, and provide additional ones from the students' class work if appropriate.

After reading each extract to the students, you may like to encourage them to consider some of the following ideas, themes and questions drawn from the extracts. Do choose on which areas you will focus. This will depend on time but more importantly on the students' level of understanding and abilities. Use your discretion and choose the themes you feel will be most beneficial for the group. You might even like to come back to some of these in the next session if time is short.

- Identification of the **story plot**, theme, **conflict** or problem, or initial event evident from this extract.

- Identification of the **immediate response/s** of the characters to the initial event.

- Identification of the **actions** of the characters to resolve the situation presented in the extract.

- Observation of any subsequent **reactions** or responses by the characters to the actions and events.

- The strength of the **story descriptions**. Were they able to visualise the characters, settings and actions of the characters from the extracts alone?

- The role of **italics** in some of the extracts – consider the role this plays in written stories. Explore with students how one would read a sentence or word in italics. Discuss what other techniques could be used in writing to show emphasis, for example, underlining, capitals, bold, other colours. Ask students to consider how we can show emphasis when we are telling stories, for example, using our voices to say a word louder or softer, quicker or slower. Using facial expression is another way of emphasising what we are saying in a story. This theme will be picked up in later sessions, but it is a good starting point here as students can see examples of what is being used for emphasis in these extracts.

- The use of the **exclamation mark (!)** and its role in written stories. How do students think you should change your expression when reading a sentence that ends with an exclamation mark?

- The role of **direct speech** in the extracts. Students might like the opportunity to read the quotes themselves as the characters. Explore with them how these words would be spoken; what type of voice would signify fear, for example, in extract 3? What would the character's facial expression be like, body language, etc? Students may also like to role play extract 12 and play the detective and witness. They might enjoy continuing the story and making up their own conclusions.

- The role of **humour** in some extracts, particularly extracts 1, 6 and 9.

- The use of **repetition** to reinforce an idea and create an effect, for example, from extract 1, 'Save him! Save him!' and 'Help! Help! Help!' and 'sucked closer and closer'. From extract 2, 'went up and up and up' and 'nearer and nearer'.

- The use of **adjectives** and **adverbs** and descriptive verbs and nouns to get meaning across more vividly.

- The choice of certain **character names**, for example, 'Mr Gloop', 'Veruca', 'Aunty Sponge', 'Aunty Spiker', 'Napoleon', 'Beauty' – and what do they make you think of?

- The choice of specific highly **descriptive and evocative** words, and the power these words have, for example: 'wretched', 'screamed', 'gasping', 'desperate', 'dangling', 'pleading', 'terrified', 'tears welling', 'confusion', 'dazed', 'barren', 'desolate', 'leap', 'furiously', 'struggled', 'swiftly', 'frantically', 'astonishing', 'boldly', 'giant', 'crunch', 'jostling', 'cautiously', 'dead stop', 'sprang', 'roaring', 'thrashing', 'blackness of despair', 'horror of remorse', 'passion of anger', 'bereft', 'enormous'.

- The use of **onomatopoeia**. Explain the meaning of this literary device to students as they will enjoy using it themselves in their own stories. It is the use of a word or words that imitate or sound like the action or objects that they refer to. So, for example, the word 'hiss' is onomatopoeic as it sounds similar to the sound made by a snake. In the case of example 6, the repetition of the word 'tap' increases its onomatopoeic quality as it sounds more like the tapping of an object – 'tap-tap-tapping'. Explore with the students how the word 'crunch' is another example of onomatopoeia from extract 9.

 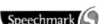

- Explore with students what is meant by '**as flat and thin and lifeless as a couple of paper dolls cut out of a picture book**' taken from extract 9. What two objects are being compared and why? What does this tell us about how Aunty Sponge and Aunty Spiker were left after being run over by the giant peach? Explain to students that this type of comparison is called a simile. You may already have introduced similes to the students in session 8. Remind them of what a simile is: a figure of speech involving the comparison of two different things which have some similarity. Remind them that a simile will always have the words 'like' or 'as' comparing the two objects. Ask students to consider why authors use similes and how effective these are for the listener or reader. Encourage them to come up with their own similes and comparisons to show how flat and lifeless the two ladies had become.

- Explore with students the meaning of '**My blood turned to ice**' from extract 7. This is another example of a comparison between two objects. What two objects are being compared, and what does this say about his blood? This figure of speech is similar to a simile but is slightly different, and is called a metaphor. A metaphor is another figure of speech which emphasises the similarities of two objects. It is different to a simile though as with a **metaphor**, the comparison is not always obvious, and it can sometimes be understood as the one object actually being the other object rather than just being compared to it. Can students see that in this example, it actually says his blood turned to ice. This is what makes it a metaphor and not a simile. If it was a simile, it would be, 'my blood is like ice'. Similes always compare two objects using the words '**as**' or '**like**', so examples of similes are: '**as quick as a tiger**', '**as strong as an ox**', '**to run like lightning**'. A metaphor is different in that it can make the same comparison, but does not use the words 'as' or 'like'. So, for example, a metaphor would be: 'The boy is a tiger', which means that he is being compared to a tiger. A definition of a metaphor is that it is a figure of speech where a word or phrase that usually means one thing is used to stand in for another thing. It is the comparison of one thing to another without the use of 'like' or 'as'. Encourage students to think of other metaphors that they might like to use. A popular metaphor that they will understand and might like to discuss is: 'the internet is an information superhighway'. Explore with students how the internet is being compared to a superhighway, and what this comparison might mean. It is a metaphor rather than a simile as it says that one object (the internet) is another object (superhighway). If it was a simile, it would read as: 'the internet is **like** a superhighway for information'.

- Explore with the students the use of **double meanings**, where the actual meaning of the words is not what they seem, or what they would usually mean. So, for example, in extract 3, when Bruno says he cannot remember how to say 'Yes': 'Bruno's mouth dropped open and he tried to remember the way you used your mouth if you wanted to say the word "yes"', he hasn't really forgotten how to form the word 'yes' in a literal sense, but it means something else here, another meaning, sometimes called a **figurative meaning** rather than a literal meaning, ie, Bruno was too scared to say 'yes', so it was as if he had forgotten how to speak. We often will come across words and sentences which have different meanings, and sometimes do not mean the obvious. Another example of this is from sayings that we often use, for example, the saying, 'it's raining cats and dogs' means it is raining a lot; it does not actually mean that cats and dogs are falling out of the sky! You might like to explore with students other double meanings and how they can be used to enhance storytelling. When unsure of the actual meaning, emphasise to the students that it can help not to always jump to the obvious meaning if it seems strange (like cats and dogs falling from the sky) but to look at the whole story or chapter. Think about what is happening in the story, what the plot is, and what the circumstances are, for example, Bruno being so very scared. This helps one interpret the words and sentences in a story correctly. Can students see how, for example, if Bruno was in a hospital being examined by a doctor, then this might have meant that he actually was physically unable to move his mouth to say 'yes'? Draw students' attention to the importance of looking for meanings by taking into account the whole story, the context, the setting and environment and the overall background. And to always check their understanding. If it doesn't make sense, then listen or read again.

- The presence of a **climax** or in what way **suspense** has been created – see, for example, extracts 11 and 12.

- Identification of the next **events or episodes, and further actions** that the characters might take.

- **Alternative ways** of responding and resolving the situations presented in the extracts.

- Identification and discussion of **complex and difficult conflicts and choices**, for example, students might like to discuss Bruno's actions in example 3.

- The success of the extract in keeping **your attention and making you want to read more…** Which extracts make the students want to get the book out of the library immediately?

Examples of story episodes and events from published works

Example 1

'"Be careful, Augustus!" shouted Mr Gloop, "You're leaning too far out!"
Mr Gloop was absolutely right. For suddenly there was a shriek and then a splash, and into the river went Augustus Gloop, and in one second he had disappeared under the brown surface. "Save him!" screamed Mrs Gloop, going white in the face, and waving her umbrella about. "He'll drown! He can't swim a yard! Save him! Save him!"
"Good heavens, woman," said Mr Gloop, "I'm not diving in there! I've got my best suit on!"
Augustus Gloop's face came up again to the surface, painted brown with chocolate. "Help! Help! Help!" he yelled. "Fish me out!"

 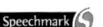

"Don't just *stand* there!" Mrs Gloop screamed at Mr Gloop. "Do something!"

"I am doing something!" said Mr Gloop, who was now taking off his jacket and getting ready to dive into the chocolate. But while he was doing this, the wretched boy was being sucked closer and closer towards the mouth of one of the great pipes that was dangling down into the river. Then all at once, the powerful suction took hold of him completely, and he was pulled under the surface and then into the mouth of the pipe.'

Charlie and the Chocolate Factory. By Roald Dahl (2008), pp98–9.

Example 2

'I went up and up and up the tower steps, gasping for breath. There was someone behind me. I could hear them getting nearer and nearer.

I kept craning back fearfully but it was so dark and I couldn't see anything. But there was a faint glimmer ahead. I was nearly at the top.

I made one last desperate effort and stepped out onto the castle battlements, my hands ready to clasp the wall…*but it wasn't there!*

I was standing on a tiny parapet, the wind whistling around me. If I took just one step forward I'd be treading thin air!'

Buried Alive. By Jacqueline Wilson (1999), p91.

Example 3

'"Have you been eating?" he asked him in a quiet voice, as if he could scarcely believe it himself.

Shmuel shook his head.

"You *have* been eating," insisted Lieutenant Kotler.

"Did you steal something from that fridge?"

Shmuel opened his mouth and closed it. He opened it again and tried to find words, but there were none. He looked towards Bruno, his eyes pleading for help.

"Answer me!" shouted Lieutenant Kotler. "Did you steal something from that fridge?"

"No sir. He gave it to me," said Shmuel, tears welling up in his eyes as he threw a sideways glance at Bruno. "He's my friend," he added.

"Your…?" began Lieutenant Kotler, looking across at Bruno in confusion. He hesitated. "What do you mean he's your friend?" he asked. "Do you know this boy, Bruno?"

Bruno's mouth dropped open and he tried to remember the way you used your mouth if you wanted to say the word "yes". He'd never seen anyone look so terrified as Shmuel did at that moment and he wanted to say the right thing to make things better, but then he realized that he couldn't; because he was feeling just as terrified himself.'

The Boy in the Striped Pyjamas. By John Boyne (2007), pp170–1.

Example 4

'Stanley felt somewhat dazed as the guard unlocked his handcuffs and led him off the bus. He'd been on the bus for over eight hours.

"Be careful," the bus driver said as Stanley walked down the steps.

Stanley wasn't sure if the bus driver meant for him to be careful going down the steps, or if he was telling him to be careful at Camp Green Lake. "Thanks for the ride," he said.

His mouth was dry and his throat hurt. He stepped onto the hard, dry dirt. There was a band of sweat around his wrist where the handcuff had been.

The land was barren and desolate. He could see a few rundown buildings and some tents. Farther away there was a cabin beneath two tall trees. These two trees were the only plant life he could see. There weren't even weeds.

The guard led Stanley to a small building. A sign on front said, YOU ARE ENTERING CAMP GREEN LAKE JUVENILE CORRECTIONAL FACILITY.'

Holes. By Louis Sachar (2000), pp11–12.

Example 5

'So back we went, and round by the crossroads; but by the time we got to the bridge it was very nearly dark, we could just see that the water was over the middle of it; but as that happened sometimes when the floods were out, master did not stop. We were going along at a good pace, but the moment my feet touched the first part of the bridge, I felt sure there was something wrong. I dare not go forward, and I made a dead stop. "Go on Beauty," said my master, and he gave me a touch with the whip, but I dare not stir; he gave me a sharp cut, I jumped, but I dare not go forward.

"There's something wrong, sir," said John, and he sprang out of the dog-cart and came to my head and looked all about. He tried to lead me forward, "Come on, Beauty, what's the matter?" Of course I could not tell him, but I knew very well that the bridge was not safe. Just then, the man at the tollgate on the other side ran out of the house, tossing a torch about like one mad. "Hoy, hoy, hoy, halloo, stop!" he cried.

"What's the matter?" shouted my master.

"The bridge is broken in the middle, and part of it is carried away, if you come on you'll be into the river." '

Black Beauty. By Anna Sewell (2001), pp88–9.

Example 6

'"All right," Veruca said, "I'll have you!"

She reached out her hands to grab the squirrel…but as she did so…in that first split second when her hands started to go forward, there was a sudden flash of movement in the room, like a flash of brown lightening, and every single squirrel around the table took a flying leap towards her and landed on her body.

Twenty-five of them caught hold of her right arm, and pinned it down.

Twenty-five more caught hold of her left arm, and pinned that down.

 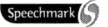

Twenty-five caught hold of her right leg and anchored it to the ground.

Twenty-four caught hold of her left leg.

And the one remaining squirrel (obviously the leader of them all) climbed up on to her shoulder and started tap-tap-tapping the wretched girl's head with its knuckles.

"Save her!" screamed Mrs Salt. "Veruca! Come back! What are they doing to her?"

"They're testing her to see if she's a bad nut," said Mr Wonka. "You watch."

Veruca struggled furiously, but the squirrels held her tight and she couldn't move. The squirrel on her shoulder went tap-tap-tapping the side of her head with his knuckles.

Then all at once, the squirrels pulled Veruca to the ground and started carrying her across the floor.'

Charlie and the Chocolate Factory. By Roald Dahl (2008), p142.

Example 7

'I began to be fascinated by these hair-scratching ladies. It is always funny when you catch someone doing something coarse and she thinks no one is looking. Nose-picking, for example, or scratching her bottom. Hair-scratching is very nearly as unattractive, especially if it goes on and on. I decided it had to be nits.

Then the most astonishing thing happened. I saw one lady pushing her fingers up *underneath the hair* on her head, and the hair, *the entire head of hair,* lifted upwards all in one piece, and the hand slid underneath the hair and went on scratching!

She was wearing a wig! She was also wearing gloves! I glanced swiftly around at the rest of the now seated audience. *Every one of them was wearing gloves!*

My blood turned to ice. I began to shake all over. I glanced frantically behind me for a back door to escape through. There wasn't one.'

The Witches. By Roald Dahl (2008), p57.

Example 8

'The very next morning the attack came. The animals were at breakfast when the look-outs came racing in with the news that Frederick and his followers had already come through the five-barred gate. Boldly enough the animals sallied forth to meet them, but this time they did not have the easy victory that they had in the Battle of the Cowshed. There were fifteen men, with half a dozen guns between them, and they opened fire as soon as they got within fifty yards. The animals could not face the terrible explosions and the stinging pellets, and in spite of the efforts of Napoleon and Boxer to rally them they were soon driven back. A number of them were already wounded. They took refuge in the farm buildings and peeped cautiously out from chinks and knot-holes. The whole of the big pasture was in the hands of the enemy.'

Animal Farm. By George Orwell (2003), pp73–4.

Example 9

'Both women swung round to look. The noise of course, had been caused by the giant peach crashing through the fence that surrounded it, and now, gathering speed every second, it came rolling across the garden towards the place where Aunt Sponge and Aunt Spiker were standing.

They gaped. They screamed. They started to run. They panicked. They both got in each other's way. They began pushing and jostling, and each one of them was thinking only about saving herself. Aunt Sponge, the fat one, tripped over a box that she'd brought along to keep the money in, and fell flat on her face. Aunt Spiker immediately tripped over Aunt Sponge and came down on top of her. They both lay on the ground, fighting and clawing and yelling and struggling frantically to get up again, but before they could do this, the mighty peach was upon them.

There was a crunch.

And then there was silence.

The peach rolled on. And behind it, Aunt Sponge and Aunt Spiker lay ironed out upon the grass as flat and thin and lifeless as a couple of paper dolls cut out of a picture book.'

James and the Giant Peach. By Roald Dahl (2008), pp56–7.

Example 10

'I came to myself in darkness, in great pain, bound hand and foot, and deafened by many unfamiliar noises. There sounded in my ears a roaring of water as of a huge mill-dam; the thrashing of heavy sprays, the thundering of the sails, and the shrill cries of seamen. The whole world now heaved giddily up, and now rushed giddily downward; and so sick and hurt was I in body, and my mind so confounded, that it took me a long while, chasing my thoughts up and down, and ever stunned again by a fresh stab of pain, to realize that I must be lying somewhere bound in the belly of that unlucky ship, and that the wind must have strengthened to a gale. With the clear perception of my plight, there fell upon me a blackness of despair, a horror of remorse at my own folly, and a passion of anger, that once more bereft me of my senses.'

Kidnapped. By Robert Louis Stevenson (2009), p57.

Example 11

'It was not very long, hardly more than a quarter of an hour, before the knock which told that the jury had come to their decision, fell as a signal for silence on every ear. It is sublime – that sudden pause of a great multitude, which tells that one soul moves in them all. Deeper and deeper the silence seemed to become, like the deepening night, while the jurymen's names were called over, and the prisoner was made to hold up her hand, and the jury were asked for their verdict.

"Guilty."'

Adam Bede. By George Eliot (2008), p474.

Example 12

'I confess at these words a shudder passed through me. There was a thrill in the doctor's voice which showed that he was himself deeply moved by that which he told us. Holmes leaned forward in his excitement and his eyes had the hard, dry glitter which shot from them when he was keenly interested.

"You saw this?"

"As clearly as I see you."

"And you said nothing?"

"What was the use?"

"How was it that no one else saw it?"

"The marks were some twenty yards from the body and no one gave them a thought. I don't suppose I should have done so had I not known this legend."

"There are many sheepdogs on the moor."

"No doubt, but this was no sheepdog."

"You say it was large."

"Enormous."

"But it had not approached the body?"

"No."

"What sort of night was it?"

"Damp and raw."'

The Hound of the Baskervilles. By Sir Arthur Conan Doyle (2006), p23

Session 12

Names of students: _____

_____

Facilitator: _____ Date: _____

School: _____

Class: _____

Aims	Method/Activities	Materials
To revise and recap concepts from the previous sessions, i.e. the middle element of the story planner. **Episode = initial event, immediate response, action, reaction.**	Group discussion recapping the main ideas from the previous session on the middle of the story, i.e. the episode and its elements: the first or initiating event (what happens), the immediate response to this initial event, the action/s that the character/s take to resolve the problem or issue that arose from the first event, and the subsequent reaction/s.	Flipchart or whiteboard, paper and pen. Story planner.
To **share with the group a main episode or event in their life** as part of their autobiography.	The students' Mission to Achieve last session was to begin thinking about their own lives and putting together an autobiography which would detail all the events thus far in their life. They were asked to focus on one or two major events that had occurred in their lives and to share these with the rest of the group. Each student gets an opportunity to share their autobiographical story with the group, focusing on describing the main events. Students should be encouraged to use their story planner when telling their story, with an emphasis on the components of the middle of the story. They should try to describe the episode in their life identifying the initiating event, the immediate responses and actions and subsequent reactions.	Story planner.
To **generate stories with exciting episodes** containing the four main	Students to take turns in the group to generate the **middle** element of stories from the action picture cards or themed story picture cards provided. Students to choose a favourite picture	Story planner. Story train track and middle carriages.

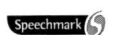

Aims	Method/Activities	Materials
elements from the story planner.	from the choices provided and tell a story based on the picture with a focus on generating an exciting middle section. For example, students choosing the picture of the boy drowning in the sea can tell the story detailing the main plot or problem and the actions taken to resolve the difficulty (ie the boy drowning). Use the story pencil or microphone and each student holding the story pencil has the opportunity to tell his or her **story episode**. The group should be encouraged to listen to every story and rate them on a rating scale from 1 to 10 on how exciting each story is. Encourage the students to add a climax to their story and show how the story they tell builds up to this climax. Students may like to role play the main events of their story.	Story F1 race track. Story football match. Story athletics race track. Story pencil or microphone. Story episodes (action pictures) included to be used as prompts to generate the middle section of their stories. Action picture prompts include: • car crash • footballer scoring goal • people boxing in a ring • lady lying in the sun • fish in water • lady at side of road with broken-down car • little boy drowning in sea • witch casting a spell • boy being bullied at school • mouse hidden in hole and taunting cat. The themed story pictures can also be used to encourage students to identify the main episodes of each picture and generate exciting

Aims	Method/Activities	Materials
		stories. The themed pictures include: • park scene • seaside scene • market scene • school cafeteria scene • gym scene.
To **revisit the examples of story plots from published works** introduced in session 11.	In the previous session, students had the opportunity to listen to a variety of story extracts from published works, and were asked to identify as many of the main elements of the episodes as possible from the extracts provided. They were also asked to consider numerous methods used by the authors to increase the interest and overall enjoyment of the story. Students evaluated the story extracts, and provided reasons for their evaluations. During this session, the facilitator might like to revisit these extracts and explore any points that had not been raised previously, or that need further discussion and expansion. It is a good opportunity, for example, for a discussion around the use of descriptive vocabulary to enhance stories (for example, the use of 'wretched' to describe Augustus Gloop in *Charlie and the Chocolate Factory* rather than the more frequently used word, 'horrible'; or the words 'giant' and 'mighty' to describe the peach rather than the more usual word, 'big', in *James and the Giant Peach*); as well as other literary devices like onomatopoeia, simile and metaphor, all of which were discussed in the previous session with examples of them illustrated in the story extracts. You might like to introduce the students to another two popular literary devices used very successfully in stories: **alliteration** and **hyperbole**. Alliteration refers to the repetition of the same beginning sound of words in a sentence. For example: 'Little Lilly loves liquorice' or 'Nasty Nick never says no!'	Story planner. Published story extracts from session 11. Teaching notes from session 11. Teaching notes from session 12.

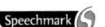

Aims	Method/Activities	Materials
	Hyperbole refers to a literary device where exaggeration is used for effect, to emphasise the point being made. For example: 'I have not slept in years' or 'I'm so hungry I could eat a horse'. Both of these statements are exaggerations, but emphasise the point you are making. It is unlikely to be true that you have not slept in years, but you say this as you want to emphasise how tired you are. Similarly, you are probably not really so hungry that you would eat a horse, but you want to emphasise how hungry you are. Discuss with the students different ways of making their stories as interesting, powerful and exciting as possible. Start with some of the examples from the teaching notes, and use the activities provided to give students opportunities to try out some of these literary devices. Encourage them to think of more examples. Help the students understand that using these devices in their stories will help make them more interesting, and will keep people's attention for longer periods of time. People will want to listen to them! It will also improve their storytelling and writing of essays in the classroom. In the next activity, where students are required to tell a story around a given plot or initiating event, they should be encouraged to use some of the identified strategies and devices to enhance their storytelling abilities. Remember to ensure they are reflecting on the use of these literary devices, and show an understanding of what devices they are using, and the effects they are hoping to achieve.	
To **expand a given story plot** into an exciting and attention-getting story.	Provide students with the list of examples of initial events/plots/conflicts given in the teaching notes. Students in pairs or groups should choose one of these initiating events/plots/conflicts and use it to build a story. The suggestions all pose potential conflicts and problems which need to be resolved. Students	Story planner. Teaching notes for session 12.

Aims	Method/Activities	Materials
	are encouraged to discuss these problems in their groups and explore ways of resolving them within the story. Attention needs to be given to the elements of the story episode/s and the actions taken by the characters to bring the story to a suitable conclusion. Encourage students to incorporate in their stories a range of literary devices discussed in the session. The other students should be able to identify the literacy devices when listening to the stories, and evaluate them.	
To **evaluate their storytelling skills**.	Students have now learned a range of skills around storytelling and should be developing into skilled storytellers. At this midway point, take some time to explore the views of students on their performance and progress. Explore how they see themselves as storytellers, and what they have got out of the programme thus far. It is a good idea for them to revisit the learning profiles they wrote at the start of the programme and assess how successful they have been at meeting some of these targets at this midway point. Encourage them to identify the areas that they still need to work on for the rest of the programme.	Student learning profiles.
To sum up and revise contents of the session.	Get volunteers from the group to summarise the main content of the session. Ask other members of the group to help, adding in the parts that may have been omitted.	Flipchart or whiteboard, paper and pen.
Mission to Achieve: Students to continue to build the autobiography of their lives, focusing this week on the past: where they have come from.	Students have begun working on their autobiographies and will have shared episodes of their autobiographies with the group earlier in the session. For this Mission to Achieve, they are being asked to focus on building up a picture of their past. This may include details about the place and time of their birth, their early life as a baby, toddler and primary school student. Students will need to find out much of this information from parents, grandparents and	Story planner. It might be helpful for students to have the story planner to help them with their autobiographies.

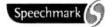

Aims	Method/Activities	Materials
	other family members. Encourage them to go further back into their past, and find out where their parents and grandparents are from, and explore their lives and their history. They should interview their family members in order to get this information, and work on putting together a family tree. At the next session, students will share stories about their early lives, with other members of the group.	

Evaluation of session/General comments

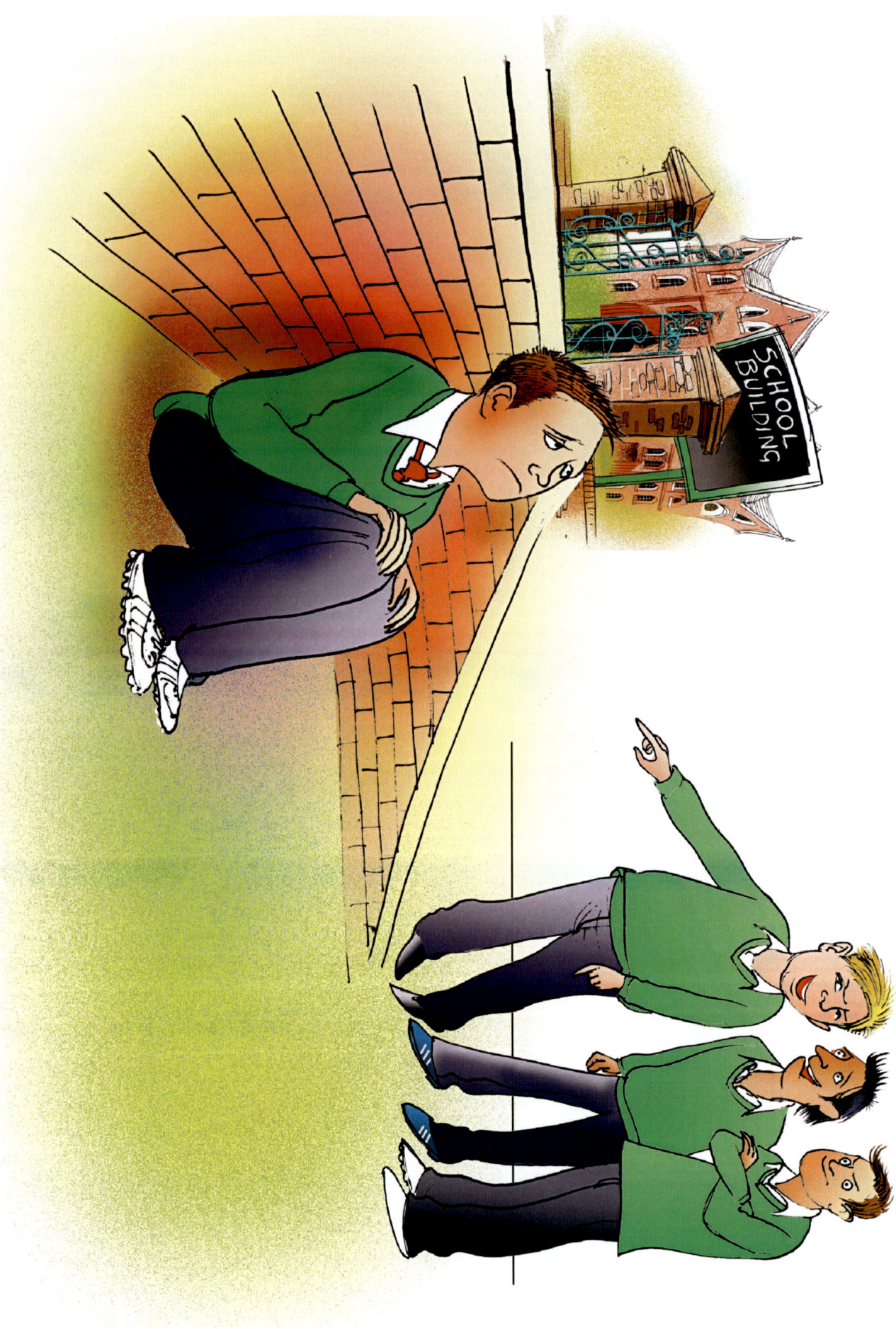

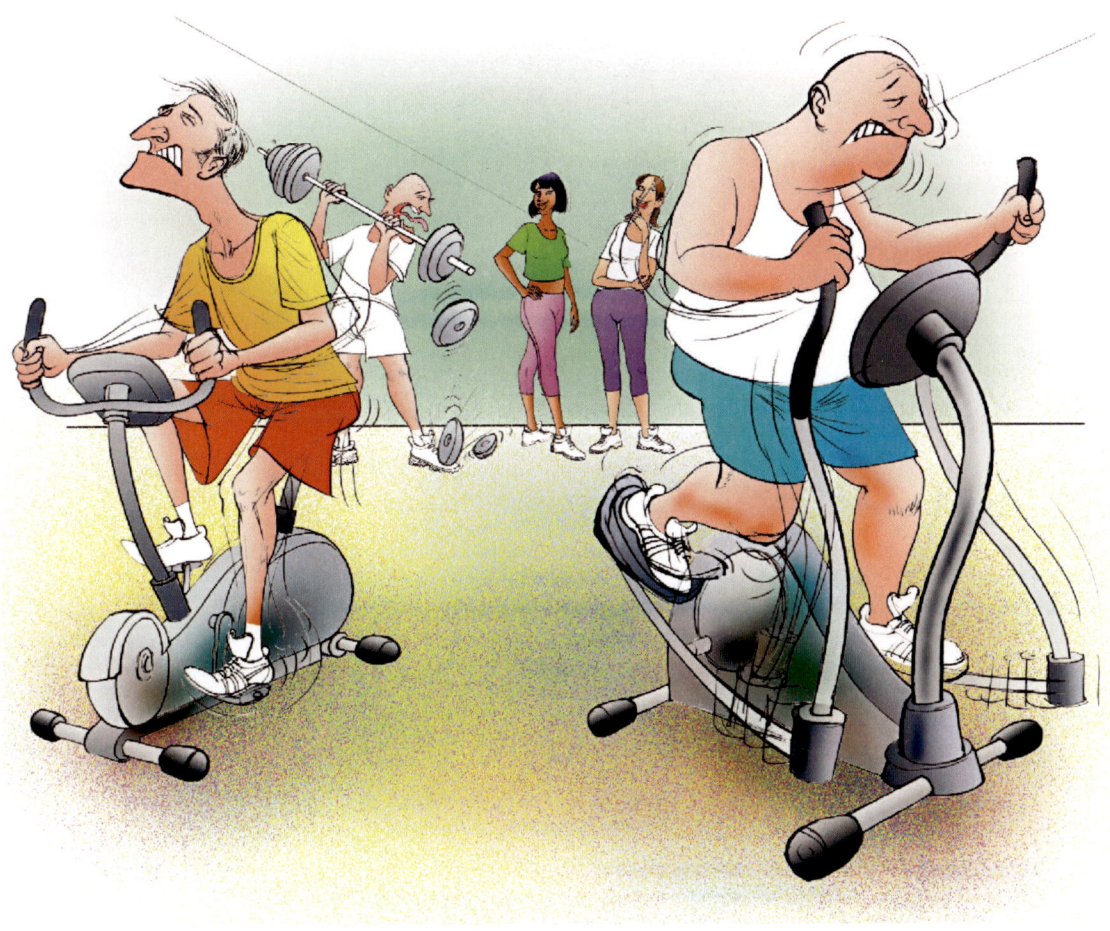

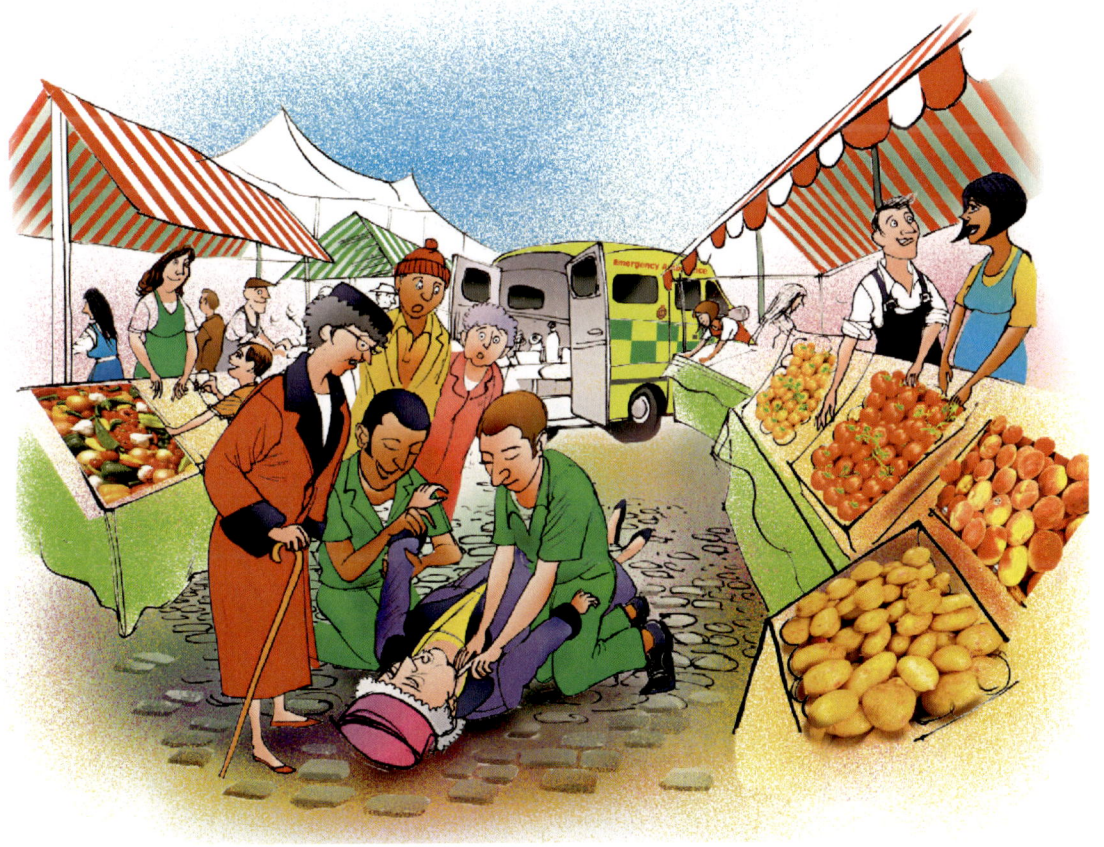

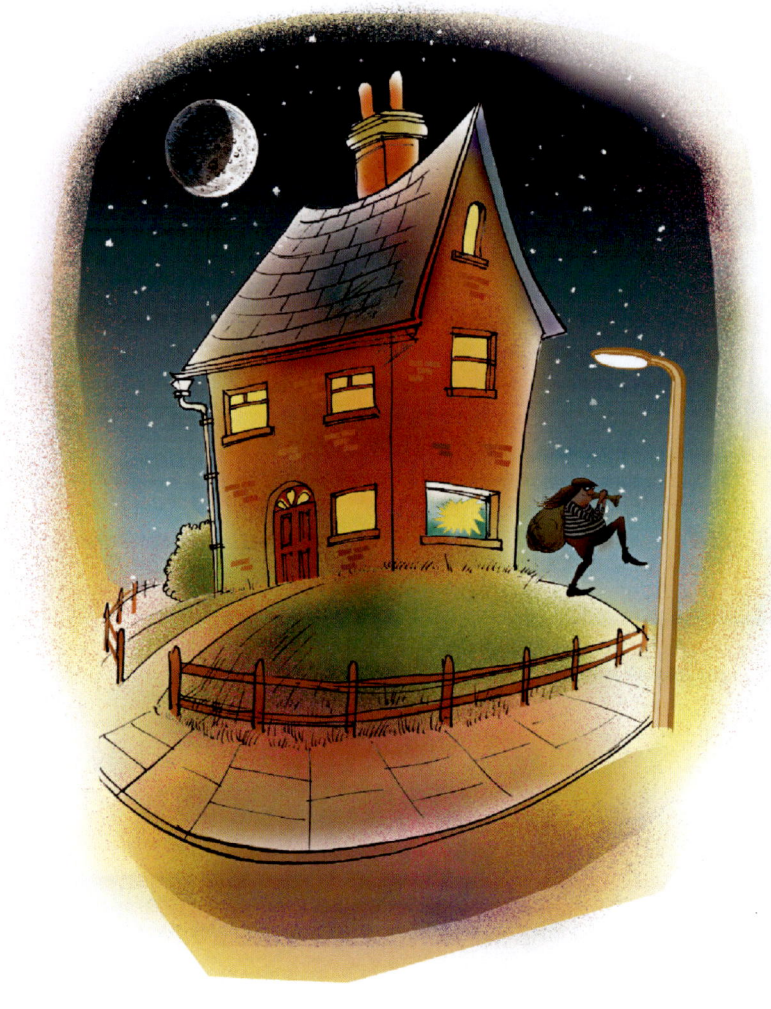

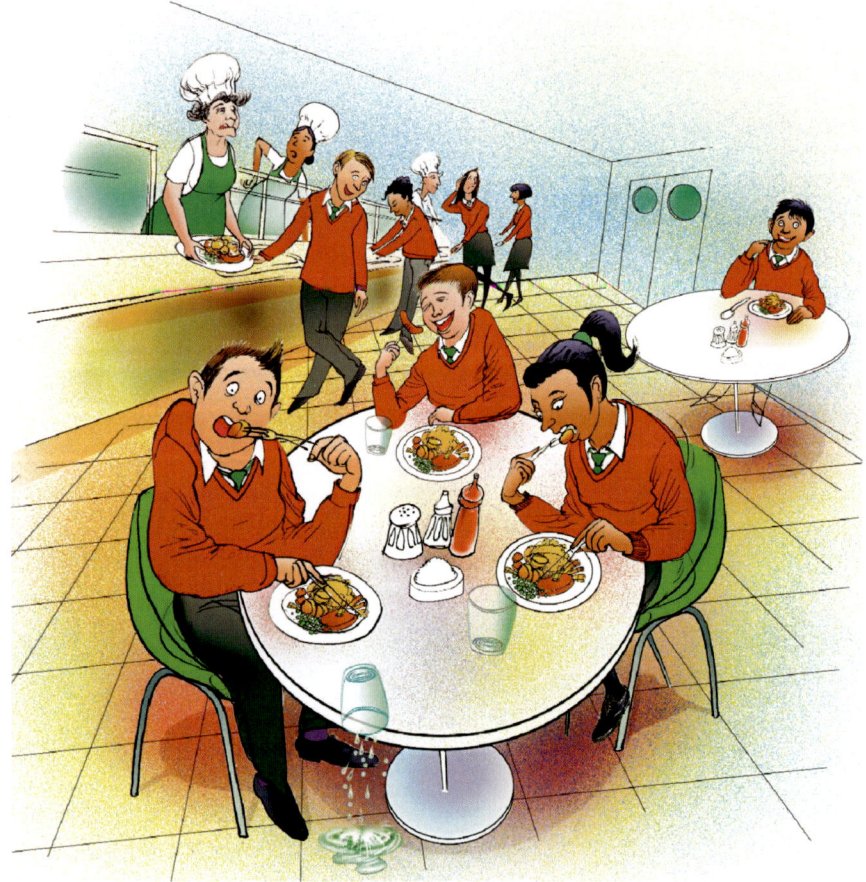

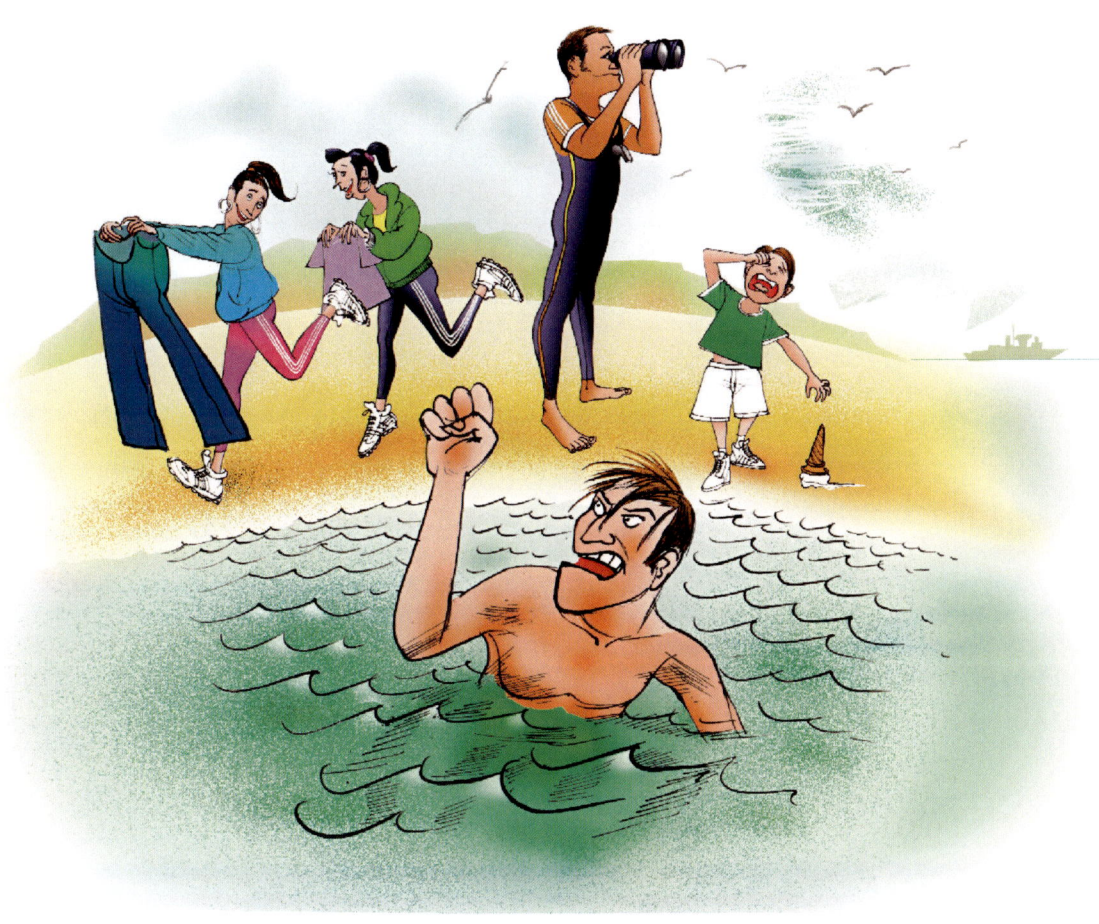

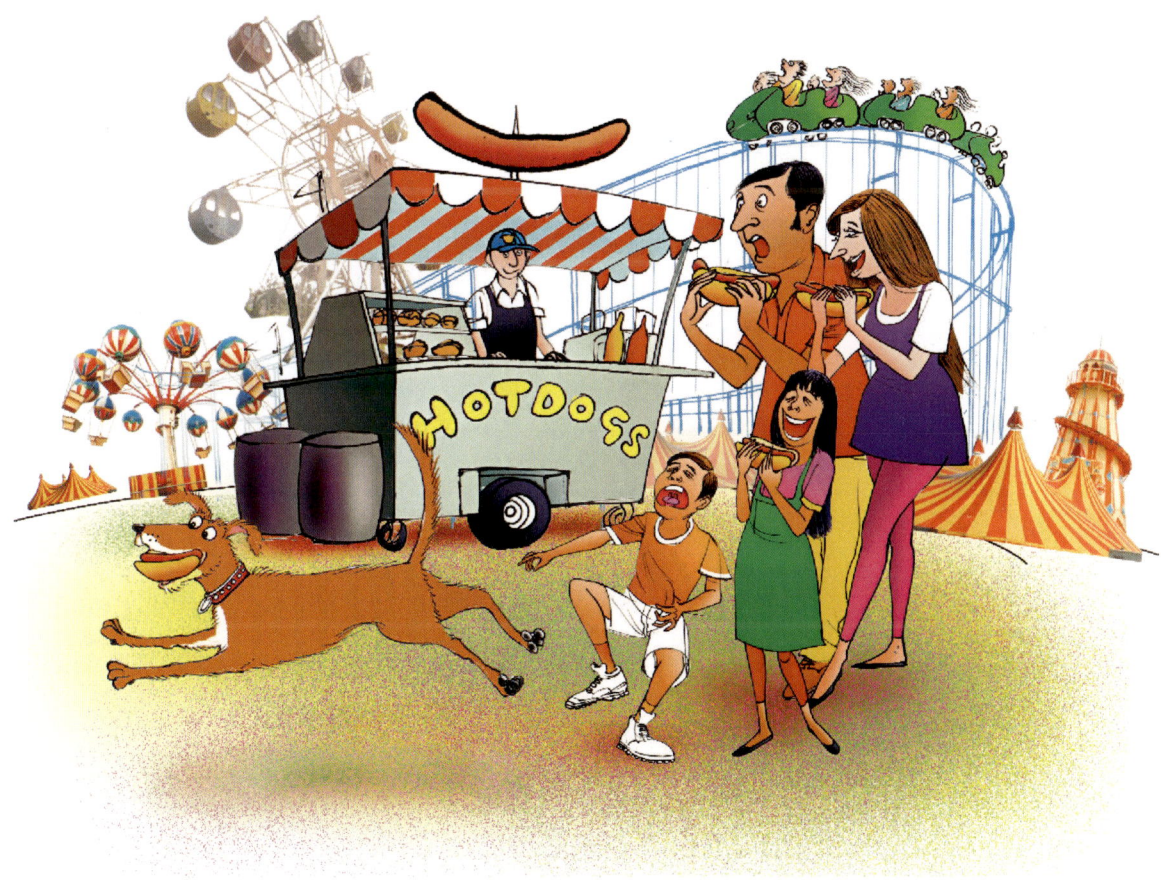

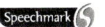

Teaching notes for Session 12

In session 11, we discussed with students a range of literary devices that could be used to enhance their storytelling abilities. We read out extracts from published books, and used these examples to show some of the devices. This is an opportunity to revise some of the devices and for students to practise using them themselves. Here is a summary of the devices, but do refer back to the teaching notes from session 11 for the more detailed explanations and examples from published texts.

- Use the story planner to help structure the story.
- Make sure your story has a beginning, middle and end.
- Introduce the characters and provide detailed information about them so the listener can understand their actions and relate to them.
- Ensure the story plot is exciting, and contains the elements of the middle of the story.
- Identify in your story a clear story plot, theme, conflict or problem, or some initial event that sets the story going.
- Include a climax in your story and try to build up suspense so that you keep the listener interested right up until the end.
- Provide a satisfying end to your story which links all the pieces of the story and provides answers to all the questions raised, or solutions to all the problems encountered, OR
- End the story with a cliffhanger or a question so that you leave the listener wanting more and waiting for the sequel.
- Use a range of descriptive words to tell your story, interesting verbs (doing words), adverbs (words that describe the verb), nouns (objects and things) and adjectives (words that describe the noun). Use the dictionary and thesaurus so that you include new and different words.
- Use direct speech to make the story more interesting and bring alive what the characters are saying. When telling the story, become the character and say their words as if you were the character.
- Include a range of literary devices in your story which make the story more captivating and people will want to listen more and more. These could include repetition, alliteration, simile, metaphor, hyperbole, onomatopoeia, figurative language or double meanings. See if students can identify any more literary devices that they may have learned about in school.
- When writing a story, use different ways of emphasising certain parts of the story, for example, use underlining, a different font, an exclamation mark, italics, bold or different colours.
- When telling a story, use your voice to emphasise the most important parts. Vary your voice, for example, make it louder or softer, speak slower or faster, whisper, and use an accent for different characters. Also use facial expression and body language to show the mood of the characters and describe the story setting and events. So, for example, show in your face that you are describing a happy or sad event, move in a depressed way and use a slow low voice when acting as a depressed character. Alternatively, move quickly and speak in a high quick voice with a broad smile if telling a story about an ecstatic lady who has just won the

lottery! These are tools that you have on you all the time. You don't need to carry them with you and can't ever leave them behind, so use them!

- Use humour in your stories.
- Think about the names you give characters and whether they can tell their own story about the characters.

Here are some activities to help students practise using some of the literary devices listed above. Some of the devices will also be followed up in subsequent sessions:

Activity 1: Choosing descriptive words

Here are some common words used frequently in everyday speech. Try and find as many words as you can which mean the same, but are more descriptive and interesting to use in your stories, for example, surely it is more interesting to say 'the furious man roared with rage' rather than 'the angry man shouted with anger'. You may find a thesaurus useful in finding new words. Have a competition to see which group member can find the most new words in a given time period. These are some examples, but do add more to the list:

- Tired
- Small
- Big
- Shouted
- Hole
- Happy
- Excited
- Push
- Box
- Pretty
- Fall
- Cry
- House
- Anger

And for the facilitator, here are some options that the students should be encouraged to find.

- Tired (exhausted, weary, worn-out, drained, drowsy, sleepy, fatigued, shattered, bushed)
- Small (tiny, minute, minuscule, little, diminutive, miniature, petite)
- Big (large, gigantic, huge, humungous, massive, immense, great, enormous, vast, whopping)
- Shouted (yelled, called, screamed, cried, bellowed, screeched, barked, bawled, hollered, roared, exclaimed.)

 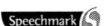

- Hole (crevasse, gap, opening, crack, break, outlet, puncture, tear, fissure, perforation, aperture, cavity, void, gulf, chasm)
- Happy (ecstatic, delirious, content, pleased, glad, cheerful, blissful, high-spirited, delighted, cheery, jovial, exultant)
- Excited (delirious, eager, animated, thrilled, enthusiastic, motivated, energised)
- Push (shove, thrust, drive, ram, force, press, propel, plunge)
- Box (crate, container, case, enclosure, carton, receptacle)
- Pretty (stunning, gorgeous, attractive, beautiful, cute, appealing)
- Fall (trip, stumble, drop, plunge, plummet, collapse, tumble)
- Cry (weep, sob, blub, blubber, snivel, whimper, howl, wail, bawl)
- House (home, dwelling, abode, residence, domicile, address, quarters, accommodation)
- Anger (annoyance, irritation, fury, rage, antagonism, resentment, exasperation).

You might also like to discuss with students the subtle differences in meaning of some of these words. So, what is the fine distinction between 'happy' and 'ecstatic'? What would make someone happy and what would need to happen for someone to be ecstatic? The same discussions can take place around the differences between 'big' and 'humungous'. Discuss with students the degrees of happiness and size, for example, using these different terms. Get them to role play the difference in, for example, being 'happy' versus being 'ecstatic', or in moving a 'big' box versus a 'gigantic' or 'humungous' box.

Provide students with the opportunity to play with words. Language is fun and they will become better storytellers and better language users if they can use words flexibly and have fun with their language.

Activity 2: Using alliteration

Get students to devise clever alliterative sentences. The sentences must make sense! Some examples include:

1 Paul Potts prayed that he would win the crazy competition.
2 Gordon the gorilla grilled great burgers.
3 Sophie saved Cyril from slipping on the pavement.
4 'Pick a poppy Polly', said Mum
5 Horrid Harry hid all Harriet's hats.

Another fun game is for students to sit in a circle, and the first student starts a sentence with the first word, and the next student in the circle adds a word to the sentence and tries to make it alliterative. Points are awarded to students who provide sensible alliterative words that fit the sentence.

Activity 3: Using simile and metaphor

Revise the difference between similes and metaphors and get students to think of clever metaphors or similes to describe the following objects. Ensure they explain why they have made such comparisons.

1   Thin Uncle Sam (so, for example, a simile the student could use might be 'as thin as a skeleton' and a metaphor would be 'Uncle Sam is a skeleton').
2   The smelly boy (the boy smelt like a skunk = simile; that skunk of a boy = metaphor).
3   The fast runner (the runner ran as fast as the speed of light = simile; he was lightning = metaphor).
4   The rough skin of grandma.
5   The shiny new car.
6   The ancient house.
7   The slippery slope.
8   The wet raincoat.
9   The deaf man.
10 The slow old lady.

Activity 4: Exploring onomatopoeia

Encourage students to think of as many words as they can which sound like the actual objects. Have a competition with the winner coming up with the most onomatopoeic words. These may include, for example:

- chatter
- buzz
- crackle
- flutter
- mumble
- jangle
- rustle
- pop
- murmur
- thud
- whizz
- squelch

See how many more students can think of…

You might also like to share with them the poem by Spike Milligan, called 'On the Ning Nang Nong', which has lots of wonderful onomatopoeic (and alliterative) words. You will find this

 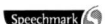

poem in *Silly Verse for Kids* (1968) by Spike Milligan, as well as, probably, in one of the poetry books in the school library.

Activity 5: Exploring hyperbole

Ask students to think up as many over-exaggerations as possible to emphasise the following.

- Love (for example: 'I love you so much I would run a million miles for you' – really, would they?)
- Hungry (just how hungry, hungry enough to eat a horse or maybe an elephant?)
- I have collected many stamps (how many? Enough to send a million letters?)
- I have so much food for the party (how much? Enough to last you forever more?)
- I was ill for such a long time (how long?)
- My headache was so bad (how bad?)
- The exam was so hard.
- The model was so gorgeous.
- The course was so easy.
- I finished the race so quickly.

Let other group members judge how effective these hyperboles are!

Teaching notes for Session 12

Practice and evaluation

Encourage students to make up stories with exciting themes and plots. Their episodes can begin with problems or conflicts and they can then describe various actions that were taken to resolve the initial problem. Let students share their stories with the group. Their stories should include expansions of the plots, conflicts or initiating events provided below, together with various actions taken by the characters to resolve the issues, as well as consequent reactions. Students should also be providing detailed character profiles of their characters in their story. Encourage students to use a range of the strategies and literacy devices that have been discussed in the last session and today. They might even like to suggest alternative (and better) ways of resolving some of the conflicts.

Here is a list of plots, conflicts or initiating events which students can use to build their story around. Allow them to choose their favourite ones to talk about. You might like to add some of your own, or the students may have their own ideas.

1   Jazz stormed in and slammed the door. It just wasn't fair! Ever since his mum had met James, nothing was the same any more. How dare he think he can swan in here pretending to be my dad? Jazz knew that he had to find a way to get rid of James – for good.

2   Lucy trembled as she stood at the gates of the tall imposing building. Clutching her bag close to her, she followed the people in front of her until she reached a window where she had to give her name and leave her passport. She hesitated. Could she really go in? What would she say? How could she tell her dad how much she loved him?; how much she missed him since he had gone to prison?

3   There was a shattering of glass and a loud piercing cry. As Mathew turned around, he saw to his horror…

4   Sunil sat down laden with drinks, snacks and all his photographs. His friends looked on expectantly. Where would he begin? Where would he start telling them about his fantastic trip to Thailand? How about from the beginning…

5   'I am very sorry,' Melissa heard Mr Pickles say, although he did not sound at all sorry, 'I have no choice but to give you detention for the next month.' Melissa's heart sank. Tomorrow she and Virginia had managed to get tickets to see the Take That concert, the first one since the return of Robbie Williams. They were planning to go to the stadium straight after school. She would have to go. Now, to think how she could get away without being missed…

6   Graham walked as quickly as he could down the road, looking back and hoping that he had finally lost sight of his brother. It was not that he did not care about Tony, and even love him in some way. And he understood why his mother had said Tony needed to stick with him at the concert. But Tony was different. He had problems walking and people often teased him. Even sometimes Graham's friends. Graham really needed to impress the guys today; otherwise they would not let him join them on holiday. 'Boo,' shouted Tony, suddenly jumping out of

 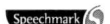

nowhere. 'Oh hell,' thought Graham, 'now I have to somehow get rid of Tony before they see him.'

7   'We love you very much and that will never change,' Paul heard his mother say, 'but we don't love each other any more.' 'It will be OK' dad said nodding fiercely, 'you and I will still see each other every day'. Paul felt tears brimming, but held them back. He somehow made his way to the front door, hauled it open and began to run. And he ran and ran and ran.

8   Anisha heard her mum in the kitchen. She was crying ever so softly, trying, Anisha knew, to hide her worries from the rest of the family. Anisha's dad had just been made redundant and there was no money to pay the rent this month. Anisha knew she had to do something to help. But what could she do?

9   The police officer was looming large in the sitting room, and Kwame's mother and father were sitting forward, concern etched on their faces. 'Kwame,' dad said sternly, 'answer the policeman, did you see anything, did you see who hit Mrs Campbell and stole her bag?' Kwame was silent. He had seen everything. He had seen how that vicious boy from his school had thrown her on the ground, and tore her bag strap off her shoulder. He had also seen the boy looking straight at him, looking at him with those venomous menacing eyes. Almost challenging him to tell the police what he knew, and then face the consequences, whatever those might be. Kwame knew he was finished if he told the police what he saw, but what else was he to do?

10 Marisa walked up the corridor and climbed the stairs. She entered the plane and turned back for one final look. This was it. This was the moment she had been working for. This was the moment she had been waiting for. There was no going back now. Her life was about to get exciting.

11 The gargantuan purple-eyed monster stretched out lazily on the pebbled beach as the sun gently poked its head through the mountains. There was so much to do and so little time that he could not afford to get much more sleep.

12 Ibrahim crept softly down the stairs balancing the heavy rucksack on his small right shoulder. His breathing was laboured and heavy, and as he turned the key and opened the front door, he took one last look behind him, and went hesitantly into the dark night.

13 There was a sudden flash of movement in the garden next door, and Monisha and her brother Raj looked at each other warily. It was cold and dark, but they knew that someone needed to go and investigate.

Evaluation

Students should now be able to provide exciting plots, in addition to having detailed characterisations and time and place information. Their storytelling skills should be developing well. This is a good opportunity to stop and explore with students how well they think they are doing. Encourage them to evaluate their storytelling skills. This may also be a good time for them to revisit the aims and targets that they set at the start of the programme.

Session 13

Names of students: _____

_____

Facilitator: _____ Date: _____

School: _____

Class: _____

Aims	Method/Activities	Materials
To revise and recap concepts from the previous sessions, i.e. the beginning and middle elements of a story, using the story planner.	Group discussion recapping the main ideas from the previous sessions on the beginning and middle of the story from the story planner.	Flipchart or whiteboard, paper and pen. Story planner.
To continue to share with the group their **autobiography** with an emphasis on past events.	The students' Mission to Achieve last session was to extend the autobiographies that they are working on and gather details from family members about their past. Students were asked to interview family members and explore their history, including where their parents and grandparents came from and the lives they lived before the student was born, and then to find out more details about their own early life, where they were born, where they lived as a baby and infant, their early schooling, etc. Each student gets an opportunity to share their autobiographical story with the group, focusing on past events. Students should be encouraged to use their story planner when telling their story and sharing their history and early life, ensuring that their story is structured with a clear beginning, middle and end. Students will be able to use the family tree they constructed to help with their narratives.	Story planner. Family tree made by students.
To focus on the final section of the story	Focus on the **end** of the story, the outcome of the story. The end of the story is represented on	Story planner.

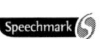

Aims	Method/Activities	Materials
planner, i.e. the end of a story.	the story planner with a picture of a chequered flag.	Story train track and end carriage.
Outcome = result and message.	Identify **outcome**, and describe what makes up the end of a story, i.e. the **results** and **message**.	Story F1 race track and end section indicated by chequered flag.
	The ending denotes the end of a story, the drawing together of all the issues, themes and/or problems raised in the story to some type of conclusion. The result refers to how the story plot ends, how the main issue, conflict or problem has been resolved. The picture on the story planner representing the result part of a story is a 'thumbs up'. This means that the result section of a story usually draws all the different parts of the story together. Emphasise to students that it does not necessarily mean that every story result is a happy one. The result can be a successful or unsuccessful resolution.	Story football match. Story athletics race track.
		Teaching notes from session 5 for examples of different story endings.
	Explain to students that not all endings are the same. Like any part of a story, there is always flexibility when making up stories. Some endings have a neat and tidy outcome which answers all the questions brought up in the story and ties up all loose ends. These are endings where all conflicts raised are resolved. They can also contain a message or moral which is a lesson that one gets from the story. However, the end of a story can also leave you wanting more information, can set up a surprise, leave you with a further mystery or even raise further questions. This serves to keep the listener interested and ensures they tune in to the next series or the next movie or read the next volume. This often occurs if there is going to be another episode or sequel to the story, for example the *Harry Potter* series. Any of these types of endings form the **result** of the story, the story outcome.	
	Can students think of stories that have these different types of endings? So, what stories can they think of that provide a clear and satisfying ending? And then what examples can they give	

Aims	Method/Activities	Materials
	where the ending raises a further question, or leaves the listener or reader in suspense and wanting more? Their examples can come from books they have read, stories they have heard, movies or television series. When endings are successful at leaving the listener or reader wanting more, they may use what we call a **cliffhanger**. This is when you are left with a mystery or an exciting event and you do not know how it will end. It is called a cliffhanger as it leaves you feeling as if you are dangling off a cliff, not knowing exactly what is underneath you and not able to move…until you find out what happens, i.e. you get the sequel! The end or outcome of the story may also contain a message or moral, something that can be learned from the characters and from their actions in resolving or dealing with the story plot, theme or conflicts. Students will sometimes have to think carefully about the underlying messages or meanings of stories. This is why the picture representing this part of the story on the story planner is of a boy thinking very hard. Revisit the teaching notes from session 5 for examples of story endings that can be read out to students. Group discussion around the endings of stories. Group members to discuss and identify their favourite endings from movies, television programmes or books and explain what makes the endings so powerful. Students can also share the endings of their favourite chosen story, and identify what type of ending it was: resolved in a satisfying way, or leaving you in suspense and with more questions.	 Remind students of their favourite story choices that they made at the start of the programme.

 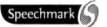

Aims	Method/Activities	Materials
To listen to and evaluate different **endings** from published works.	Provide examples from published stories on 'story endings' in the following teaching notes. Read these story endings to students and encourage them to evaluate how exciting or satisfying the ending is. Get them to compare and contrast the different story endings and identify those that leave the listener with further questions versus those that provide solutions. How, for example, do the endings of a 'mystery' versus an 'adventure' versus a 'romantic' novel differ? Discuss whether these endings appear to tie all loose ends up or rather create more suspense. Explore whether students would like to read these books after having read the endings.	Examples of different story endings from publications in the teaching notes for this session.
To identify specific phrases and sentences which are commonly used for story **endings**.	Provide students with commonly used phrases and sentences for **story endings**. These include: • And they all lived happily ever after • And finally • In the end, all went according to plan • Finally • Eventually • That was an important lesson we all learned • And the moral of the story is… • At last • Their dreams had finally come true • They would never ever talk about this again • The mystery was finally solved • And it was all so exciting, that I decided to write it as a story • She took one look back, and went on, never to be seen again. Students to take turns to generate their own ideas for ways of ending a story. Encourage them to think specifically about endings which are full of suspense and leave the listener with further questions, for example: • He had managed to keep the secret for now. But for how long would it last?	Flipchart or whiteboard, pen and paper.

Aims	Method/Activities	Materials
	• Slowly in the very deepest darkest depths of the earth, the creature began to stir again. • The policeman turned the microphone off. He had told the town that the gang had been caught and apprehended. They didn't need to know that the leader, and most violent, of the gang had escaped. • The prison doors closed behind the prisoner as he was locked up for life. How could he prove that he was innocent, and that the real murderer was still at large? • The virus was halted, for now!	
To identify the **message, moral** or **theme** from stories.	Discuss with students how some stories end with a moral, message or lesson for the listener or reader. Explore whether students have examples of any stories they know which leave you with something to think about, a message, or some advice for how to live your life. This is often called a moral, which is another word for lesson. Ask students what they think the moral or lesson is of their chosen favourite story, if there was one. Introduce students to **fables**, short stories which usually teach a lesson or moral. Fables often involve stories of animals as the main characters with human-like qualities, so the animals are often seen to be behaving like human beings in that they talk, feel and act like humans. The most popular fables are written by a Greek author called Aesop (check students remember that the meaning of author = person who has written the story). Aesop's famous fables are very well known and are short fables, or stories, and most of them feature familiar animals as the characters. It is not known how old Aesop's fables are, as they were originally handed down from one generation to the next. It is	Fables provided in the teaching notes.

 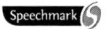

Aims	Method/Activities	Materials
	thought that Aesop lived from about 620 to 560 BC. Students take turns identifying the **themes** and **messages** from the fables provided in the teaching notes. Students usually really enjoy reading the fables and you might like to encourage them to identify not only the endings, but also the main characters in the fable, and the main story components: setting, episode/s and outcome. Play a game where students are encouraged to think of different story endings for the fables and different morals or themes for each one.	
To generate different **story endings** for nursery rhymes and fairytales and other favourite stories.	Share some popular nursery rhymes with students. Identify the endings for each one. Students take turns to provide a different **ending** for these common nursery rhymes and fairytales. These could include: • 'Humpty Dumpty' • 'Little Miss Muffett' • 'Mary had a Little Lamb' • 'Jack and Jill' • 'Baa Baa Black Sheep' • 'The Three Little Pigs' • 'Cinderella' • 'Little Red Riding Hood' • 'Hansel and Gretel' • 'Beauty and the Beast' • 'Goldilocks and the Three Bears'. The above are only suggestions and students may have their own favourites. Each story should be recounted with its traditional ending first, so students remember how they typically end, for example, '… All the king's horses and all the king's men couldn't put Humpty together again'. Then the students suggest completely different endings, so for example, a doctor	Story planner with focus on end section. Story pencil or microphone – group member with story pencil/microphone is the person who holds the floor and talks. The other members are encouraged to listen carefully. Revisit group rules if necessary.

Aims	Method/Activities	Materials
	arrives by the wall just in time to take Humpty to the hospital and manages to save him. This is always great fun for students. They should be encouraged to be as silly as they like and have fun suggesting different endings. They might also like to think about adding a moral or message to these nursery rhymes or fairytales. So continuing the 'Humpty Dumpty' theme where the doctor comes just in time to save him, what might the moral or message be of this 'new' story? Some suggestions might be: (1) Never sit on walls, or (2) never rely on the king's men to make you better again! Or maybe even that a good doctor can always put anyone together again! Students can also suggest alternative endings for their own favourite stories, as well as any other stories with which they are familiar, for example, the *Harry Potter* books. The group may also enjoy changing the endings of their favourite movies and television programmes.	
To produce different **endings** for various stories.	Students pair up and make up a story of their own between them. They then share the story with the rest of the group members. Another group then takes that story and decides on a completely different ending, with both a result and a meaning or moral. That group then shares the new story with the group. Each group member is to have a chance in a group to make up and tell a story and to add a completely different ending to another group's story. Students should then evaluate which made the better story, the original ending, or the one after the change was made. Remind students to adhere to the group rules and take turns when sharing their stories.	Story planner. Story pencil or microphone.
To sum up and revise contents of the session.	Get volunteers from the group to summarise the main content of the session. Ask other members of the group to help, adding in the parts that may have been omitted.	Flipchart or whiteboard, paper and pen.

 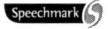

Aims	Method/Activities	Materials
Mission to Achieve: Students to use their story planner to structure one story which they have learned during their lessons in school.	Students have now covered all the elements of the story planner and should have a clear idea about the necessary components that make up an interesting and captivating story. Students learn about many different stories, fictional and non-fictional, in school. In this task, they will be asked to choose one story from any of their lessons, and break up the story into its story component parts using the story planner. Students can choose any subject area that they like, and any story. They can either write the different components of the story on the story planner and bring this in with them to the next session; or alternatively, can use the story planner as a memoryaid, and share with the group the different components of their chosen story, if they would prefer not to write anything down.	Story planner.

Evaluation of session/General comments

Teaching notes for Session 13

Examples of story endings from published works

Read the following story endings to the students and encourage comments on each one. Discuss how powerful, evocative and interesting each story ending is. Get the students to compare and contrast each one, comparing, for example, the end of one type of story with another. Ask students whether the ending is satisfying, i.e. does it answer their questions or perhaps raise anticipation for the next instalment of the story? Can they identify any cliffhangers which the authors have used to leave the listener or reader wondering what happened next?

Example 1

'Father and mother sat together, quietly re-living the first chapter of the romance which for them began some twenty years ago. Amy was drawing the lovers, who sat apart in a beautiful world of their own, the light of which touched their faces with a grace the little artist could not copy. Beth lay on her sofa, talking cheerily with her old friend, who held her little hand as if he felt it possessed the power to lead him along the peaceful way she walked. Jo lounged in her favourite low seat, with the grave, quiet look which best became her; and Laurie, leaning on the back of her chair, his chin on a level with her curly head, smiled with his friendliest aspect, and nodded at her in the long glass which reflected them both.

So grouped, the curtain falls upon Meg, Jo, Beth and Amy. Whether it ever rises again, depends upon the reception given to the first act of the domestic drama called "LITTLE WOMEN". '

Little Women. By Louisa May Alcott (2003), pp282–3.

Example 2

'Matilda leapt into Miss Honey's arms and hugged her, and Miss Honey hugged her back, and then the mother and father and brother were inside the car and the car was pulling away with the tyres screaming. The brother gave a wave through the rear window, but the other two didn't even look back. Miss Honey was still hugging the tiny girl in her arms and neither of them said a word as they stood there watching the big black car tearing round the corner at the end of the road and disappearing for ever into the distance.'

Matilda. By Roald Dahl (2008), p232.

Example 3

'No limits, Jonathan? He thought. Well, then, the time's not distant when I'm going to appear out of thin air on your beach, and show you a thing or two about flying!

And though he tried to look properly severe for his students, Fletcher Seagull suddenly saw them all as they really were, just for a moment, and he more than liked, he loved what it was he saw. No limits, Jonathan? He thought, and he smiled. His race to learn had begun.

Jonathan Livingston Seagull. A Story. By Richard Bach (1973), p93.

Example 4

' "We'll keep in touch," Dennis said. He raised his hand to check his bowtie. "Yes," she said. "Maybe we'll go to a movie some time." "That would be nice," she said, "Or at least go for a hamburger." They both laughed. "Remember Primitive Love and the Wambesi?" Dennis asked. They laughed again. "Good-bye, Dennis", she said. He looked at her again but didn't speak. She kissed him quickly on the cheek. "I'll always remember you," she said, and she started down the hall.'

My Darling My Hamburger. By Paul Zindel (1978) pp125–6.

Example 5

' "Then there was no window cleaner?" cried Rhoda. "Nobody saw him?"

"I saw," said Poirot. "With the eyes of the mind one can see more than with the eyes of the body. One leans back and closes the eyes – "

Despard said cheerfully:

"Let's stab him, Rhoda, and see if his ghost can come back and find out who did it."

Cards on the Table. By Agatha Christie (2001), p320.

Example 6

'I have walked that long road to freedom. I have tried not to falter; I have made missteps along the way. But I have discovered the secret that after climbing a great hill, one only finds that there are many more hills to climb. I have taken a moment here to rest, to steal a view of the glorious vista that surrounds me, to look back on the distance I have come. But I can rest only for a moment, for with freedom come responsibilities, and I dare not linger, for my walk is not yet ended.'

Long Walk to Freedom. The Autobiography of Nelson Mandela. By Nelson Mandela (1994), p617.

Example 7

'I see that child who lay upon her bosom and who bore my name, a man, winning his way up in that path of life which once was mine. I see him winning it so well, that my name is made illustrious there by the light of his. I see the blots I threw upon it, faded away. I see him, foremost of just judges and honoured men, bringing a boy of my name, with a forehead that I know and golden hair, to this place – then fair to look upon, with not a trace of this day's disfigurement – and I hear him tell the child my story, with a tender and a faltering voice.

It is a far, far better thing that I do, than I have ever done; it is a far far better rest that I go to, than I have ever known.'

A Tale of Two Cities. By Charles Dickens (2000), p390.

Example 8

'Every day of the week, hundreds and hundreds of children from far and near came pouring into the City to see the marvellous peach stone in the Park. And James Henry Trotter, who once,

 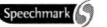

if you remember, had been the saddest and loneliest little boy that you could find, now had all the friends and playmates in the world. And because so many of them were always begging him to tell and tell again the story of his adventures on the peach, he thought it would be nice if one day he sat down and wrote it as a book.

So he did.

And that is what you have just finished reading.

James and the Giant Peach. By Roald Dahl (2008), p156.

Example 9

'But they had not gone twenty yards when they stopped short. An uproar of voices was coming from the farmhouse. They rushed back and looked through the window again. Yes, a violent quarrel was in progress. There were shoutings, bangings on the table, sharp suspicious glances, furious denials. The source of the trouble appeared to be that Napoleon and Mr Pilkington had each played an ace of spades simultaneously.

Twelve voices were shouting in anger, and they were all alike. No question, now, what had happened to the faces of the pigs. The creatures outside looked from pig to man, and from man to pig, and from pig to man again; but already it was impossible to say which was which.'

Animal Farm. By George Orwell (2003), p102.

Example 10

'There was nothing particularly special about this place, or different, but then he did a little exploration of his own and discovered that the base of the fence here was not properly attached to the ground as it was everywhere else and that, when lifted, it left a large gap large enough for a very small person (such as a little boy) to crawl underneath. He looked into the distance then and followed it through logically, step by step by step, and when he did he found that his legs seemed to stop working right – as if they couldn't hold his body up any longer – and he ended up sitting on the ground in almost exactly the same position as Bruno had every afternoon for a year, although he didn't cross his legs beneath him.

A few months after that some other soldiers came to Out-With and Father was ordered to go with them, and he went without complaint and he was happy to do so because he didn't really mind what they did to him any more.

And that's the end of the story about Bruno and his family. Of course all this happened a long time ago and nothing like that could ever happen again.

Not in this day and age.'

The Boy in the Striped Pyjamas. By John Boyne (2007), pp214–15.

Example 11

'They both felt that their souls were being lifted to the stars as an angelic choir sang the praises of their love.

"You have always had my love and my heart. Now you possess my very soul – forever in this world and the next," Robert whispered to her.

And Viola knew that her new life in the Castle of Dreams would indeed be Heaven itself.'
  A Castle of Dreams. By Barbara Cartland (2009), p146.

Example 12

'I have now lived in this happy place a whole year. Joe is the best and kindest of grooms. My work is easy and pleasant, and I feel my strength and spirits all coming back again. Mr Thoroughgood said to Joe the other day, "In your place he will last till he is twenty years old – perhaps more."
Willie always speaks to me when he can, and treats me as his special friend. My ladies have promised that I shall never be sold, and so I have nothing to fear; and here my story ends. My troubles are all over, and I am at home; and often before I am quite awake, I fancy I am still in the orchard at Birtwick, standing with my old friends under the apple trees.'
  Black Beauty. By Anna Sewell (2001), pp344–6.

Example 13

'Dear reader! It rests with you and me, whether, in our two fields of action, similar things shall be or not. Let them be! We shall sit with lighter bosoms on the hearth, to see the ashes of our fires turn grey and cold.'
  Hard Times. By Charles Dickens (2003), p288.

Example 14

'He had no further intercourse with Spirits, but lived upon the Total Abstinence Principle, ever afterwards; and it was always said of him, that he knew how to keep Christmas well, if any man alive possessed the knowledge. May that be truly said of us and all of us! And so, as Tiny Tim observed, G-d bless Us, Every One!'
  A Christmas Carol. By Charles Dickens (1979), pp158–9.

 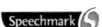

Teaching notes for Session 13

The moral/message of the story

Here are some common fables with which the students may be familiar. Recap each fable and get students to suggest the main lessons, moral or message from each fable. At the end of each fable is the moral. Do not read the moral immediately to the students. Encourage students to guess at what it may be before giving them the answer. You may also like to draw their attention to the traditional manner in which each fable begins, for example, 'Once upon a time'.

After they have identified the message, students can identify the characters and different story elements. They might also like to try thinking up a different ending and a different message for each one.

These fables were accessed from an online collection of Aesop's fables: http://aesopfables.com. There are more fables that you may like to look at the same website.

1 The Hare and the Tortoise

'The Hare was once boasting of his speed before the other animals. "I have never yet been beaten," said he, "when I put forth my full speed. I challenge any one here to race with me." The Tortoise said quietly, "I accept your challenge."
 "That is a good joke," said the Hare; "I could dance round you all the way."
"Keep your boasting till you've beaten," answered the Tortoise. "Shall we race?"
So a course was fixed and a start was made. The Hare darted almost out of sight at once, but soon stopped and, to show his contempt for the Tortoise, lay down to have a nap. The Tortoise plodded on and plodded on, and when the Hare awoke from his nap, he saw the Tortoise just near the winning-post and could not run up in time to save the race. Then said the Tortoise: "Plodding wins the race."'

MORAL: Slow and steady wins the race. Work steadily and you will get to your goal in the end.

2 The Shepherd's Boy and the Wolf (The Boy who Cried Wolf)

'A Shepherd-boy, who watched a flock of sheep near a village, brought out the villagers three or four times by crying out, "Wolf! Wolf!" and when his neighbors came to help him, laughed at them for their pains. The Wolf, however, did truly come at last. The Shepherd-boy, now really alarmed, shouted in an agony of terror: "Pray, do come and help me; the Wolf is killing the sheep"; but no one paid any heed to his cries, nor rendered any assistance. The Wolf, having no cause of fear, at his leisure lacerated or destroyed the whole flock.'

MORAL: There is no believing a liar, even when he speaks the truth. So do not lie.

3 The Lion and the Mouse

'Once when a Lion was asleep a little Mouse began running up and down upon him; this soon wakened the Lion, who placed his huge paw upon him, and opened his big jaws to swallow him. "Pardon, O King," cried the little Mouse: "forgive me this time, I shall never forget it: who knows but what I may be able to do you a turn some of these days?" The Lion was so tickled at the idea of the Mouse being able to help him, that he lifted up his paw and let him go. Some time after the Lion was caught in a trap, and the hunters who desired to carry him alive to the King, tied him to a tree while they went in search of a wagon to carry him on. Just then the little Mouse happened to pass by, and seeing the sad plight in which the Lion was, went up to him and soon gnawed away the ropes that bound the King of the Beasts. "Was I not right?" said the little Mouse.'

MORAL: Little friends may prove great friends. Be kind and help everyone as you never know who will be in a position to help you later on.

4 The Fox and the Grapes

'One hot summer's day a Fox was strolling through an orchard till he came to a bunch of Grapes just ripening on a vine which had been trained over a lofty branch. "Just the thing to quench my thirst," quoth he. Drawing back a few paces, he took a run and a jump, and just missed the bunch. Turning round again with a One, Two, Three, he jumped up, but with no greater success. Again and again he tried after the tempting morsel, but at last had to give it up, and walked away with his nose in the air, saying: "I am sure they are sour." '

MORAL: It's easy to look down and despise what you cannot have.

5 The Goose with the Golden Eggs

'One day a countryman going to the nest of his Goose found there an egg all yellow and glittering. When he took it up it was as heavy as lead and he was going to throw it away, because he thought a trick had been played upon him. But he took it home on second thoughts, and soon found to his delight that it was an egg of pure gold. Every morning the same thing occurred, and he soon became rich by selling his eggs. As he grew rich he grew greedy; and thinking to get at once all the gold the Goose could give, he killed it and opened it only to find nothing.'

MORAL: Greed often overreaches itself. Don't be greedy as it often results in you losing everything.

 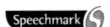

6 The Ant and the Dove

'An ant went to the bank of a river to quench its thirst, and being carried away by the rush of the stream, was on the point of drowning. A dove sitting on a tree overhanging the water plucked a leaf and let it fall into the stream close to her. The ant climbed onto it and floated in safety to the bank. Shortly afterwards a birdcatcher came and stood under the tree, and laid his lime-twigs for the dove, which sat in the branches. The ant, perceiving his design, stung him in the foot. In pain the birdcatcher threw down the twigs, and the noise made the dove take wing.'

MORAL: One good turn deserves another.

7 The Father and his Two Daughters

'A man had two daughters, the one married to a gardener, and the other to a tilemaker. After a time he went to the daughter who had married the gardener, and inquired how she was and how all things went with her. She said, "All things are prospering with me, and I have only one wish, that there may be a heavy fall of rain, in order that the plants may be well watered." Not long after, he went to the daughter who had married the tilemaker, and likewise inquired of her how she fared; she replied, "I want for nothing, and have only one wish, that the dry weather may continue, and the sun shine hot and bright, so that the bricks might be dried." He said to her, "If your sister wishes for rain, and you for dry weather, with which of the two am I to join my wishes?" '

MORAL: You can't please everybody.

8 The Wolf in Sheep's Clothing

'A Wolf found great difficulty in getting at the sheep owing to the vigilance of the shepherd and his dogs. But one day it found the skin of a sheep that had been flayed and thrown aside, so it put it on over its own pelt and strolled down among the sheep. The Lamb that belonged to the sheep, whose skin the Wolf was wearing, began to follow the Wolf in the Sheep's clothing; so, leading the Lamb a little apart, he soon made a meal off her, and for some time he succeeded in deceiving the sheep, and enjoying hearty meals.'

MORAL: Appearances are deceptive.

9 Mercury and the Woodman

'A Woodman was felling a tree on the bank of a river, when his axe, glancing off the trunk, flew out of his hands and fell into the water. As he stood by the water's edge lamenting his loss, Mercury appeared and asked him the reason for his grief. On learning what had happened,

Speechmark

out of pity for his distress, Mercury dived into the river and, bringing up a golden axe, asked him if that was the one he had lost. The Woodman replied that it was not, and Mercury then dived a second time, and, bringing up a silver axe, asked if that was his. "No, that is not mine either," said the Woodman. Once more Mercury dived into the river, and brought up the missing axe. The Woodman was overjoyed at recovering his property, and thanked his benefactor warmly; and the latter was so pleased with his honesty that he made him a present of the other two axes. When the Woodman told the story to his companions, one of these was filled with envy of his good fortune and determined to try his luck for himself. So he went and began to fell a tree at the edge of the river, and presently contrived to let his axe drop into the water. Mercury appeared as before, and, on learning that his axe had fallen in, he dived and brought up a golden axe, as he had done on the previous occasion. Without waiting to be asked whether it was his or not, the fellow cried, "That's mine, that's mine," and stretched out his hand eagerly for the prize: but Mercury was so disgusted at his dishonesty that he not only declined to give him the golden axe, but also refused to recover for him the one he had let fall into the stream.'

MORAL: Honesty is the best policy.

10 The Ant and the Grasshopper

'In a field one summer's day a Grasshopper was hopping about, chirping and singing to its heart's content. An Ant passed by, bearing along with great toil an ear of corn he was taking to the nest.
"Why not come and chat with me," said the Grasshopper, "instead of toiling and moiling in that way?"
"I am helping to lay up food for the winter," said the Ant, "and recommend you to do the same."
"Why bother about winter?" said the Grasshopper; we have got plenty of food at present." But the Ant went on its way and continued its toil. When the winter came the Grasshopper had no food and found itself dying of hunger, while it saw the ants distributing every day corn and grain from the stores they had collected in the summer. Then the Grasshopper knew: It is best to prepare for the days of necessity'.

MORAL: It is best to prepare for the days ahead. Always be well prepared for the future. Plan ahead!

Session 14

Names of students: _____

_____

Facilitator: _____ Date: _____

School: _____

Class: _____

Aims	Method/Activities	Materials
To revise and recap concepts from the previous sessions, i.e. the entire story planner including all main elements: **beginning, middle and end**.	Group discussion recapping the main ideas from the previous sessions. Revise all three main story elements and their component parts through discussion using the story planner.	Flipchart or whiteboard, paper and pen. Story planner.
Students to show the different story components of their chosen story from one of their lessons in school.	This is an opportunity for students to practise using the story planner in the classroom with the school curriculum. Students have the opportunity to share with the group the story they have chosen from class, to explain what lesson and subject the story is from, and why they chose it. They are then asked to tell the story identifying clearly the different story elements, including: 1 Beginning – **setting** (character, time, place) 2 Middle – **episode** (initial event, happening; immediate response, action, reaction) 3 End – **outcome** (result and message/moral). Students are to be encouraged to use their story planner to help them identify the story components. Discuss with students the role of the story planner in the classroom, and explore with them how they might be able to use the story planner to help them to understand	Individual story planners detailing elements of the stories chosen by students from their classes.

 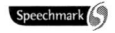

Aims	Method/Activities	Materials
	lessons, to write stories and to complete homework tasks.	
To introduce the concept of order and **sequencing** and to create an awareness of the importance of correct sequencing when story telling.	The main focus of the session is on sequencing of stories. Students are to be encouraged to think about the importance of **order and sequencing**. The story train track and beginning, middle and end carriages should be revisited to emphasise the importance of sequencing. Discuss with group what would happen if the end of the train was at the front, or if the middle of the train was at the end. Create an awareness of how confusion would ensue and the story would not have a logical sequence.	Story train track and train carriages.
To complete the **'what happened next'** sentences and short stories to emphasise the importance of sequencing and order.	Students are required to take turns completing the short stories in the teaching notes and recounting what happens next. It is important to highlight to them the importance of the correct ordering of the sentences which reflect the order of the sequences of each story. For example, the lady washes the breakfast dishes after breakfast. Discuss how silly it would be to say that the lady washes the breakfast dishes and then has breakfast.	What happened next scenarios for completion – in teaching notes for session 14.
To **sequence** in correct order a range of sequence cards per story. To then tell the story once the sequence cards have been arranged in the correct sequence using all elements of the story planner.	The focus of this activity is on **story sequencing** and story progression. Students to be presented with different sequence stories supplied in the story resource. There are a range of sequence stories with a different number of sequence cards per story. Begin at the most basic level, i.e. with the story with 4 sequence cards, and build up progressively to the sequence story with 8, 10 or 11 sequence cards per story. The students are to order the cards correctly and then tell the story. Place the sequence cards down in a random order on the table without telling the story. The students take turns in putting the sequence cards in their correct order. Once they have done this, they then take	Story planner. Story pencil or microphone. Range of sequence stories with various numbers of sequence cards per story, contained in the resource.

Aims	Method/Activities	Materials
	turns (using the story pencil) to tell the story from the sequence cards that they have put in the correct order. They should be encouraged to pick up any mistakes in their ordering of the pictures when they attempt to tell the story. They should then correct the ordering as and when it is necessary. Encourage the use of all elements of the story planner when they are telling the story. When students are sequencing the sequence cards, encourage them to use the story template forms. This will help them sequence the cards in the correct order. Introduce the students to the story template forms which break up stories into five sequential parts and are an alternative to the story planner, for structuring their stories. There are two different forms, both of which are organised into five sections, each introduced by different words or phrases. The students should be encouraged to use the story templates to help them structure their story sequentially. Story template 1 has five parts which are introduced by the following words or phrases: **First** – corresponds to story beginning **Next** – corresponds either to story beginning or story middle **And then** – corresponds to story middle **After that** – corresponds to story middle **Finally** – corresponds to story end. Draw students' attention to how the different parts of the story template map on to the elements of the story planner. Story template 2 also has five parts which are introduced by the following words or phrases: **Once upon a time** – corresponding to story beginning **On a cold afternoon** – corresponds either to story beginning or story middle **To his shock** – corresponds to story middle	Story template form 1 and story template form 2.

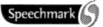

Aims	Method/Activities	Materials
	But then – corresponds to story middle **Eventually** – corresponds to story end. Draw students' attention to how the different parts of the story template map on to the elements of the story planner. These story templates are to help students sequence their ideas more coherently into logically ordered stories and will assist them to sequence the sequence cards correctly. Encourage them to physically place each sequence card on to the appropriate part of the story templates, for example, the first sequence card could be placed on the first rectangle which begins with the word '**First**' for story template 1 or '**Once upon a time**' for story template 2. The last sequence card would be placed on the fifth rectangle of story template 1 which has the word, '**Finally**', etc. Since most of the sequence stories have more than five sequence cards, more than one sequence card may correspond to each part of the story template. Draw attention to how the different colours on the word template match with the different components on the story planner. Discuss with students how they can use these story templates during the classroom when writing or constructing stories, as well as for homework.	
To **construct stories** with story elements missing or incorrectly sequenced.	This is a fun activity where students have the opportunity to produce poorly sequenced stories, or stories with a clear omission of one main story element, so, for example, telling a story with the resolution of the problem given before the listeners have been told about the problem, or telling a story with the introduction given only at the end of the story. The facilitator should begin with a poorly sequenced story, or with a story missing a main story element like, for example, the main	Story pencil or microphone. Story planner. Story template forms 1 and 2.

Aims	Method/Activities	Materials
	character. Group members are then asked to evaluate the story, identifying the problem with the story and improving it by adding in the omitted element or sequencing the story more correctly. They are then to take turns making up stories themselves which have some sequential errors, and other members then take it in turns to identify what is wrong with the story and how it can be improved. This is a good opportunity to draw the students' awareness to the confusion that can arise when stories are constructed with poor sequencing, or with missing story elements.	
To sum up and revise contents of the session.	Get volunteers from the group to summarise the main content of the session. Ask other members of the group to help, adding in the parts that may have been omitted.	Flipchart or whiteboard, paper and pen.
Mission to Achieve: Students are required to construct a simple written story using the story template forms showing the sequencing and ordering of events.	Students are encouraged to write a short story on anything they like using the story template forms which they used in the previous activity. They are to follow the words and phrases on the story template 1 **(First, Next, And then, After that, Finally)** or story template 2 **(Once upon a time, On a cold afternoon, To his shock, But then, Eventually)** and take care with the sequencing of their ideas. Allow students to choose from the story template form 1 or 2.	Photocopy story template forms for students to take home.

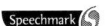

Evaluation of session/General comments

Story Template Form 1

First

Next

And then

After that

Finally

Story Template Form 2

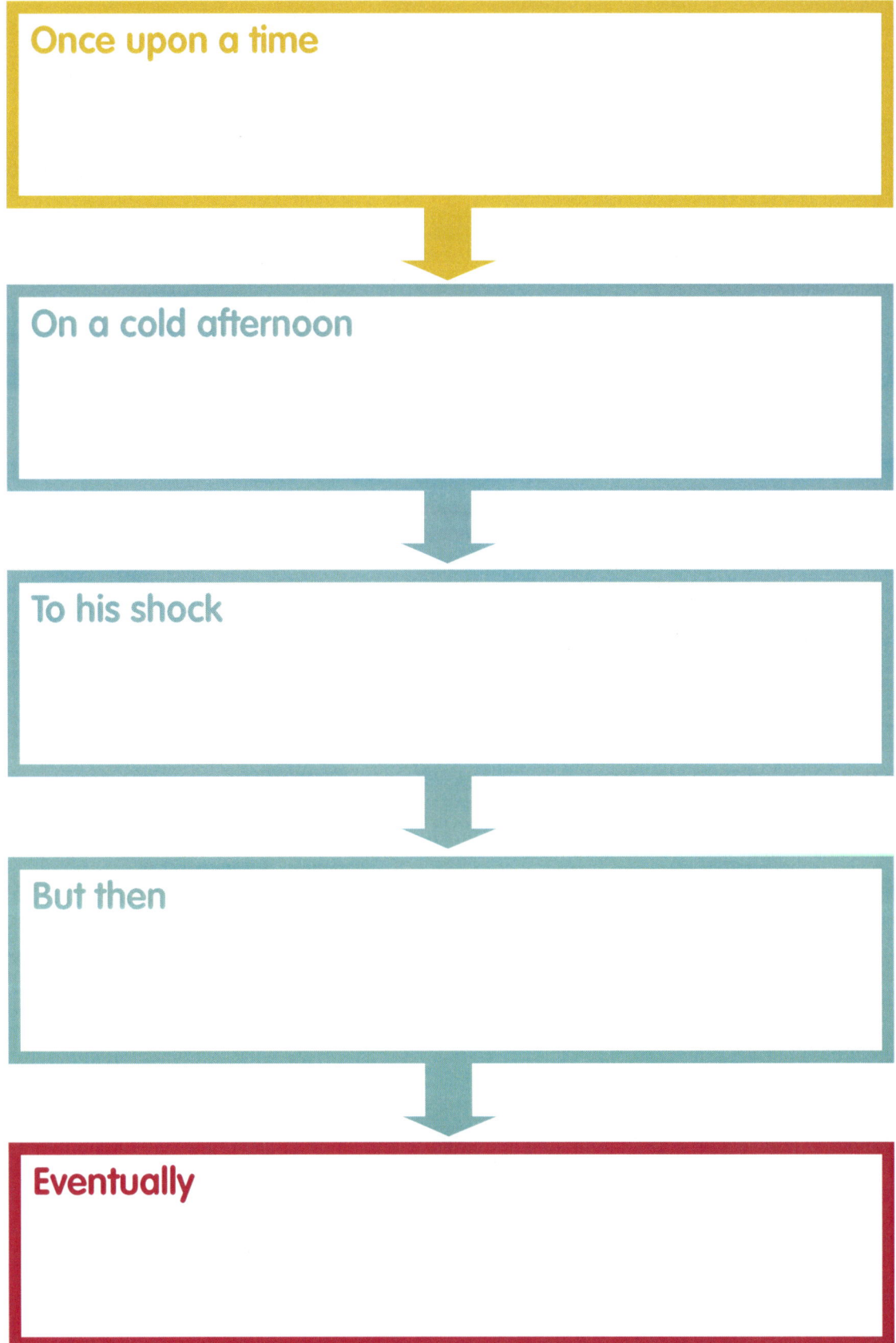

Once upon a time

On a cold afternoon

To his shock

But then

Eventually

Teaching notes for Session 14

What happened next? activity

In this task, the first sentence is read to students, who are then asked to come up with ideas about what may happen next. The main aim of this task is to ensure students understand the importance of the logical ordering of sentences and how the first sentence needs to come first, and the sentence following it, is the logical consequence of the first sentence.

If events in the story are not told in a coherent logical fashion, then the story will be confusing and very difficult to follow. This is an important lesson for students and should be the main focus of this session.

Example:

The man crashed his car into the central island. What happened next?

In this example, students are encouraged to provide suggestions for what might come after this first sentence. Suggestions may include that **he calls for the police on his mobile phone**, or that **he walks to the nearest garage to get help**. These suggestions all logically follow from the first sentence. An illogical sentence would be that **the man was talking on his mobile phone and did not see the central island ahead of him**. This sentence would clearly come before the first sentence rather than after. Provide this example for the students and ensure they understand the importance of logically sequencing ideas and concepts when telling a story.

Use the following sentences to provide the students with more opportunities to generate logical sequences to follow these events. It is fine to get them to produce illogical sequences for fun; as long as it is clear that they understand how silly these are.

1   The baker dropped all the eggs on the kitchen floor. **What happened next?**

2   The teacher ran out of ink as she began to mark the essays. **What happened next?**

3   David forgot to charge his mobile phone before he left for work. **What happened next?**

4   The businessman arrived at the airport without his passport. **What happened next?**

5   The model fell fast asleep in the hot midday sun. **What happened next?**

6   Mrs Simpson left the chicken in the oven all day and completely forgot about it. **What happened next?**

7   The children missed the school bus. **What happened next?**

8   The runner began to have serious stomach cramps midway through the race. **What happened next?**

 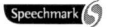

9   The footballer ran up to the penalty spot to take the final all-important penalty. **What happened next?**

10   The model fell over her long dress as she was walking down the ramp. **What happened next?**

11   As the *X Factor* contestant was about to start singing, there was a sudden power failure. **What happened next?**

12   Charlie watched as the boy hit the old lady and took her bag. **What happened next?**

13   The Australian tourist was sitting on the tube with her handbag open. **What happened next?**

14   Kieran was about to leave for the party when his jeans split. **What happened next?**

15   The children sat down in the hall to take their science exam. **What happened next?**

Teaching notes for Session 14

Sequence stories

You will find a number of sequence stories with different sequence cards per story. Begin with the easiest story, i.e. with the least number of cards (four) and build up to the stories with more sequence cards (8–11). Present each story separately to the students. For each story, place the sequence cards on the table in front of the students and get them to arrange the sequence cards in their correct order.

The students should then take turns telling the story using everything they have learned about storytelling. This includes using all the elements of the story planner, as well as using all the techniques and strategies that they have learned about making their story more interesting and exciting. Remind those listening to the students, to listen actively using the active listening behaviours identified in session 2.

Please remember that the students are to generate their own stories from the pictures. The details of the stories provided below should not be read to the students. This is for your information only and can help to check that students are including all details when they tell their stories from the picture cards. Students should also be encouraged to devise their own title for each story.

Sequence story 1

Running for the bus

Picture 1: Boy walking to bus stop.
Picture 2: Boy sees bus coming in distance and runs for bus; there is a banana skin lying ahead of him on the pavement.
Picture 3: Boy slips on banana skin and falls.
Picture 4: Boy gets up slowly and bus goes off without him, so he misses the bus and looks angry.

Sequence story 2

The wasted shopping trip

Picture 1: Man leaves house in morning with coat.
Picture 2: Man is walking across road with money slowly falling out of pocket into road.
Picture 3: Man now walking in high street, money still falling out of coat pocket.
Picture 4: Man in shop picking up newspaper and milk.
Picture 5: Man standing at checkout looking for money and finds he has no money and an empty pocket.

Sequence story 3

Having fun at the cinema

Picture 1:   Boy and girl waiting in line to buy cinema tickets.

Picture 2:   Boy and girl get to front of line and purchase cinema tickets.

Picture 3:   Boy and girl buy drinks and popcorn at cinema kiosk.

Picture 4:   Boy and girl sitting in cinema laughing at movie.

Picture 5:   Boy and girl coming out of cinema laughing and having a great time.

Sequence story 4

The escape of the lucky mouse

Picture 1:   Cat sleeping peacefully on floor next to his food.

Picture 2:   Mouse scurries past, and slowly approaches the cat and his food.

Picture 3:   Mouse is about to eat some of the cat's food, and cat wakes up and opens his eyes.

Picture 4:   Mouse runs away with cat chasing it.

Picture 5:   Mouse disappears through hole in wall.

Picture 6:   Cat peering into small hole, mouse taunting cat.

Picture 7:   Cat sitting outside hole looking puzzled and frustrated – there is nothing that he can do but wait and wait and wait…

Sequence story 5

The cat's dinner party

Picture 1:   Lady cooking in kitchen.

Picture 2:   Lady sets table for dinner.

Picture 3:   Table is set and lady continues to prepare the food for dinner.

Picture 4:   Lady puts food on table.

Picture 5:   Table is now full of food and lady is cooking with her back to the table.

Picture 6:   Cat is on table eating the food; lady's back is to table.

Picture 7:   Lady turns around and is horrified when she sees all food has been eaten by cat.

Picture 8:   Lady runs after cat with stick, shouting and waving arms – very angry.

Sequence story 6

The missing ladder

Picture 1: Man in overalls outside front of house, opening can of paint with ladder resting on side of wall.

Picture 2: Man begins painting outside wall of house.

Picture 3: Man climbs up a little bit on ladder and paints upper part of wall.

Picture 4: Man climbs up to top of ladder.

Picture 5: Man is seen working on top of roof with back to ladder resting on side of house.

Picture 6: Some young boys seen walking down road passing the house laughing and pointing at ladder.

Picture 7: One of the boys picks up ladder with other boys watching.

Picture 8: Boys running away from the house with the ladder.

Picture 9: Man on roof ready to come down and looks for ladder realising it is gone.

Picture 10: Man looks shocked and starts shouting for help and waving arms around.

Sequence story 7

The race

Picture 1: Lady wakes up in the morning.

Picture 2: Lady gets dressed in sports gear with trainers.

Picture 3: Lady eats breakfast, healthy cereal.

Picture 4: Lady is then travelling on train.

Picture 5: Lady arrives at a sports stadium where there are a lot of other people.

Picture 6: Lady stands at beginning of race with others, and man is there with gun to begin the race.

Picture 7: Everyone running race, picture of lady running with crowd.

Picture 8: Lady coming towards end of race, chequered flag is in sight.

Picture 9: Lady runs past chequered flag; hands held high in victory.

Picture 10: Lady limping home holding her trainers in hand with medal around her neck.

Picture 11: Lady lying on sofa at home eating a chocolate, with no shoes and blisters on feet.

Sequence story 2: **The wasted shopping trip**

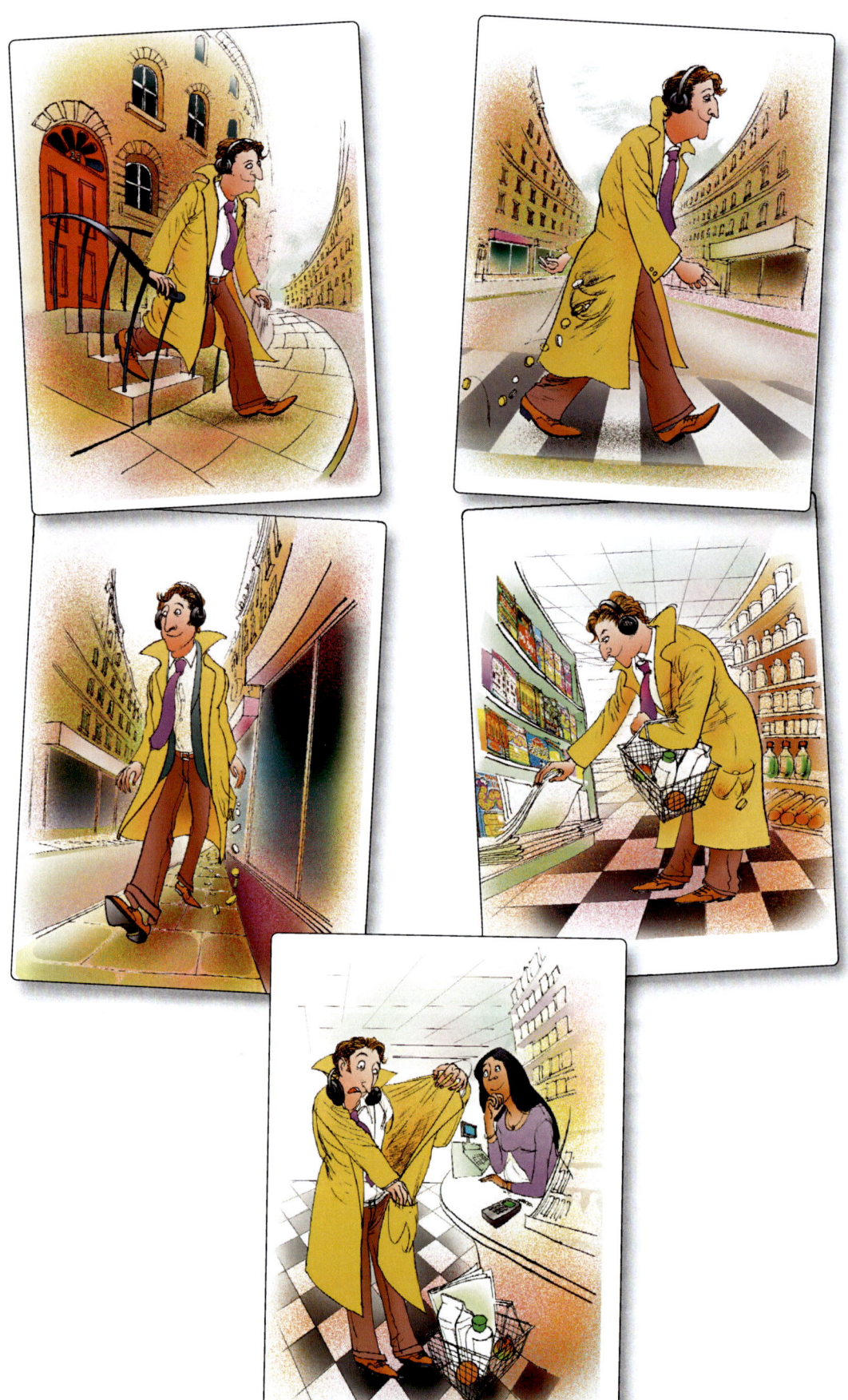

Sequence story 3: **Having fun at the cinema**

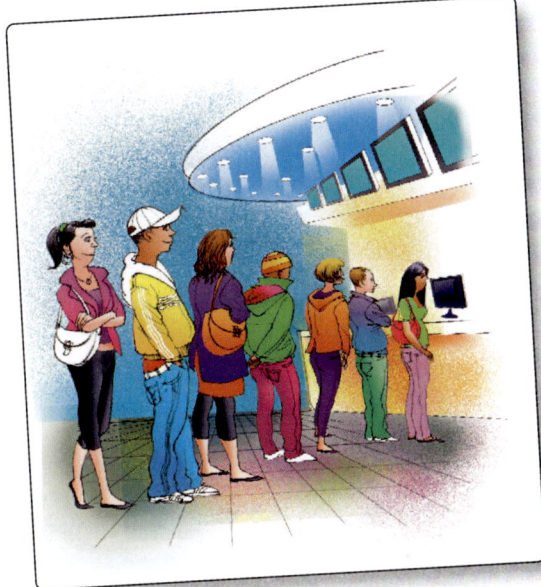

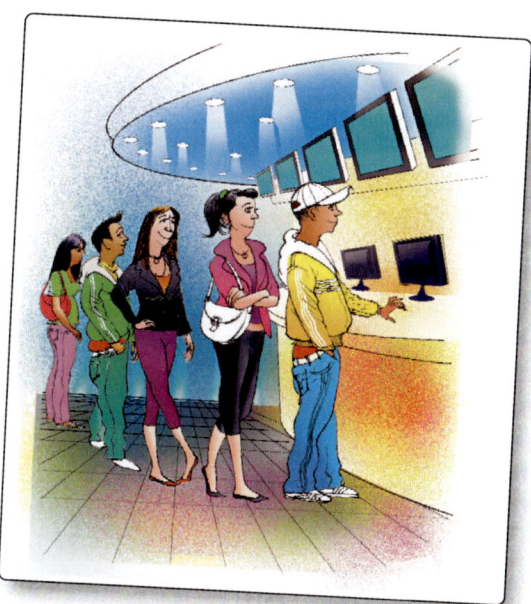

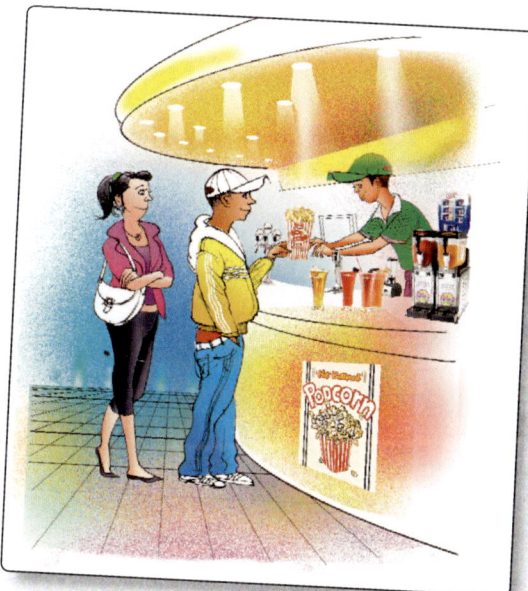

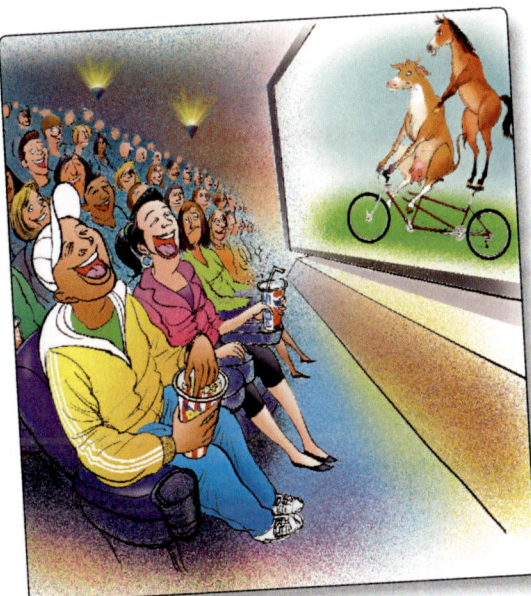

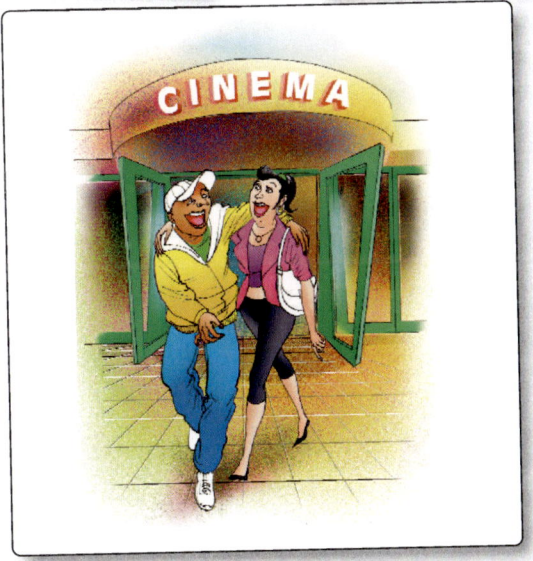

Sequence story 6: The missing ladder

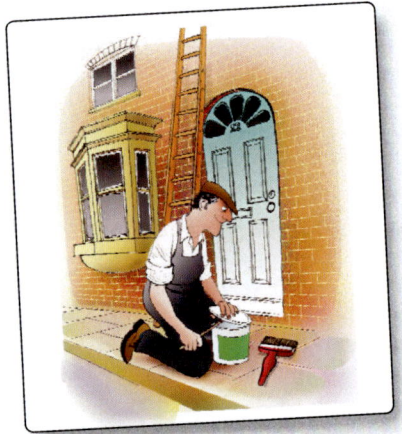
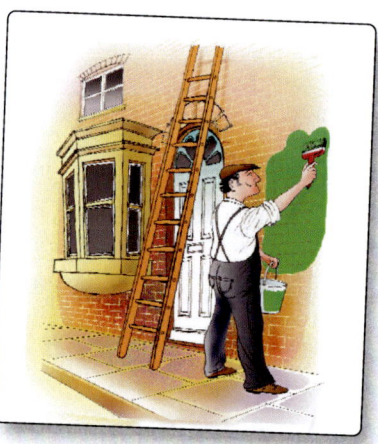
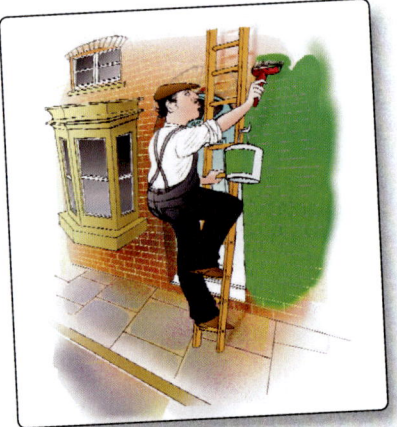
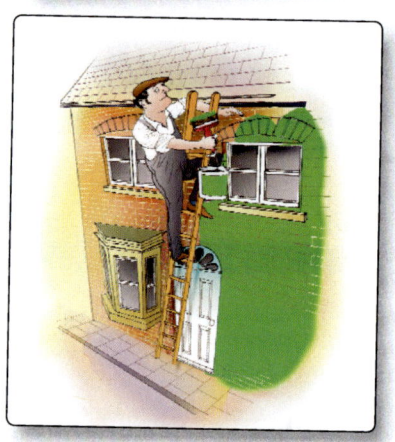
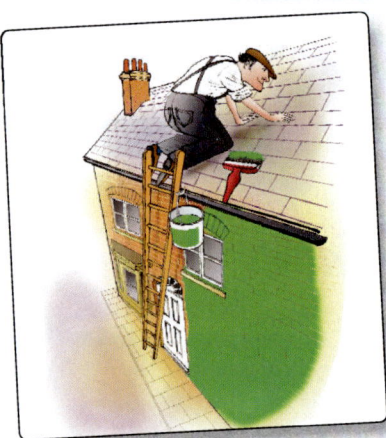
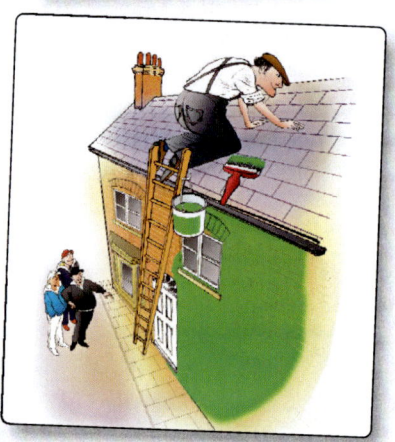
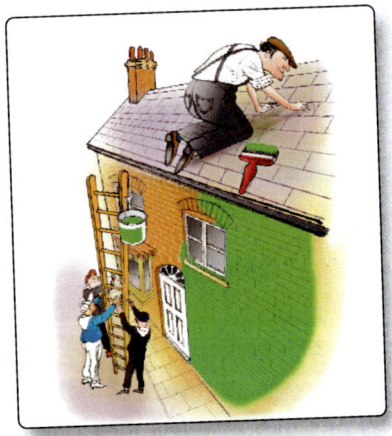
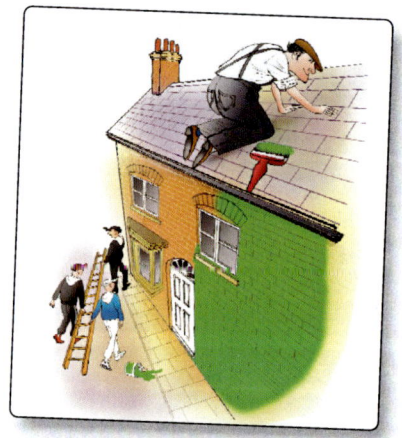
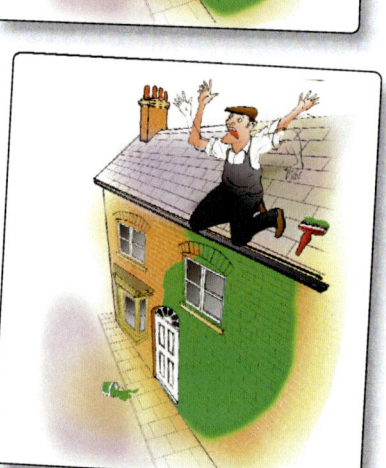

Session 15

15

Names of students: _____

_____

Facilitator: _____ Date: _____

School: _____

Class: _____

Aims	Method/Activities	Materials
To revise and recap concepts from the previous sessions, i.e. the entire story planner including all main elements: **beginning, middle** and **end**.	Group discussion recapping the main ideas from the previous sessions. Students have now covered all aspects of the story planner and are able to construct a story with all main story elements. Revise all three main elements and their parts through discussion using the story planner, story race track and story train track.	Flipchart or whiteboard, paper and pen. Story planner. Story F1 race track. Story train track and train carriages. Story football match. Story athletics race track.
To discuss the Mission to Achieve from the previous session, drawing attention to the logical sequencing of events in a story.	In this activity, continue to focus attention on the logical **sequencing** and progression of events in a story. Each student has the opportunity to show their story template and tell the story they have constructed for homework from the last session. The group are to evaluate the story and comment on the sequential order of the events. Students are to focus particular attention on the ordering of events in the story they hear.	Story pencil or microphone. Story template with written story produced by the students for their Mission to Achieve from last session.
To **evaluate stories** and **explore the reasons for evaluation**.	Throughout the programme, students have been encouraged to evaluate their own storytelling skills, as well as the storytelling skills of the other group members. In this session, we provide students with a list of possible questions that they can use to assess the quality of the stories they hear and tell. Encourage students to think about the	Flipchart or whiteboard, paper and pen. Evaluative questions in teaching notes for this session.

Aims	Method/Activities	Materials
	questions, and to add any more when hearing a story. Establish with students why it is important to self-evaluate. Brainstorm with them the reasons for evaluation. Explore with them the importance of knowing what you are good at, and what you need to work on, and discuss why this is so important. Ask students how they can ever repeat what they are best at, if they are unable to recognise what this may be. Similarly, if they do not reflect on what is difficult for them and what might need more work, how then will they ever improve on these aspects? Discuss the importance of evaluating the stories of other members of the group and explore the most appropriate ways of doing this. Ask students why they are evaluating others. Encourage them to think about the importance of learning from their peers and sharing their skills. Discuss how they would like someone to evaluate them. Identify with students the importance of constructive feedback, of making sure there is positive feedback first, and of ensuring that the constructive feedback contains practical suggestions for improvement. This will ensure that all students keep developing and improving their storytelling skills and are sensitive in their evaluations.	
To make up and share complete well structured and exciting stories to the group using the story planner.	Individually, or in pairs, students are given some time to prepare a complete and well structured story using all the components of the story planner. The story should contain a detailed **beginning** with detailed **character**, **time** and **place** information; a **middle** with one or more **episodes** containing a main initiating **happening** or first event, an **immediate response,** an **action** and a **reaction**; and an **ending** with an **outcome** containing a **result** and **message**. Students can either choose their own topic, or facilitators can choose to give them a topic.	Flipchart or whiteboard paper and pen. Story planner. Use story pencil or microphone to indicate turns. Topic areas from teaching notes for session 15.

Aims	Method/Activities	Materials
	Some suggested topic areas are provided in the teaching notes.	
	This is the first opportunity for students to construct and tell their own stories using all of the components of the story planner that they have learned about in the programme. Students should be encouraged to use as many of the storytelling devices we have covered previously in their stories as possible. These may include direct speech, simile, alliteration, repetition, onomatopoeia, etc.	
	The rest of the group are encouraged to listen to each student and to evaluate their story. The students are to rate each story on a 1–10 rating scale giving reasons for their ratings (1 = poor and 10 = excellent). It is important to ensure that positive points are made first and students give suggestions on how stories can be improved. Each story should contain all parts of the story planner and those listening should identify the different parts from the story planner after they have listened to the story.	
	The person with the highest score is named the story king or queen for the session.	
To choose an appropriate **title** for each story.	After listening to the stories, the rest of the group are to choose an appropriate title for each one. This should not be the **title** that they were given by the facilitator, but a different title of their own. Discuss with the students how the title might reflect the contents of the story. Explore what makes a good title which captures the attention of the reader or listener, for example, a short concise title, a clear title, a title that reflects the story, or a title that teases the audience. Not all titles, however, tell us much about what the story is about. Discuss with the students titles of books that they might know and what these titles evoke for them, for example, *Buried Alive*, by Jacqueline Wilson; *Holes*, by Louis Sachar and *The Twits* by	

 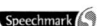

Aims	Method/Activities	Materials
	Roald Dahl. Explore with students their own examples of favourite and funny titles. Titles can sometimes help you get a feeling about what the book will be about. Some titles will describe perfectly the contents of the story, for example, *The Witches* by Roald Dahl is a book about witches. Even the title *Holes* describes to some degree what happens in the story, i.e. there is a lot of digging of holes! With some titles, however, it is much less clear what the story is about; for example, *Lord of the Flies* by William Golding is a difficult title to interpret if you have not read the book. The same could be said about Jacqueline Wilson's book entitled *Double Act*, although here one might take a guess that it is a story about twins.	
To **construct different stories** by adding or changing different elements of the story planner.	Each student now retells their **story**, but this time they have to add a **character** and change the **setting** of the story. Each student chooses one character to add to their story. Place the character cards face down on the desk and students choose one character card which they then have to incorporate into their original story. In addition to this, each student chooses a setting card (also placed face down on the table) and is required to change their original story to accommodate the new setting. For example, if their original story is about a footballer playing a match in a football stadium, and the student chooses a new character card of a 'tramp' and a new setting card of a 'bedroom', then the student has to alter their original story by incorporating the tramp and bedroom into their original story about the footballer. They now have to think about a story which still incorporates the footballer, but this time the setting is the bedroom, and there is an additional character, a tramp. This is both fun and challenging! Students are to be encouraged to be bold with their stories and have fun adding in different characters and settings. They can even change	Story planner. Character picture cards included in the resource. Setting picture cards included in the resource.

Aims	Method/Activities	Materials
	the endings of their stories if they wish. The facilitator can add more changes if appropriate and should vary the instructions and level of complexity depending on the emerging narrative skills of the students. This session is to emphasise how they are in control over the stories they tell and how flexible and fun storytelling can be.	
To sum up and revise contents of the session.	Get volunteers from the group to summarise the main content of the session. Ask other members of the group to help, adding in the parts that may have been omitted.	Flipchart or whiteboard, paper and pen.
Mission to Achieve: Students to make up a character using the character word map and bring the word map to the next session, together with one item of clothing which the character will wear.	Students are asked to provide a detailed character profile using the character word map to assist them. They can make up any character they wish, and in the next session, will construct a story with this character. They should bring along with them one item of clothing that belongs to this character, and which they feel shows something about their character. For example, if their character is flamboyant, they may bring a pink bowtie with them. Alternatively, if they are describing an old frail man, they might choose to bring a walking stick with them.	Story planner. Character story map.

 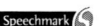

Evaluation of session/General comments

P This page may be photocopied for instructional use only. © Victoria Joffe Speechmark

Teaching notes for Session 15

Evaluation of stories produced

Throughout the sessions, students have been encouraged to evaluate their own and other people's stories. There are a number of questions that they can ask to help their evaluations and ensure that the stories have all the features that have been discussed in this programme. Some suggested questions follow, but students should be encouraged to generate more questions themselves.

Discuss with students the importance and role of self-evaluation in their learning and continual development. Explore the ways they can provide feedback and learn from other members of the group, the importance of giving positive feedback first, and making sure all feedback is constructive and consists of suggestions for improvement. Remind them that it is not helpful to be negative, when evaluating either themselves or others.

To evaluate a story that you hear, you may like to consider the following:

1 What was the story about?

2 Did the story contain all the elements of the story planner?

3 Who were the main characters in the story?

4 Where did the story take place?

5 When did the story take place?

6 How many details were given about each character?

7 How many details were given about the time and place of the story?

8 How well can you visualise the characters, time and place of the story?

9 Do you identify with the characters in the story?

10 How well do you feel you know the characters from the character profiles you were given?

11 What was the main event, problem or plot of the story?

12 What did the character/s do to solve the problem or conflict?

13 How did the characters behave in the story?

 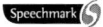

14 How did the characters feel in the story?

15 Did the characters' feelings and/or behaviour change during the course of the story? If so, how and why?

16 How exciting was the overall story?

17 Did the story have an exiting climax?

18 What did the character's actions tell you about him or her?

19 What was the outcome of the story?

20 How exciting was the ending?

21 Did the ending contain a cliffhanger?

22 Was the ending satisfying?

23 What did you learn from the story?

24 Did the story contain any direct speech?

25 Did the story include any story devices to make it more interesting, such as alliteration, hyperbole, humour, double meaning, simile, rhyme, onomatopoeia?

26 How well was the story told?

27 Did the storyteller hold your attention throughout?

28 Did the storyteller use his/her voice, facial expression and body language in different ways to make the story more exciting?

29 Did the storyteller use role play, pictures or other prompts to make the story more exciting?

30 Did the title of the story capture your attention and interest before you heard the story?

31 Would you like to listen to another story by the same storyteller?

Teaching notes for Session 15

Here are some topic areas which the students can use to build their stories around. Feel free to add you own, or even better, get the students to come up with their own ideas. Remind students that they are now telling a fictional or made-up story, but that does not mean it can be unstructured and all over the place! Their story needs to be captivating, exciting and well structured with all the three main elements of the story planner which we have now completed.

1 My biggest regret and how it changed my life

2 If I only knew then, what I know now, I would never have accepted the money

3 It should have been the happiest day of my life

4 The best decision I have ever made

5 A memorable journey

6 I told you so!

7 The greatest memory of my life

8 The most embarrassing thing that has ever happened to me

9 The neighbour from hell

10 The road to nowhere

11 The best invention ever

12 A tragedy that could so easily have been avoided

13 The harmless boy who caused such devastation

14 Murder on Bus No 22

15 It was nothing short of a miracle

16 Catch me if you can

17 Poison was the murder weapon of choice

18 The proudest moment of my life

19 It was never meant to be this way

20 The stranger at the door

21 The missing lottery ticket

22 If only…

23 …And suddenly, I woke up

24 The message in the bottle read, 'HELP ME'

25 Shipwrecked.

 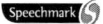

Session 16

16

Names of students: _____

_____

Facilitator: _____ Date: _____

School: _____

Class: _____

Aims	Method/Activities	Materials
To revise and recap the main concepts from the previous sessions, i.e. the **story planner**.	Group discussion recapping the main ideas from the previous sessions on the story planner.	Flipchart or whiteboard, paper and pen. Story planner.
Students to **introduce their characters** from their Mission to Achieve activity and tell a story with this character, using all story elements of the story planner.	Each student has the opportunity to introduce their character using the character word map which they completed for their Mission to Achieve task. They are to provide a detailed character description of their character and explain how their chosen item of clothing for their character provides more information about who their character is. So, for example, if the chosen item of clothing they have brought in is an old, torn, worn jersey, what might this say about their character? Contrast this with a pearl necklace or dazzling high-heeled shoes which another student may have brought in. Students are to explore what the items they have brought in tell us about their characters. The group might like to explore further what 'objects' or 'appearances' say about us as characters, and whether 'appearances can be deceptive'. What, for example, do we think the character wearing the torn, worn, old jersey is like, and on what are we basing this judgement? Students are then asked to get into small groups and construct stories with their main characters. They are to find ways of integrating	Story planner. Story pencil or microphone. Character word map of individual characters. Items of clothing brought in by students for their individual characters.

 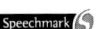

Aims	Method/Activities	Materials
	all their chosen characters in each story told per group, and ensure that they weave into the story, and into their character, the details and history behind their chosen item of clothing. So, for example, the story may divulge what happened to the character wearing the torn, worn, old jersey. Students should be reminded to tell exciting and well structured stories using all the components of the story planner that have been covered in previous sessions.	
To revise and revisit what makes an exciting story, with a particular focus on the **delivery** of the story.	Through group discussion, explore what makes an interesting and exciting story. Revisit the points from the teaching notes from sessions 3, 11 and 12 and brainstorm with students different ways of making a story more captivating and exciting. Revisit and revise all the different strategies that students can draw upon which have been covered in previous sessions, and are summarised in the teaching notes in this session, to enhance storytelling in both oral and written forms. Focus attention on the (oral) telling of stories and encourage the group to brainstorm all ways available to make stories sound more interesting and exciting, and ways of getting and keeping their audience's attention. Describe for students vocal variety and all the different things we can do with our voices alone to show a range of emotions and feelings and enhance our storytelling, including varying volume, speed and intensity. Encourage them to think of all the different ways we can use not only our voices, but also our faces and entire bodies to communicate our meaning. Emphasise the importance of matching the words we use to the different ways we use our voices, faces and bodies to further impart our message.	Teaching notes from sessions 3, 11 and 12 on how to make a story more interesting. Flipchart or whiteboard, paper and pen. Teaching notes for this session with explanations about paralinguistic features and suggestions for enhancing the delivery of stories.

Aims	Method/Activities	Materials
	Create awareness for students of the powerful role that their voices, faces and body language play in storytelling. Ask students to think about how, for example, they recognise when their teacher is angry, or in a bad mood, when their mum or dad is in a particularly good mood, etc. Ask them to identify how they recognise the moods of people, and what cues they use to do this.	
	Focus their attention on the changes in voices, facial expressions and body language, and how all three of these communicate a message on their own.	
	Explore with them the importance of using vocal features, facial expressions and body language that match the feelings they are trying to show. Discuss, for example, how confusing it is if the character is recounting some very sad news, but the person telling the story or acting out the character is using a loud voice, talking quickly with a big smile on their face. Discuss the importance of congruence in the words we say, in how we say them, in the message we are imparting, the facial expressions we use and our body language. The messages we give using all parts of our body should be congruent and communicate the same thing.	
	Identify with students a range of facial expressions and body postures that may impart different messages. Get students to identify the different messages you can give through facial expressions (smile, frown, furrowed forehead, steely half-shut eyes, eyes to the ground, eyes shifting from side to side) and body language (bent over, standing tall, chest and elbows out, walking with a limp, walking slowly, walking quickly, head up and confident, head lowered, body turned away or facing the group), etc.	

 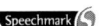

Aims	Method/Activities	Materials
	Define for students the meaning of **paralinguistic features**. **Paralinguistic features** refer to aspects of spoken communication which are not part of the actual word or words we speak, but are important at influencing the overall meaning of what we say. They include intonation, volume, pitch, rate and stress, and non-verbal behaviour, including facial expression. Further definitions on each example are provided in the teaching notes for this session. Explain these terms for students using the definitions and show them how varying these aspects of the voice can increase the overall excitement of the story and make it sound much more interesting. The facilitator may like to first give an example of telling or reading aloud a story using a monotonous voice with no vocal variety at all. Students are to evaluate this way of telling a story and to discuss how interesting it was and how easy or difficult it was to listen to. The facilitator should then retell the same story, but this time using interesting vocal variety, direct speech, facial expression and any other story features that are appropriate. The students are to compare and contrast the two ways of telling a story and discuss how using the voice, and face and body, can greatly enhance the telling of a story. See the teaching notes that follow for further ideas and suggestions.	
To practise **varying the voice and observe how this impacts on overall meaning**.	Students are to be encouraged to try out the suggestions for **vocal variety** using the activities in the teaching notes. Students take turns saying the given sentences, emphasising the different words in bold in different ways, using vocal variety and focusing on the change in the meaning of the sentence resulting from the change in emphasis.	Sentences from the teaching notes with different words in bold for emphasis.

Aims	Method/Activities	Materials
To **depict a range of emotions using vocal variety, facial expression and body language**.	In the previous tasks, students have had the opportunity to focus their attention on the role of the voice, facial expression and body language, and how all three of these communicate a message on their own. In this activity, each student randomly chooses one emotion from a range provided by the facilitator. The emotions are written face down on pieces of paper to ensure that no one knows what emotion they are choosing. The students are then required to act out the emotion using the voice, facial expression or body language. They should first try to use just one of these forms of communication to depict the emotion, and the rest of the group try and guess the emotion. If the group members cannot guess, the student then adds other means of communication, for example, tries to depict the emotion using voice and facial expression, and then adds some form of body language if the group are still unable to guess the emotion. The winner of this game is the student who manages to act out the emotion, using the least number of different forms of communication, allowing the group to correctly guess the emotion in question.

Students should discuss and explore how successful they were at guessing the emotion; and explore what the student did to show the specific emotion effectively. So, for example, what facial expression, type of voice or body language depicted the emotion of depression? Was it a slow, low voice, or a slow laboured walk, or a bent posture or a face with a deep frown and a furrowed forehead? Allow students the opportunity to depict these different feelings and emotions and see how many different voices, body movements and facial expressions they can use to illustrate these feelings. | List of emotions from the teaching notes. Each emotion needs to be written down by the facilitator on individual cards to be chosen, blind, by each group member. |
| Students to explore ways of **increasing** | Group to consider how to make a story exciting in the written format. | Revisit story extracts provided in session 11 as examples of |

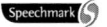

Aims	Method/Activities	Materials
interest and excitement with a written story.	Discuss, for example, the use of punctuation (an exclamation mark for emphasis) underlining key words, using different colour pens, writing in larger letters, using capitals, italics, bold, different fonts, etc. Remind students, for example, of the use of italics and exclamation marks used for effect in the story extracts provided in session 11. Encourage more suggestions from the students on ways of making written stories more exciting. Ask them to think about how articles are written in their favourite magazines and in newspapers. How do these popular magazines and newspapers catch the public's attention? What print font do they use, what size and type and how frequently do they vary these? Explore with students the use of pictures to enhance the story. Discuss the role of the heading or headline and how this can be used to capture attention. Draw attention, for example, to how in newspapers and magazines, headlines are short, using only key words to explain the content of the article; how these headlines often use double meaning, humour or some other type of literary device, such as repetition or rhyme, to capture attention; and how the headings are always in bigger type, and often in a different font to the rest of the article. See if students can think of any other ways to make the word in print more interesting to the reader.	the use of italics, exclamation marks, direct speech and other story devices which serve to enhance stories in the written format. Teaching notes for session 16.
To **construct and share a story** using all the elements from the story planner and techniques learned about how to make the story more interesting.	The students take turns to **integrate all the knowledge** they have gathered from previous sessions and each student tells a story with all the elements from the story planner, using as many techniques as possible to make their story interesting. The story pencil or microphone is used to indicate turns. Copies of the story planner should be provided to each student as a reminder of the elements needed for each story. Use the character, place and time word maps to facilitate a detailed description of the setting and characterisation. Check that stories contain all key elements of the story planner:	Story planner. Story pencil or microphone. Character, time and place word maps. List of behaviours indicating active listening from session 2, as a reminder to students.

Aims	Method/Activities	Materials
	Setting: character/s, time, place **Episode:** initial event or first happening, immediate response, actions, reactions **Outcome:** result, message. The stories are to be generated from the themed story picture cards enclosed in the resource. Each of these descriptive pictures show various exciting events which can be woven into an exciting story. Students should focus attention on what has been covered in this session around using other modes of communication in addition to words and sentences (voices, facial expression, body language) to make their stories more captivating and interesting. Students are encouraged to listen carefully to each story using the active listening behaviours and to evaluate each story, providing positive comments and suggestions for improvement. Students to rate each story on a 1–10 rating scale using the evaluation questions from session 15. At the end of the session the story king or queen is announced, i.e. the person with the highest score.	List of possible ways of making a story more interesting. The themed story picture cards enclosed in the resource: • park scene • seaside scene • market scene • school cafeteria scene • gym scene • burglary scene.
To **revise all the contents** of the resource using a story square spiral puzzle.	If time allows in this session, use the story square spiral puzzle included in the teaching notes for session 17 to help to revise all the main content areas covered in the resource. This is a fun activity which students will enjoy, and at the same time they will be revising and consolidating new concepts and knowledge.	Story square spiral puzzle included in teaching notes for session 17.
To sum up and revise contents of the session.	Get volunteers from the group to summarise the main content of the session. Ask other members of the group to help, adding in the parts that may have been omitted.	
Mission to Achieve: Students to cut out and bring two examples of a story from their favourite magazine and	Students are asked to bring with them an article from their favourite magazine and an article from the newspaper that they most frequently read. They are asked to identify the main story components from each story using the story planner.	Flipchart or whiteboard, paper and pen. Story planner.

 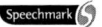

Aims	Method/Activities	Materials
newspaper and identify the key story components using the story planner, as well as the story devices that have been used to enhance meaning and capture attention.	They should also identify the main story strategies that the author has used to capture the reader's attention. Each story should include the written story, the title of the story and name of the author. If the story has an accompanying picture, then the picture should be attached to the story and the name of the illustrator (person who drew the picture) should also be identified.	

Evaluation of session/General comments

Teaching notes for Session 16

This is how we make our stories more interesting and exciting...

Some suggestions have already been given to students in sessions 3 and 12 on ways of making a story more interesting. Revisit these examples and explore each one in more detail with the students and encourage them to try out these suggestions when telling their own stories, and to add their own ideas.

- Tell a story with which others can identify, for example, tell a story about current issues that students face in school when talking to a group of school students, for example, bullying, preparing for exams, or getting a part-time job.

- Use prompts, for example, when describing a tramp as your main character, put on an old coat or a threadbare hat, or when involving an elderly lady as a character, use a walking stick.

- Use role play, so act out as if you are the tramp, with perhaps a limp and shuffle, or walk slowly and doubled over as the elderly lady.

- Use direct speech. This means speak as if you are the actual character. So if you were telling a story about a tramp, you might say in a trembling weak voice, 'Excuse me sir, do you have some spare change for a cup of coffee?'

- Use different voices to indicate different characters in the story. So speak like the horrible character who kicks the tramp and refuses to give him any money. Think about how the voice will change depending on whether your character is an elderly lady or a young man.

- Make your voice as interesting as you can. Do not speak in one way all the time. Try and vary your voice by changing your loudness levels (loud and soft), the speed at which you talk (fast and slow) and the pitch (high, middle and low) – see the following teaching notes for further ideas on delivery.

- Use all the elements of the story planner. Include detailed descriptions of the character, place and time; include exciting episodes with a climax and different actions taken to resolve the story conflict. Provide a satisfying end to the story, including a cliffhanger if you wish and/or a moral to the story.

- Use a variety of story features which have been discussed in previous sessions, including: metaphor, simile, rhyme, alliteration, hyperbole, repetition, onomatopoeia.

- Include humour: humorous stories are fun to listen to and always get a reaction.

- Include your own personal experiences when you can. So if you are telling a story about bullying, and you have had some experience of it, then use this experience when telling the story. It will make it seem more real.

- Include the emotions, thoughts and feelings of the different characters in addition to their actions as this will bring alive the characters for your listener and will help them understand why the characters are acting in certain ways.

- Use interesting and different words, for example, use a variety of different adjectives to describe the characters and or settings. So, for example, instead of saying 'the angry boy spoke', you may like to say, 'the irate incensed teenager spat out his words in fury' and instead of saying 'it was summer', you could say, 'it was a warm balmy summer's evening with the humidity clinging to every pore'. Similarly, students may like to comment on their favourite meal as being a tasty, mouth-watering, delicious cacophony of scrumptious tastes!

- Think about the names you give to places and the characters in your story and see if they can in some way add something to the story. So, for example, consider Roald Dahl's use of 'Mr and Mrs Gloop' and 'Veruca' in *Charlie and the Chocolate Factory* and how this adds to our understanding of the characters and general enjoyment of the story. And what about the names of some of your favourite characters in the *Harry Potter* books, for example, Albus Dumbledore, Susan Bones and The Bloody Baron! See if students can name some more.

 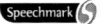

Teaching notes for Session 16

Varying the delivery of telling the story

There are many different ways that we can make our voices and faces more interesting and vary our vocal delivery. Discuss the following with the students and encourage them to try out the different options. Options include:

- The use of different facial expressions – try to show on your face what the characters are experiencing, or mirror the mood of the settings. Get the students to practise showing different feelings and emotions through their facial expressions, for example, compare the facial expressions of sad, happy, angry and frustrated.

- Use language in different ways, for example, include interesting adjectives and use all five senses to describe characters and time and place settings.

- Use repetition to emphasise the important part/s of the story.

- Use gesture to emphasise main concepts of the story, for example, shake your fist to show that a character is threatening violence, or show by using both hands the size of an object you are describing in the story.

- Exaggerate the most important part/s of a story. You can exaggerate using your voice, by speaking louder, for example, or by using gesture or facial expression.

- Vary paralinguistic features – this refers to using the voice in different ways and includes the following:

  ➤ **Volume:** this refers to the loudness levels of the voice and can vary from very soft to very loud. Encourage students to think about how varying the loudness of their voices can impact on overall understanding. For example, what mood or feeling is created when using a whisper, versus shouting? Give an example to students about how whispering increases the tension in a story and is therefore a good technique to use when telling a scary part of a story.

  ➤ **Rate:** this refers to the speed of the voice, how quickly we speak, and can vary from very slow to very fast. Again, allow students to consider how changes in rate can enhance different meanings. An elderly man may, for example, use a very slow soft voice, while a busy young businessman may talk quickly using a loud booming voice.

  ➤ **Pitch:** this refers to how high or low the voice is. Men have lower pitches than women. One can use pitch changes to enhance storytelling, for example, use a very high-pitched voice for a witch or an elderly man, and a low pitch for a bear or monster.

> ➤ **Intonation:** this refers to the rise and fall of the voice. For example, when making a simple statement, like 'the bread is on the table', then the sentence ends with a falling intonation. If however you are asking a question, you will usually end the question with a rising intonation showing that you are waiting for an answer.

> ➤ **Tone:** We can vary our voice in many ways to reflect different tones, for example, a critical tone versus a happy tone versus a sarcastic tone. Get the students to play around with their voices to indicate these different emotions.

Practise saying the following sentences, emphasising the bold word using any of the suggested ways of varying your voice, including varying the loudness, pitch, rate or intonation. Get the students to practise varying their voice using these sentences and using the voice to emphasise the bold word. Show the students how changes in the emphasis of different words in the sentence can change the meaning. Discuss how the use of vocal variety makes the sentence more interesting.

Practice sentence 1

- **Get** your black socks out of the green cabinet before you go to football training.

- Get **your** black socks out of the green cabinet before you go to football training.

- Get your **black** socks out of the green cabinet before you go to football training.

- Get your black **socks** out of the green cabinet before you go to football training.

- Get your black socks out of the **green** cabinet before you go to football training.

- Get your black socks out of the green **cabinet** before you go to football training.

- Get your black socks out of the green cabinet **before** you go to football training.

- Get your black socks out of the green cabinet before **you** go to football training.

- Get your black socks out of the green cabinet before you **go** to football training.

- Get your black socks out of the green cabinet before you go to **football** training.

 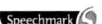

Practice sentence 2

- **I** will not drink this bowl of soup on the kitchen counter.

- I will **not** drink this bowl of soup on the kitchen counter.

- I will not **drink** this bowl of soup on the kitchen counter.

- I will not drink **this** bowl of soup on the kitchen counter.

- I will not drink this **bowl** of soup on the kitchen counter.

- I will not drink this bowl of **soup** on the kitchen counter.

- I will not drink this bowl of soup **on** the kitchen counter.

- I will not drink this bowl of soup on the **kitchen counter**.

Practice sentence 3

- **Take** your filthy football boots off my marble table immediately!

- Take **your** filthy football boots off my marble table immediately!

- Take your **filthy** football boots off my marble table immediately!

- Take your filthy **football** boots off my marble table immediately!

- Take your filthy football **boots** off my marble table immediately!

- Take your filthy football boots **off** my marble table immediately!

- Take your filthy football boots off **my** marble table immediately!

- Take your filthy football boots off my **marble** table immediately!

- Take your filthy football boots off my marble **table** immediately!

- Take your filthy football boots off my marble table **immediately**!

Teaching notes for Session 16

Let's show how we feel using different means of communication

Write each of these emotions on a separate card and get each student to choose one. They are then required to act out the emotion using one form of communication: voice, facial expression or body language. They should act out the emotion without explicitly articulating how they are feeling or labelling the emotion (for example, saying 'I am sad'). The rest of the group are to try and guess what emotion the student is acting out. If they cannot guess on the first attempt, then the student should add other means of communication, so, for example, using voice plus facial expression on the second attempt. No words describing or labelling the emotion are allowed, but they can talk and use their voice to reflect a specific feeling. Students should try to depict the emotion so clearly that the group are able to guess correctly with the smallest number of clues. Once the group have guessed the emotion correctly, they are to identify what communication the student used to reflect the specific emotion, and evaluate why it was or was not effective.

Some emotions you might like to use include:

ecstatic	worried
frightened	excited
depressed	guilty
surprised	angry
disgusted	aggressive
disappointed	delighted
relieved	embarrassed
envious	horrified
dejected	fearful
sad	

And feel free to add your own…

 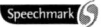

Teaching notes for Session 16

Written stories

You can also vary the delivery of a story and make it more exciting and appealing when using print or written language. You will not be able to use the voice, but you can use variations in the written form. Consider how to make a story more exciting when using the written word. Here are some suggestions, and elicit more from the students. Students should think about how their favourite authors use words, fonts, scripts, etc to make their stories more exciting.

- The use of punctuation, for example, the exclamation mark – 'Oh no!' she shouted.

- The use of the comma (,) or semi-colon (;) to show the need to pause between words or phrases and to show where to pause.

- The use of direct speech, for example, write the actual words that the character is saying: '"**I'll huff and I'll puff and I'll blow the house down**," boomed the scary wolf.'

- Use of a range of different descriptive words.

- Addition of pictures or diagrams to add or support meaning.

- Use a heading or headline which grabs the audience's attention; make it short and concise, play with words, i.e. use double meaning, humour, etc.

- Write the story in different shapes on the page, so, for example, if your story is about a ship, write the story in the shape of a ship.

- Change the print/writing in various ways, including:

  - Size – use smaller or bigger letters

  - Different fonts

  - Use capitals for emphasis

  - Italics

  - Bold

  - Underline key words

  - Different colour fonts or pens.

Session 17

Names of students: _____

_____

Facilitator: _____ Date: _____

School: _____

Class: _____

Aims	Method/Activities	Materials
To revise and recap concepts from the previous sessions, i.e. the entire story planner including all main elements: **beginning, middle** and **end**. Focus on the **delivery of a story** and different means of communication to make the story more interesting.	Group discussion recapping the main ideas from the previous sessions. Students have now covered all aspects of the story planner and are able to construct a story with all main elements. Revise all three main story elements and their component parts through discussion using the story planner, story F1 race track, story train track, story football match or story athletics race track. Revise different means of communication that can be used to enhance storytelling.	Flipchart or whiteboard, paper and pen. Story planner. Story F1 race track. Story train track and train carriages. Story football match. Story athletics race track.
To discuss the two magazine and newspaper articles brought in by students as part of their Mission to Achieve from the previous session, drawing attention to **the main story components**, the **title** of the story, the main **plot** of each story, the **author** and **illustrator** of the story and different ways that the author has used the written word	Each student has the opportunity to show the chosen newspaper and magazine article that they have brought in. The student summarises the article, providing an overview of the main story elements using the story planner. The **title** and **heading/s** of the article are shared with the group. The student evaluates the stories and identifies the features used which enhance its overall readability. A discussion is held on the suitability of each title, any additional headings, and whether it captivates the readers' attention and reflects accurately the contents of each story. The group to consider whether they have a better title or headline for each article. The students are also to identify the main **plot** of each article.	Flipchart or whiteboard. Pen and paper. Teaching notes for session 17. Magazine and newspaper articles brought in by the students.

 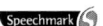

Aims	Method/Activities	Materials
to increase audience attention.	Each student is encouraged to provide the name/s of the **author** of the article and the **illustrator** if the article has a photograph or other illustration. Differentiate for the students the role of the author and illustrator. Explore with the students the role of any pictures or photographs and whether they effectively add something to the overall enjoyment of and interest in the article.	
To introduce and discuss **poetry** with a focus on **narrative or story poems**. Differentiate between **prose** and **poetry**.	Up until this point, the focus of the sessions has been on different types of stories or story genres. We have discussed stories that appear in books, stories from movies and television, stories that take the form of articles in newspapers and magazines, fables and fairytales, as well as stories that we have made up and shared. These types of stories are referred to as prose, the language used in everyday life. In this session, we introduce students to poetry and differentiate poetry from the stories we have covered up to this point. Brainstorm with students the difference between stories that we have discussed from books, magazines, on television and in the cinema, and poetry. Explore with students their ideas about poetry and what the features are in a poem. Use the following teaching notes to discuss and explain the main features of poetry and compare and contrast prose and poetry. Invite students to identify poems that they know and like, poems that they have learned as children and poems that they are covering in lessons. Explore with students the stories that these poems tell and to what extent they contain the elements of the typical stories that we have discussed previously. Introduce to students the idea of the narrative poem or story poem. The narrative poem is the name given to poems which tell a story.	Flipchart or whiteboard. Pen and paper. Teaching notes for session 17.
Provide examples of **narrative poems** for the students and	The students are given the opportunity to listen to a range of popular and powerful story poems. These story poems, in the teaching	Story planner. Poetry examples in

Aims	Method/Activities	Materials
identify the **literary devices** used in each poem.	notes, are read to the students. Each poem is different and uses a variety of literacy devices to develop its story content and theme. Students are supported in identifying the main theme of the poem and the literary devices used in each one, as well as the main story elements using the story planner. The students are invited to comment on each poem and discuss which poems they enjoyed the most, which was their most and least favourite and provide reasons for these choices. Each poem presented in the teaching notes is followed by some initial points of discussion which the facilitator can use to begin to explore the poems. Each poem has been chosen for specific reasons including its frequency and use in schools, its popularity, beauty of language, relevance, fun quality, unique story content, use of literary devices and identifiable story elements which students can map on to the story planner. Facilitators may like to read all the poems and choose a couple of the students' favourite ones to explore in more detail. Each poem can be discussed in more detail with regards to literary devices and story structure and content. The depth and breadth of the discussion will depend on the ability and interest of the students and is left to the discretion of the facilitator. The teaching notes contain all the suggested story poems with some main pointers for discussion which can serve as a good starting point. The facilitator may choose to bring other examples to the session, and may use specific examples of story poems being taught in the classroom.	the teaching notes for session 17.
To revise main areas of narrative covered in the resource through the **story square spiral puzzle**.	The students take turns answering the questions from the story square spiral puzzle. The answer to every question or clue begins with the last letter of the preceding answer. The content areas span all topics covered in the	Story square spiral puzzle in teaching notes for session 17.

 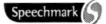

Aims	Method/Activities	Materials
To sum up and revise contents of the session.	narrative programme. Get volunteers from the group to summarise the main content of the session. Ask other members of the group to help, adding in the parts that may have been omitted.	Flipchart or whiteboard, paper and pen.
Mission to Achieve: Students **to continue to build their autobiography of their lives, but this time focusing on their future and how they would like their future to unfold**.	Students have begun working on their autobiographies and will have shared episodes of their autobiographies with the group earlier in the programme. For this Mission to Achieve, they are being asked to focus on building up a picture of their future. This may include details about where they would like to see themselves in ten years' time, what country, what town, what they would like to see themselves doing, who they will be friends with, how they will act and feel, etc. This is an opportunity for students to build a story about their hopes and wishes for their future. Get them to think about their hopes and aspirations for the future so they can share some of these with members of the group next session.	Story planner. It might be helpful for students to have the story planner to help them with their autobiographies.

Evaluation of session/General comments

Teaching notes for Session 17

What is the difference between prose and poetry?

In this session, we want to explore with the students the features of poetry and how it differs from the literature we have already been discussing, i.e. prose. Prose is the name given for the stories we have been talking about thus far in this programme, the stories of books, films and television which can be fiction or non-fiction. There are many similarities between prose and poetry, which we are going to talk about in this session.

Both prose and poetry are expressions, either spoken or written. Poetry is usually written in a more structured way and has a specific rhythm, like a song, and a beat like a drum. Rhythm, a continuous and reoccurring beat, is a feature of all poems.

Prose is the language of everyday and ordinary speech. It is used by speakers and is the language we come across most frequently and use when talking to each other throughout the day, and when telling stories. Prose is a very broad term and refers to many different types of writing and forms of spoken language. Up until this point, we have focused on prose. One can say that the main aim of prose is to convey a message or meaning. Poetry also can convey a meaning; however its main aim is to entertain and evoke feelings in the listener through the use of a range of literary devices.

Poetry is more structured and rhythmical than prose, with a greater variety of literary devices. Most, but not all, poems rhyme, and many of them contain a variety of literary devices that we have already identified in some of the stories we have discussed. Even though these literary devices, like rhyme, metaphor and alliteration, can and do occur in prose (stories), they are more frequently seen in poetry.

What is poetry?

A poem is a verbal composition designed to convey an experience, idea or emotion in a vivid and imaginative way using language that has been specifically chosen for its sound, beauty, and power to evoke deep feelings and emotions. It can also be characterised by its use of literary techniques, for example, metre (the rhythm), metaphor and rhyme. It is a piece of writing which has an intensity or beauty of language and its main focus is typically on the use of language and the beauty it invokes. In poetry, language is used first and foremost for its beauty and power to invoke deep and intense feelings. Poems have a rhythm and beat to them, and many of them contain rhyming words, i.e. words that end with the same rhyming sounds, for example, 'boat' and 'coat'; 'sun' and 'bun'; 'slip' and 'trip'.

We call the person who writes poetry a poet. This is different from the person who writes prose, who we refer to as an author.

The facilitator might like to ask students to provide some examples of their favourite poems, or poems with which they are familiar from the classroom.

The narrative poem

There are poems which have all the features of poetry, i.e. the use of specific literary devices to convey beauty, rhythm and the use of language in vivid and imaginative ways, but also tell a story. These poems are called story or narrative poems.

Narrative poetry is a genre (or type) of poetry that tells a story. In this respect, it is the same as the stories we have already talked about. The narrative poem has a plot. The poems may be long or short, but all will tell a story. In this session, we will introduce the students to some popular narrative poems. The facilitator should encourage the students to sit back and enjoy listening to these story poems. It is advisable for them to be read aloud on more than one occasion to give the students the opportunity to take in their full effect and impact. Students should be encouraged to explore and discuss the following in each poem:

- Identification of the main themes and plot
- Identification of the main story components – beginning, middle, end
- Identification of the characters, time and place
- Identification of the episodes: initial event, immediate response, action/s and reactions
- Identification of any climax or conflict
- Identification of the means taken to resolve the issues
- Identification of the end result and any moral or messages from the poem
- Use of literary devices and their effectiveness
- Use of humour
- The relevance of the theme to life today and key messages that can be learned from the poem.

Evaluate the poems and explore their favourites and the reasons for their choice.

Please read the following narrative poems to the students. You may have your own favourites which you would like to add, or bring along some story poems that are frequently used in class.

Narrative poem 1

'Matilda told such Dreadful Lies,
It made one Gasp and Stretch one's Eyes;
Her Aunt, who, from her Earliest Youth,
Had kept a Strict Regard for Truth,
Attempted to Believe Matilda:
The effort very nearly killed her,
And would have done so, had not She
Discovered this Infirmity.
For once, towards the Close of Day,
Matilda, growing tired of play,

 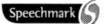

And finding she was left alone,
Went tiptoe to the Telephone
And summoned the Immediate Aid
Of London's Noble Fire-Brigade.
Within an hour the Gallant Band
Were pouring in on every hand,
From Putney, Hackney Downs, and Bow.
With Courage high and Hearts a-glow,
They galloped, roaring through the Town,
"Matilda's House is Burning Down!"
Inspired by British Cheers and Loud
Proceeding from the Frenzied Crowd,
They ran their ladders through a score
Of windows on the Ball Room Floor;
And took Peculiar Pains to Souse
The Pictures up and down the House,
Until Matilda's Aunt succeeded
In showing them they were not needed;
And even then she had to pay
To get the Men to go away!

It happened that a few Weeks later
Her Aunt was off to the Theatre
To see that Interesting Play
The Second Mrs. Tanqueray.
She had refused to take her Niece
To hear this Entertaining Piece:
A Deprivation Just and Wise
To Punish her for Telling Lies.
That Night a Fire *did* break out
You should have heard Matilda Shout!
You should have heard her Scream and Bawl,
And throw the window up and call
To People passing in the Street –
(The rapidly increasing Heat
Encouraging her to obtain
Their confidence) – but all in vain!
For every time she shouted "Fire!"
They only answered "Little Liar!"
And therefore when her Aunt returned,
Matilda, and the House, were Burned.'

'Matilda Who Told Lies, and was Burned to Death'. By Hilaire Belloc, from *The Nation's Favourite Poems of Childhood* (2000), pp60–1.

Some initial areas for discussion include:

- Identify the story of the poem
- Explore main themes of the poem
- Role of humour
- Use of rhyme (for example: 'town' and 'gown'; 'fire' and 'liar')
- Use of direct speech – 'Matilda's House is Burning Down'
- Use of literary device, alliteration (for example: 'Peculiar Pains')
- Use of descriptive words (for example: 'Scream and Bawl')
- Characterisation of the character, Matilda
- Overall message and moral of the poem.

Narrative poem 2

'I wander'd lonely as a cloud
That floats on high o'er vales and hills,
When all at once I saw a crowd,
A host, of golden daffodils;
Beside the lake, beneath the trees,
Fluttering and dancing in the breeze.
Continuous as the stars that shine
And twinkle on the Milky Way,
They stretch'd in never-ending line
Along the margin of a bay:
Ten thousand saw I at a glance,
Tossing their heads in sprightly dance.
The waves beside them danced; but they
Out-did the sparkling waves in glee:
A poet could not but be gay,
In such a jocund company:
I gazed – and gazed – but little thought
What wealth the show to me had brought:
For oft, when on my couch I lie
In vacant or in pensive mood,
They flash upon that inward eye
Which is the bliss of solitude;
And then my heart with pleasure fills,
And dances with the daffodils.'

'Daffodils'. By William Wordsworth, from *The Nation's Favourite Poems* (1996), p17.

Some initial areas for discussion include:

- Identify the story of the poem
- Explore main themes of the poem
- Discuss the way the poet evokes feelings of joy and beauty
- Use of rhyme (for example: 'trees' and 'breeze'; 'glance' and 'dance')
- Use of literary device, simile (for example: 'I wandered lonely as a cloud') – explore with students the comparison between the poet and a cloud
- Use of literary device, personification. Personification is a new literary device that we have not discussed before. It is a device where objects or non-human things are given human qualities. For example: 'Tossing their heads in sprightly dance.' Here, the daffodils, which are non-human, are given the actions of humans, so they toss their heads and dance
- Use of descriptive words (for example: 'sparkling waves in glee')
- Visualisation: Explore with students what they see when they close their eyes and visualise the scene of daffodils. How vivid is their picture, and what makes this poem so powerful and evocative?

Narrative poem 3

'Bent double, like old beggars under sacks,
Knock-kneed, coughing like hags, we cursed through sludge,
Till on the haunting flares we turned our backs
And towards our distant rest began to trudge.
Men marched asleep. Many had lost their boots
But limped on, blood-shod. All went lame; all blind;
Drunk with fatigue; deaf even to the hoots
Of tired, outstripped Five-Nines that dropped behind.
Gas! Gas! Quick, boys! – An ecstasy of fumbling,
Fitting the clumsy helmets just in time;
But someone still was yelling out and stumbling,
And flound'ring like a man in fire or lime ...
Dim, through the misty panes and thick green light,
As under a green sea, I saw him drowning.
In all my dreams, before my helpless sight,
He plunges at me, guttering, choking, drowning.
If in some smothering dreams you too could pace
Behind the wagon that we flung him in,
And watch the white eyes writhing in his face,
His hanging face, like a devil's sick of sin;
If you could hear, at every jolt, the blood
Come gargling from the froth-corrupted lungs,
Obscene as cancer, bitter as the cud
Of vile, incurable sores on innocent tongues,
My friend, you would not tell with such high zest

To children ardent for some desperate glory,
The old Lie; Dulce et Decorum est
Pro patria mori.'

'Dulce Et Decorum Est'. By Wilfred Owen, from *The Nation's Favourite Poems* (1996), p20.

Some initial areas for discussion include:

- Identify the story of the poem
- Explore main theme of the poem
- Discuss the relevance of this theme today: war never being justified
- Explore the feelings that this poem evokes
- Discuss the way the poet evokes feelings of desolation, desperation, death, and terror
- Use of rhyme (for example: 'pace' and 'face'; 'fumbling' and 'stumbling')
- Use of literary device, simile – (for example: 'like old beggars under sacks') – explore with students the comparison between beggars and sacks
- Use of powerful descriptive words (for example: 'vile incurable sores' and 'white eyes writhing in his face')
- Explore with students some of the meanings of words used, (for example: 'drunk with fatigue'; 'smothering dreams' and 'hanging face'
- Visualisation: explore with students what they see when they close their eyes and visualise the scene of war. How vivid is their picture, and what makes this poem so powerful and evocative?

You may also like to read another poem by Wilfred Owen, 'Anthem for Doomed Youth', which is also about the experiences of war. Encourage students to compare and contrast the two poems.

Narrative poem 4

'This morning I was kidnapped
By three masked men.
They stopped me on the side walk,
And offered me some candy,
And when I wouldn't take it
They grabbed me by the collar,
And pinned my arms behind me,
And shoved me in a backseat
Of this big black limousine and
Tied my hands behind my back
With sharp and rusty wire.
Then they put a blindfold on me
So I couldn't see where they took me,
And plugged up my ears with cotton

So I couldn't hear their voices.
And drove for 20 miles or
At least for 20 minutes, and then
Dragged me from the car down to
Some cold and moldy basement,
Where they stuck me in a corner
And went off to get the ransom
Leaving one of them to guard me
With a shotgun pointed at me,
Tied up sitting on a stool...
That's why I'm late for school!'

'Kidnapped!!!' By Shel Silverstein, from *The New Faber Book of Children's Poems*, edited by Matthew Sweeney (2001), p136.

Some initial areas for discussion include:

- Identify the story of the poem
- Explore main themes of the poem
- Role of humour
- Use of rhyme (for example: 'stool' and 'school')
- Use of alliteration (for example: 'big black' and 'masked men')
- Use of descriptive words (for example: 'cold and moldy basement')
- Explore with students whether the poet is being serious in the poem and whether he really was kidnapped. Discuss with them what it means to write or say something with 'tongue in cheek'! This means saying something in a serious way which should be taken as a joke or in a light-hearted manner. It is meant in an ironic way, not to be taken too seriously
- Overall message and moral of the poem
- Use of exclamation mark at the end of the poem
- Explore with students their best excuse for being late for school!

Narrative poem 5

'It is eighteen years ago, almost to the day –
A sunny day with leaves just turning,
The touch-lines new-ruled – since I watched you play
Your first game of football, then, like a satellite
Wrenched from its orbit, go drifting away.

Behind a scatter of boys. I can see
You walking away from me towards the school
With the pathos of a half-fledged thing set free
Into a wilderness, the gait of one
Who finds no path where the path should be.

That hesitant figure, eddying away
Like a winged seed loosened from its parent stem,
Has something I never quite grasp to convey
About nature's give-and-take – the small, the scorching
Ordeals which fire one's irresolute clay.

I have had worse partings, but none that so
Gnaws at my mind still. Perhaps it is roughly
Saying what God alone could perfectly show –
How selfhood begins with a walking away,
And love is proved in the letting go.'

'Walking Away. For Sean'. By C. Day Lewis, from *The Nation's Favourite Poems of Childhood* (2000), p44.

Some initial areas for discussion include:

- Identify the story of the poem
- Explore main themes of the poem
- Discuss with students who 'Sean' is in relation to the poet
- Explore with students the idea that 'love is proved in the letting go'. Do they agree with this sentiment?
- Describe the time and place of the poem and give reasons for their answer
- Explore the feelings that this poem evokes and the feelings of the poet as the father
- Explore how Sean might be feeling and how they felt as students starting a new school
- Compare these feelings with the feelings they have about starting anything new and scary
- Discuss with students the following simile: 'Like a winged seed loosened from its parent stem' – discuss what is being compared to what, and what information this gives us. Why is this such a powerful image that has been created for us?
- Use of rhyme (for example: 'day' and 'play' and 'away'; 'see', 'free' and 'be')
- Use of literary device, simile (for example: 'like a satellite') – explore with students what is being compared to a satellite.

Narrative poem 6

'Gust becos I cud not spel
It did not mean I was daft
When the boys in school red my riting
Some of them laffed

But now I am the dictater
They have to rite like me
Utherwise they cannot pas
Ther GCSE

Some of the girls were ok
But those who laffed a lot
Have al bean rownded up
And hav recintly bean shot

The teecher who corrected my speling
As not been shot at al
But four the last fifteen howers
As bean standing up against a wal

He has to stand ther until he can spel
Figgymisgrugifooniyn the rite way
I think he will stand ther for ever
I just inventid it today'

'Gust Becos I Could Not Spel'. By Brian Patten, from *The Nation's Favourite Poems of Childhood* (2000), p54.

Some initial areas for discussion include:

- Identify the story of the poem
- Explore main themes of the poem
- Discuss the feeling of struggling academically in school and the feelings that the poet is experiencing
- Role of humour
- Discuss the style of the poem and use of spelling errors
- Explore with students what they would do if they were dictator of the world for a day.

Narrative poem 7

I
'The wind was a torrent of darkness among the gusty trees,
The moon was a ghostly galleon tossed upon cloudy seas,
The road was a ribbon of moonlight over the purple moor,
And the highwayman came riding
    Riding–riding–
The highwayman came riding, up to the old inn-door.

He'd a French cocked-hat on his forehead, a bunch of lace at his chin,
A coat of the claret velvet, and breeches of brown doe-skin.
They fitted with never a wrinkle. His boots were up to the thigh.
And he rode with a jewelled twinkle,
    His pistol butts a-twinkle,
His rapier hilt a-twinkle, under the jewelled sky.

Over the cobbles he clattered and clashed in the dark inn-yard,
And he tapped with his whip on the shutters, but all was locked and barred.
He whistled a tune to the window, and who should be waiting there
But the landlord's black-eyed daughter,
    Bess, the landlord's daughter,
Plaiting a dark red love-knot into her long black hair.

And dark in the dark old inn-yard a stable-wicket creaked
Where Tim the ostler listened. His face was white and peaked.
His eyes were hollows of madness, his hair like mouldy hay,
But he loved the landlord's daughter,
    The landlord's red-lipped daughter,
Dumb as a dog he listened, and he heard the robber say–

"One kiss, my bonny sweetheart, I'm after a prize to-night,
But I shall be back with the yellow gold before the morning light;
Yet, if they press me sharply, and harry me through the day,
Then look for me by moonlight,
    Watch for me by moonlight,
I'll come to thee by moonlight, though hell should bar the way."

He rose upright in the stirrups. He scarce could reach her hand,
But she loosened her hair i' the casement. His face burnt like a brand
As the black cascade of perfume came tumbling over his breast;
And he kissed its waves in the moonlight,
    (Oh, sweet, black waves in the moonlight!)
Then he tugged at his rein in the moonlight, and galloped away to the West.

II

He did not come in the dawning. He did not come at noon;
And out o' the tawny sunset, before the rise o' the moon,
When the road was a gypsy's ribbon, looping the purple moor,
A red-coat troop came marching–
    Marching–marching–
King George's men came matching, up to the old inn-door.

They said no word to the landlord. They drank his ale instead.
But they gagged his daughter, and bound her to the foot of her narrow bed;
Two of them knelt at her casement, with muskets at their side!
There was death at every window;
    And hell at one dark window;
For Bess could see, through her casement, the road that *he* would ride.

 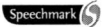

They had tied her up to attention, with many a sniggering jest.
They had bound a musket beside her, with the barrel beneath her breast!
"Now, keep good watch!" and they kissed her.
    She heard the dead man say–
Look for me by moonlight;
    Watch for me by moonlight;
I'll come to thee by moonlight, though hell should bar the way!

She twisted her hands behind her; but all the knots held good!
She writhed her hands till her fingers were wet with sweat or blood!
They stretched and strained in the darkness, and the hours crawled by like years,
Till, now, on the stroke of midnight,
    Cold, on the stroke of midnight,
The tip of one finger touched it! The trigger at least was hers!

The tip of one finger touched it. She strove no more for the rest.
Up, she stood up to attention, with the muzzle beneath her breast,
She would not risk their hearing; she would not strive again;
For the road lay bare in the moonlight;
    Blank and bare in the moonlight;
And the blood of her veins in the moonlight throbbed to her love's refrain .

Tlot-tlot; tlot-tlot! Had they heard it? The horse-hoofs ringing clear;
Tlot-tlot, tlot-tlot, in the distance! Were they deaf that they did not hear?
Down the ribbon of moonlight, over the brow of the hill,
The highwayman came riding,
    Riding, riding!
The red-coats looked to their priming! She stood up, straight and still!

Tlot-tlot, in the frosty silence! *Tlot-tlot*, in the echoing night!
Nearer he came and nearer! Her face was like a light!
Her eyes grew wide for a moment; she drew one last deep breath,
Then her finger moved in the moonlight,
Her musket shattered the moonlight,
Shattered her breast in the moonlight and warned him–with her death.

He turned; he spurred to the West; he did not know who stood
Bowed, with her head o'er the musket, drenched with her own red blood!
Not till the dawn he heard it, his face grew grey to hear
How Bess, the landlord's daughter,
    The landlord's black-eyed daughter,
Had watched for her love in the moonlight, and died in the darkness there.

Back, he spurred like a madman, shouting a curse to the sky,
With the white road smoking behind him and his rapier brandished high!
Blood-red were his spurs i' the golden noon; wine-red was his velvet coat;
When they shot him down on the highway,
    Down like a dog on the highway,
And he lay in his blood on the highway, with the bunch of lace at his throat.

And still of a winter's night, they say, when the wind is in the trees,
When the moon is a ghostly galleon tossed upon cloudy seas,
When the road is a ribbon of moonlight over the purple moor,
A highwayman comes riding–
    Riding–riding–
A highwayman comes riding, up to the old inn-door.

Over the cobbles he clatters and clangs in the dark inn-yard.
He taps with his whip on the shutters, but all is locked and barred.
He whistles a tune to the window, and who should be waiting there
But the landlord's black-eyed daughter,
    Bess, the landlord's daughter,
Plaiting a dark red love-knot into her long black hair.'

    'The Highwayman'. By Alfred Noyes, from *The Nation's Favourite Poems* (1996), pp33–6.

Some initial areas for discussion include:

- Identify the story of the poem
- Explore main themes of the poem
- Explore the vivid setting that the poem details (for example: 'wind was a torrent of darkness')
- Discuss the strong and detailed characterisation of the highwayman and Bess, for example: 'He'd a French cocked-hat on his forehead' and 'The landlord's red-lipped daughter'
- Explore the feelings that this poem evokes: love, sorrow, loss. In what way does the poem evoke these feelings?
- Explore with the group the idea of sacrifice and sacrificing for love. Who made a sacrifice in this poem and how did this happen?
- Discuss the following description of Tim: 'His eyes were hollows of madness'. What was making him appear 'mad'?
- Compare this poem with the poem discussed previously, 'Walking Away. For Sean', which also explores the theme of loss, but in a very different way. How different?
- Use of rhyme (for example: 'coat' and 'throat'; 'moor' and 'door'; 'rest' and 'breast')
- Use of literary device, simile (for example: 'dumb as a dog he listened') – explore with students the comparison between Tim and a dog
- Use of literary device, onomatopoeia (for example: 'clattered and clashed')
- Use of literary device, metaphor (for example: 'road was a ribbon of moonlight') – explore with students the comparison between the road and a ribbon. Discuss with them why this is an example of a metaphor and how it is different to a simile

 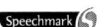

- Use of direct speech, the robber talking directly to Bess
- Use of literary device, alliteration (for example: 'ghostly galleon')
- Use of literary device, repetition (for example: 'A highwayman comes riding–
  Riding–riding–A highwayman comes riding'
- Use of powerful descriptive words (for example: 'gusty trees' and 'drenched with her own red blood')
- The rhythm of the poem and how its speed and beat creates the movement of the highwayman's horses and urgency of the poem
- Visualisation: explore with students what they see when they close their eyes and visualise the scene of blood and death. How vividly can they create this picture of love and loss?
- Contrast the feelings of Tim with those of Bess and the highwayman. Explore with students the emotion of jealousy.

Narrative poem 8

'When I am an old woman I shall wear purple
With a red hat which doesn't go, and doesn't suit me.
And I shall spend my pension on brandy and summer gloves
And satin sandals, and say we've no money for butter.
I shall sit down on the pavement when I'm tired
And gobble up samples in shops and press alarm bells
And run my stick along the public railings
And make up for the sobriety of my youth.
I shall go out in my slippers in the rain
And pick flowers in other people's gardens
And learn to spit.

You can wear terrible shirts and grow more fat
And eat three pounds of sausages at a go
Or only bread and pickle for a week
And hoard pens and pencils and beermats and things in boxes.

But now we must have clothes that keep us dry
And pay our rent and not swear in the street
And set a good example for the children.
We must have friends to dinner and read the papers.

But maybe I ought to practise a little now?
So people who know me are not too shocked and surprised
When suddenly I am old, and start to wear purple.'

'Warning'. By Jenny Joseph, from *The Nation's Favourite Poems* (1996), p45.

Some initial areas for discussion include:

- Identify the story of the poem
- Explore main themes of the poem
- Role of humour
- Discuss with students the age of the poet and encourage them to give reasons for their answer
- Explore what behaviours and activities they would choose to do, when they are old, which would shock
- Explore with students what they think the character is like at present and what her behaviour is like. Is it conventional or eccentric, and how do they know?
- Discuss the use of the literary device, alliteration (for example: 'satin sandals')
- Explore use of descriptive words (for example: 'gobble up' and 'hoard pens and pencils')
- Are students able to visualise the character dressed in purple with a red hat?

Narrative poem 9

'I saw a jolly hunter
with a jolly gun
Walking in the country
In the jolly sun.

In the jolly meadow
sat a jolly hare.
Saw the jolly hunter.
Took jolly care.

Hunter jolly eager –
Sight of jolly prey.
Forgot gun pointing
wrong jolly way

Jolly hunter jolly head
over heels gone.
Jolly old safety catch.
not jolly on.

Bang! went the jolly gun.
Hunter jolly dead.
Jolly hare got clean away.
Jolly good, I said.'

> 'I saw a jolly hunter'. By Charles Causley, from *The Nation's Favourite Twentieth Century Poems*, Edited by Griff Rhys-Jones (1999), p125.

 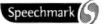

Some initial areas for discussion include:

- Identify the story of the poem
- Explore main themes of the poem
- Discuss the view of the poet towards hunting
- Explore with students their own views about hunting
- Role and type of humour. Explore with students how this is dark or black humour and in what way' Black humour is humour which deals with the more unpleasant things in life in an ironic way. Discuss with students how this poem is an example of black humour
- Comment on style of poem: use of unusual and abbreviated sentences (for example: 'Hunter jolly eager' and 'forgot gun pointing'
- Use of literary device, repetition (for example: repetition of the word 'jolly')
- Explore the use of 'double meanings' and words not always meaning what they usually mean. For example, discuss the use of 'jolly' throughout this poem and whether it is in fact being used to mean cheerful and fun. Discuss the use of the word 'jolly' in the phrase 'jolly dead'. In what different ways is the poet using the word 'jolly'? Explore with students the use of irony, which is the use of words to convey a meaning that is the opposite of its literal meaning. How does the poet use 'jolly' in this poem?
- The rhythm of the poem
- Discuss the use of the exclamation mark at the end of the 16th line.

Narrative poem 10

'Augustus Gloop! Augustus Gloop!
The great big greedy nincompoop!
How long could we allow this beast
To gorge and guzzle, feed and feast
On everything he wanted to?
Great Scott! It simply wouldn't do!
However long this pig might live,
We're positive he'd never give
Even the smallest bit of fun
Or happiness to anyone.
So what we do in cases such
As this, we use the gentle touch,
And carefully we take the brat
And turn him into something that
Will give great pleasure to us all—
A doll, for instance, or a ball,
Or marbles or a rocking horse.
But this revolting boy, of course,
Was so unutterably vile,
So greedy, foul, and infantile
He left a most disgusting taste

Inside our mouths, and so in haste
We chose a thing that, come what may,
Would take the nasty taste away.
"Come on!" we cried, "The time is ripe
To send him shooting up the pipe!
He has to go! It has to be!"
And very soon, he's going to see
Inside the room to which he's gone
Some funny things are going on.
But don't, dear children, be alarmed;
Augustus Gloop will not be harmed,
Although, of course, we must admit
He will be altered quite a bit.
He'll be quite changed from what he's been,
When he goes through the fudge machine:
Slowly, the wheels go round and round,
The cogs begin to grind and pound;
A hundred knives go slice, slice, slice;
We add some sugar, cream, and spice;
We boil him for a minute more,
Until we're absolutely sure
That all the greed and all the gall
Is boiled away for once and all.
Then out he comes! And now! By grace!
A miracle has taken place!
This boy, who only just before
Was loathed by men from shore to shore,
This greedy brute, this louse's ear,
Is loved by people everywhere!
For who could hate or bear a grudge
Against a luscious bit of fudge?'

Extract from *Charlie and the Chocolate Factory*. By Roald Dahl (2008), pp104–5.

Some initial areas for discussion include:

- Identify the story where the extract has come from
- What or who is this poem about?
- Explore main themes of the poem
- Role of humour
- Discuss the strong characterisation of the boy, Augustus Gloop. Question whether students feel they have a strong picture of this boy in their minds. Perhaps even get them to draw Augustus Gloop as they see him
- Explore the name 'Gloop' and what visual image it evokes for the students

- Use of rhyme (for example: 'beast' and 'feast'; 'slice' and 'spice'; 'grudge' and 'fudge')
- The use of strong descriptive words and adjectives (for example: 'The great big greedy nincompoop')
- Use of direct speech – 'Come on!' we cried, 'The time is ripe To send him shooting up the pipe! He has to go! It has to be!'
- Use and effect of the exclamation mark
- Use of literary device, alliteration (for example: 'feed and feast' and 'gorge and guzzle')
- Use of powerful words and synonyms (for example: eat – 'gorge', 'guzzle', 'feed', 'feast')
- Use of the literary device, metaphor. Encourage students to try and find the metaphor. Provide them with clues. Augustus is being compared to an animal, but which one? Get students to identify the metaphor of Augustus being compared to a pig. Discuss why this is a metaphor rather than a simile
- The use of the literary device, repetition (for example: 'A hundred knives go slice, slice, slice')
- Discuss with students the eventual fate of Augustus
- The rhythm of the poem
- Encourage students to list all the many adjectives that have been used to describe Augustus
- Overall message and moral of the poem.

Narrative poem 11

'Two roads diverged in a yellow wood,
And sorry I could not travel both
And be one traveler, long I stood
And looked down one as far as I could
To where it bent in the undergrowth;

Then took the other, as just as fair,
And having perhaps the better claim
Because it was grassy and wanted wear,
Though as for that the passing there
Had worn them really about the same,

And both that morning equally lay
In leaves no step had trodden black.
Oh, I marked the first for another day!
Yet knowing how way leads on to way
I doubted if I should ever come back.

I shall be telling this with a sigh
Somewhere ages and ages hence:
Two roads diverged in a wood, and I,
I took the one less traveled by,
And that has made all the difference'.

'The Road not Taken'. By Robert Frost, from *The Nation's Favourite Poems* (1996), p77.

Some initial areas for discussion include:

- Identify the story of the poem
- Explore main themes of the poem
- Discuss with students what the poet is taking about when he refers to 'two roads'. Explore with students what 'roads' are representing in this poem
- Explore with students the meaning of the road 'less traveled by'
- Discuss with students whether the poet is saying that there is a right and wrong way, or whether there are just a range of choices that we can take. Encourage them to give reasons for their answer
- Describe the time and place of the poem and give reasons for your answer
- Discuss the use of the first person and the impact this has on overall meaning
- Use of rhyme (for example: 'wood' and 'could'; 'day', 'way' and 'lay')
- Discuss with students why taking the road less travelled has 'made all the difference' for him in his life
- Overall message and moral of the poem
- Allow students the opportunity to share when in their own lives they have had a difficult choice to make. What choice did they make and did it work out to be the right choice for that time?

Narrative poem 12

'I leant upon a coppice gate
When Frost was spectre-gray,
And Winter's dregs made desolate
The weakening eye of day.
The tangled bine-stems scored the sky
Like strings of broken lyres,
And all mankind that haunted nigh
Had sought their household fires.

The land's sharp features seemed to be
The Century's corpse outleant,
His crypt the cloudy canopy,
The wind his death-lament.
The ancient pulse of germ and birth
Was shrunken hard and dry,
And every spirit upon earth
Seemed fervourless as I.

At once a voice arose among
The bleak twigs overhead
In a full-hearted evensong
Of joy unlimited;

An aged thrush, frail, gaunt, and small,
In blast-beruffled plume,
Had chosen thus to fling his soul
Upon the growing gloom.
So little cause for carolings
Of such ecstatic sound
Was written on terrestrial things
Afar or nigh around,
That I could think there trembled through
His happy good-night air
Some blessed Hope, whereof he knew
And I was unaware.'

‘The Darkling Thrush’. By Thomas Hardy, from *The Nation’s Favourite Poems* (1996), p67.

Some initial areas for discussion include:

- Identify the story of the poem

- Explore main themes of the poem

- Discuss the ethos and mood created by the poem

- Explore the ways the poet manages to evoke the opposing feelings of desolation and hope

- Identify what he uses to signify hope

- Identify and describe the main character

- Explore the setting (place and time) described powerfully by chosen words and phrases (for example: ‘Frost was spectre-gray’; ‘Winter’s dregs’ and ‘shrunken hard and dry’)

- Identify the literary device of simile: ‘The tangled bine-stems scored the sky
  Like strings of broken lyres’ – discuss the comparison between the stems and strings of a lyre

- Use of rhyme (for example: ‘day’ and ‘gray’; ‘plume’ and ‘gloom’)

- Use of literary device, alliteration (for example: ‘His crypt the cloudy canopy’)

- Use of the first person to narrate the poem

- Use of powerful descriptive words (for example: ‘dregs made desolate’ and ‘shrunken hard and dry’).

- Explore with students some of the meanings of words and phrases used (for example, what do the following phrases mean: ‘weakening eye of day’ and ‘land’s sharp features’?)

- Visualisation: Explore with students what they see when they close their eyes and visualise the winter scene of bleakness and desolation. Can students listen carefully to hear the singing of the thrush? How vivid are the pictures and sounds from this poem and how does the poet succeed in making these images so powerful and evocative?

There are many other poems that you may like to share with the students, poems that tell powerful or funny stories. Try looking at poetry anthologies in the school or public library. For example, you might like to read the poem 'chocs' by Carol Ann Duffy. The story poem is about someone eating their way happily through a box of chocolates, an activity probably experienced by many of the students themselves!

Here are some points for discussion on this poem:
- Identify the story of the poem
- Explore main theme of the poem
- Role of humour
- Discuss the use of the abbreviation 'chocs' for the title
- Discuss with students what this phrase in the poem refers to: 'five finger-piglets'
- Explore the use of some descriptive words used, for example: 'electrifying rustle' and 'dark and glamorous scent'
- Identify use of synonyms for the word, 'eat': 'chomped', 'gorged', 'stuffed my face' – in what way do these words differ from 'eat'. How are they more powerful?
- Discuss the style of the poem and use of the first person to narrate the poem
- Discuss with students whether this is a scenario they experience in their daily lives too
- Which chocolates in their homes always get left in the box?

 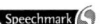

Teaching notes for Session 17

Narrative story square spiral

Write the answers to each clue in the square spiral below, but be careful, the last letter of one answer is the first letter of the next! All answers have something to do with stories and the themes covered, so you should be able to answer them all!

Clues

1   Name of person who writes a book (6 letters)

2   One of the elements of the middle part of the story, one part of the episode (8 letters)

3   The last part of a story (3 letters)

4   A literary device (2 words, 12 letters)

5   Exaggeration (9 letters)

6   Middle part of a story (7 letters)

7   Listening tools (4 letters)

8   Comparing like with like (6 letters)

9   Here's looking at you (2 words, 10 letters)

10   Heading (5 letters)

11   The setting where we and all other living things live (5 letters)

12   A famous and popular character from a fantasy series of books also made into movies (2 words, 11 letters)

13   Type of story genre (7 letters)

14   Always ask questions and look at your strengths and weaknesses (10 letters)

15   A story (9 letters)

16   One uses vocal variety and facial expression to create this and make something stand out (8 letters)

17   Beginning of story on the story planner (7 letters)

18   Another word meaning 'story type' (5 letters)

19   Another adjective meaning 'very very happy' (8 letters)

20   Willy Wonka is one of these in *Charlie and the Chocolate Factory* (9 letters)

21   What you do with a book (4 letters)

22   Words that provide a lot of interesting detail and are illustrative and imaginative are said to be this (11 letters)

23   Later time of day (7 letters)

24   Surname of Augustus from *Charlie and the Chocolate Factory* (5 letters)

25 The main theme or action of a story (4 letters).

26 A component of the setting of a story (4 letters)

27 Another word for 'talk' (7 letters)

28 Framework that we are using in the programme to help us make up exciting stories (2 words, 12 letters)

29 The beat in music or in poetry (6 letters)

30 Aha! A part of the end of a story (5 letters)

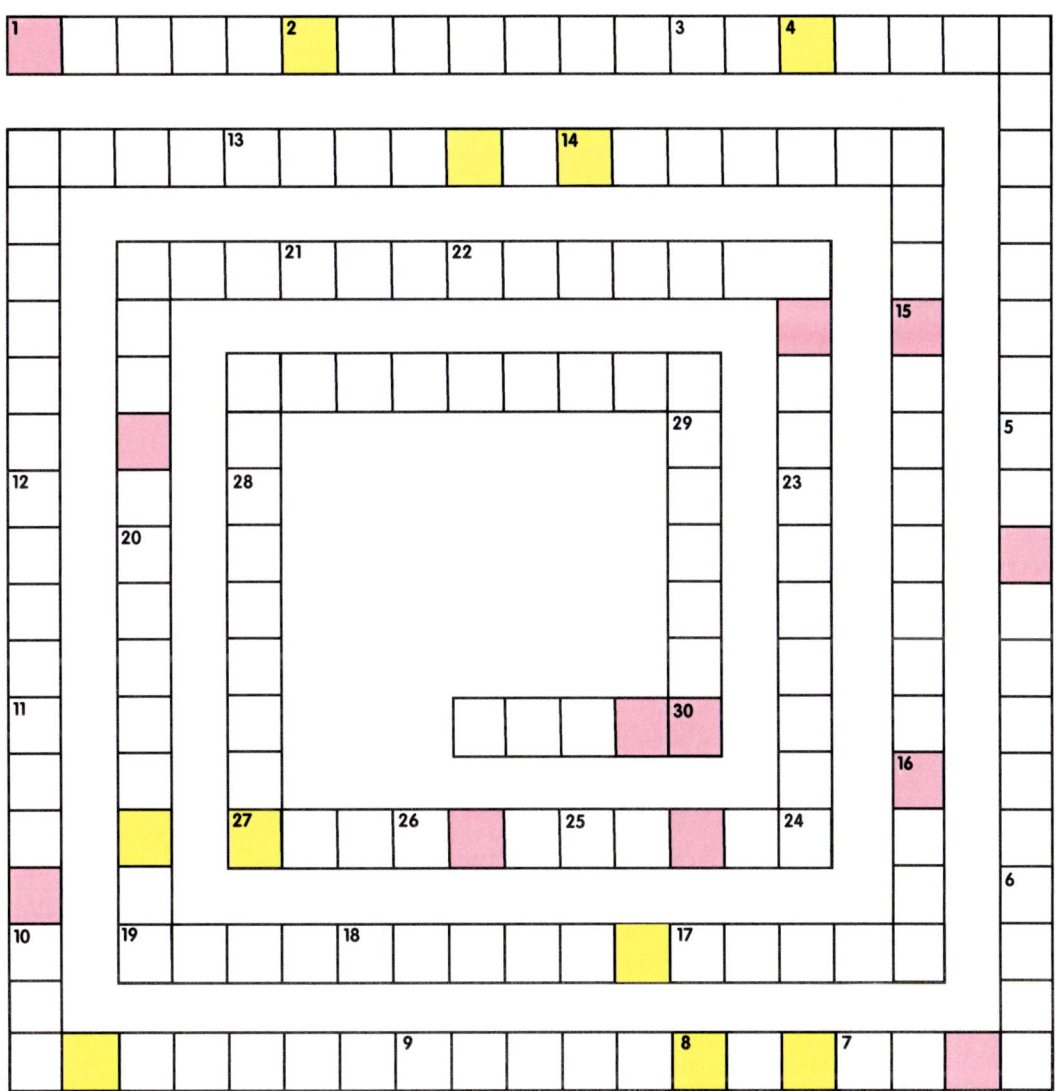

Answers:

*A*UTHO**R** – RESPONSE – END – **D**IRECT SPEECH – HY*P*ERBOLE – EPIS*O*DE – E**A**RS – **S**IMILE –

EYE CON**T**ACT – T*I*TLE – EARTH – HARRY POTTER – ROMA**N**CE – **E**VALUATION – *N*ARRATIV**E** –

EMPHASIS – S**E**TTING – GENRE – EC**S**TATIC – CH*A*RACTER – READ – DESCRIP*T*IVE – EVENI NG –

GL*O*OP – PL*O*T – TIM*E* – EXPRESS – STORY PLANNER – RHYTH*M* – M*O*RAL.

Once the students have completed the story square spiral, take the letters in the yellow shaded squares (or bold) to make a mystery word (a popular television series)[5] and the letters in the pink squares (or italic) to make another literary device[6]. Can students guess what these may be?

---

[5] The answer is *EastEnders*.   [6] The answer is onomatopoeia.

298

18

Session 18

Names of students: _____

_____

Facilitator: _____ Date: _____

School: _____

Class: _____

Aims	Method/Activities	Materials
To revise and recap concepts from the previous sessions, i.e. the entire story planner including all main elements: **beginning**, **middle** and **end**.	Group discussion recapping the main ideas from the previous sessions. Students have now covered all aspects of the story planner and are able to construct a story with all main elements. Revise all three main story elements and their component parts through discussion using the story planner, story F1 race track, story train track, story football match or story athletics race track.	Flipchart or whiteboard, paper and pen. Story planner. Story F1 race track. Story train track and train carriages. Story football match. Story athletics race track.
To revise differences between **prose** and **poetry**.	Review elements of a poem and compare with prose. Ask students to name three of the poems discussed in the previous session.	
Students to **share** their **autobiography** with the group, focusing on their **future story**.	Students have been working on their autobiographies during the programme, and were asked as part of their Mission to Achieve from the last session to consider how they would like their 'stories' to look in the future and to think about how they would like to see their future. They were asked to think about their stories, focusing on their wishes and aspirations for the future. Where do they see themselves in ten years? What will they be doing? Where will they be living? Who will they be spending time with? This is an opportunity for students to share their wishes and aspirations. In the session, they will each have a chance to share their 'future' story with other members of the group. They will	Story planner. It might be helpful for students to have the story planner to help them with their autobiographies.

Aims	Method/Activities	Materials
	have entered into the time capsule and be looking at themselves and their lives in ten years' time. They will tell this story to the group and provide descriptions of the setting that they see themselves in, including time and place. They will also provide a detailed description of themselves as the main protagonist or character of this story. So, who have they become, what type of person are they? They will provide details of the other characters, sharing their life, and recount the main episodes taking place for them at this future time. Students should be reminded that even though this has not happened yet, and they are telling a story about the future, they should make it as real as possible, rather than a fantasy. The aim of this activity is to get students to realistically think about where they are going in their life, about their hopes and dreams, and where they would most like to be in ten years' time. Once all students have shared their 'future story', they can compare them and see how many of their hopes and aspirations are shared. Allow discussion during this activity on how these dreams and aspirations can be achieved so as to ensure the future story becomes a reality and is non-fiction rather than fiction. Facilitate discussions around the steps that students need to take to make their dreams a reality. Explore what they can be doing NOW which may help to make their aspirations come true in the future. Discuss how what they are doing at the moment really matters, and is the perfect preparation for what they will be doing in the future. For example, if one of the students wants to be a lawyer and work in court, explore with the group what needs to happen in school now to prepare him or her for that future. You might like to use an analogy here of a runner or football player. So,	

Aims	Method/Activities	Materials
	for example, neither a runner nor a football player will just get up one morning and run a marathon, or play in a World Cup football final. They will require many months of planning, preparation and hard work if they are going to be successful. This is the same for us all. Students will have a chance to make their 'future stories' realistic and true rather than fantasy or fiction, if they can clearly identify their future goals and aspirations, and are prepared to work hard and do the planning and preparation in the present.	
	Facilitators should be prepared to support discussion around the reality of students' hopes and aspirations. If a student five feet tall, for example, includes in his 'future story' the plan to become a basketball player, this is a good opportunity to discuss the reality of this dream in a safe and supportive environment. Allow students the opportunity to evaluate their own goals and future aspirations and to identify the steps they will need to take to make these dreams a reality. Discuss with students the importance of looking realistically at their dreams and assessing whether the steps they need to take are realistic or impossible. So, for example, having to work really hard to get good grades so that you can study further is a more realistic and achievable aim than planning to grow ten inches in the next year to enable you to become a basketball player!	
	Discuss with students the 'unrealistic' parts of their story and explore other ways of achieving their hopes. For example, if you will never become a basketball player because of your size, is there another future story you can tell which sees you being involved in some other way in basketball, for example, as a sports editor or writer, or manager or coach of the team? One student who wanted to be a footballer, but knew he was not good enough,	

 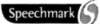

Aims	Method/Activities	Materials
	told a future story where he worked at Wembley stadium maintaining the ground and leading tours around the stadium. That was his future story. Find out what your students' future stories are and encourage them to share them with each other. Why not even share your own future story with them?	
To introduce the students to limericks and discuss them in relation to stories and poetry.	The students are now introduced to another very popular literary form which tells a story: the limerick. Explain to students what limericks are, their structure and typical content. In the last session we introduced poetry to the group and focused on the narrative poem, the poem that tells a story. We will now look at another type of poem which is very popular with many people, even those who don't enjoy poetry! That is, the limerick. A **limerick** is a special type of poem which is made up of five lines with a very strict structure and rhyming sequence. The rhyming sequence is **AABBA**. This means that the first two lines and last line of a limerick rhyme and the middle two lines rhyme with each other. Limericks are usually very funny and humorous, which is probably the reason why they are so popular with many young people. They also have a strict rhythmical structure with the first, second and fifth line having seven to ten syllables and the middle third and fourth sentences having five to seven syllables. A **syllable** is a sound unit with one vowel and one, two or more consonants. You will find more details and a greater description in the teaching notes that follow. Discuss with students the origins of the limerick, its structure and typical content areas. See teaching notes for session 18 for further information about limericks.	Flipchart or whiteboard, paper and pen. The story planner to assist in identifying the main story components of the limerick. Teaching notes for session 18.

Aims	Method/Activities	Materials
Students to **listen to a range of popular published limericks.**	The students are given the opportunity to listen to a range of different published limericks. They are encouraged to identify the main story or plot of each one, and recognise the different story components and the rhyme sequences. Allow discussion of the role of humour in limericks and invite students to evaluate the limericks they hear. Emphasise for students that even a piece of writing as short as a limerick, i.e. five lines, tells a story. Encourage students to identify the different parts of the story, the beginning with the characters, place and time details; the middle, with the main plot and story theme; and the end with the result and message. Not every limerick will have each of these components, but get students to use the story planner to identify which elements of a story each limerick they hear does have. Discuss how humorous they are, which ones tell the funniest or most exciting story, which are their favourites and reasons for their choice. Students should be encouraged to enjoy the limericks and have fun with them! Encourage the students to try to play with words and language, which is what the limericks give them the opportunity to do. Encourage students to identify the word play, rhyme and rhythm by repeating the limericks, allowing them to say their favourite ones out loud, writing them on the whiteboard and circling the rhyming patterns and other literary devices identified.	Story planner for the identification of story components. Examples of published limericks to be read to students.
Students to **devise their own limericks and share them** with the group.	Students now have the opportunity to create their own limericks. They can do this individually, in pairs or in groups. Invite them to think of a main theme that their limerick will be about and remind them to keep to the strict limit of five sentences and to adhere to the structured rhyming sequence.	Flipchart, whiteboard, paper and pen. Story planner to help students write the limerick.

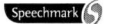

Aims	Method/Activities	Materials
	Read the top tips for writing limericks which are included in the teaching notes. Students need to be reminded to choose their words very carefully as they need to try say a lot in a very short poem of five lines only! Encourage the use of a dictionary, thesaurus and rhyming dictionary, if available, to assist them with this task. Once each student has made up their limerick, they are to read it to the rest of the group. The group discuss and evaluate each limerick in the positive and constructive way that they have been undertaking their evaluations throughout the programme. Students might also like to draw a diagram to depict the main plot or theme of their story.	Examples of published limericks from teaching notes. Dictionary and thesaurus to help students devise their own limericks. Tips on writing limericks in the teaching notes.
To sum up and revise contents of the session.	Get volunteers from the group to summarise the main content of the session. Ask other members of the group to help, adding in the bits that may have been omitted.	Flipchart or whiteboard, paper and pen.
Mission to Achieve: Students are asked to **identify the story components of their favourite songs using the story planner**. Students to bring to the next session the words of their chosen song.	Students are asked to think about their very favourite song and listen carefully to the words. They should consider the story that the song is telling, and identify the different story elements of the song using the story planner. They are to bring in the words of their favourite song to the next session, together with the completed story planner of the song. Note for the facilitator: In the next session we will discuss story songs. The teaching notes for session 19 contain a recommended list of story songs for discussion.	Story planner for each student to use to identify the main story elements from their favourite songs. Story template forms 1 and 2.

Evaluation of session/General comments

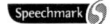

Teaching notes for Session 18

What is a limerick?

A limerick is a popular form of poetry which is often comical, nonsensical or silly and sometimes even rude. It is by its very nature simple and short. It has a very strict structure which makes it a very recognisable form of poetry. A limerick is typically made up of five lines. It has a strict rhyme scheme and a catchy and bouncy rhythm.

The rhyme scheme follows the following sequence:

LINE 1: Rhyming A
LINE 2: Rhyming A
LINE 3: Rhyming B
LINE 4: Rhyming B
LINE 5: Rhyming A

As evident from the above explanation, the first two lines and final fifth line of the limerick all rhyme, i.e. the word endings have the same sound and therefore rhyme with each other; and the two middle lines, the third and fourth line, also rhyme with each other. The final fifth line may sometimes simply repeat the first line.

The limerick follows a specific rhythm, called an anapestic rhythm. This means that the rhyming lines 1, 2 and 5 have seven to ten syllables; and the rhyming lines 3 and 4, have five to seven syllables.

A syllable is a sound structure with one vowel and one or more consonants. For example, the word 'pat' has one syllable, and the word 'patter' has two syllables. Here are some more examples of syllable counting. It may help you to get students to clap as they say the word, as the number of claps will follow the rhythm of the word and will usually coincide with the number of syllables.

- Dog   one syllable
- Ladder   two syllables
- Spaghetti   three syllables
- Caterpillar   four syllables
- Pronunciation   five syllables.

Some additional syllabification exercises

1 Ask students to give you some more examples of one-, two-, three-, four- and five- syllable words.

2   Get students to count how many syllables there are in the following words:

- Ball
- Geography
- History
- Education
- Butterfly
- Hippopotamus
- Tennis
- Cat
- Up
- Happy

Our jaw-dropping technique

Some students may find it quite hard to count the number of syllables in words. Some of our teaching assistants came up with a great way to help them count syllables, a strategy we called the jaw-dropping technique! Basically, students were told to count the number of times that their jaw dropped when saying a word, and that this number would correspond to the number of syllables in the word. Students were encouraged to hold a flat hand, palm down, just below their chin. As they said a word, they counted the number of times their jaw hit their hand. This would usually indicate the number of syllables in a word. No, it is not magic! But every time your mouth gets in the position to make a new vowel, the jaw moves downwards. And if you recall, a syllable will have one vowel and one or more consonants. So, counting how often your mouth moves to form a vowel is actually counting how many syllables there are in that word. So get them doing the jaw-dropping technique if there is any syllable counting confusion!

The limerick typically has the following rhythmical structure:

'da da **DUM** da da **DUM** da da **DUM**
da da **DUM** da da **DUM** da da **DUM**
da da **DUM** da da **DUM**
da da **DUM** da da **DUM**
da da **DUM** da da **DUM** da da **DUM**'.

The limerick has a long history and dates back to the fourteenth century. The word limerick comes from the Irish town of Limerick.

It was a very popular form of poetry used for nursery rhymes and poems for children. Even Shakespeare wrote some limericks. You will find his limericks in his plays *Othello* and *King Lear*. Limericks are usually very funny and witty. They use words in a clever way, often including double meanings, which we have discussed before, where the obvious meaning is not what is intended. Making up limericks is a great opportunity to play around with words and their structure and meanings. Limericks often end with a punch line or surprise ending.

 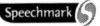

Teaching notes for Session 18

Examples of popular limericks

Here are some examples of limericks. Read them a few times to the students and encourage them to comment on their typical rhyme and rhythmic structure, and invite them to identify the different story components using their story planner.

Most of the limericks will stick to the guidelines given above, but remember as with everything, there are exceptions and some of the limericks will change the rules a little. Get students to check each limerick and see whether they have adhered to the rules of the limerick. If not, get them to identify what is different.

Encourage students to isolate the character and place or time where the limerick is set. Students should identify the main theme and plot of each limerick, the conflict or problem for the character, and the actions taken to get it resolved. Support students to identify all the literary devices that are being used and evaluate their success. Use a group discussion to choose the most and least favourite limericks of the group and identify the reasons for these choices. And most importantly, enjoy reading the limericks and the students will enjoy listening to them. They might even like to read one or two of them aloud themselves.

Limerick example 1

'There was an Old Man with a beard,
Who said, "It is just as I feared! –
Two Owls and a Hen,
Four Larks and a Wren,
Have all built their nests in my beard!" '

   By Edward Lear, from *The Nonsense Verse of Edward Lear* (1984), p27.

Limerick example 2

'There was an Old Man in a tree,
Who was horribly bored by a bee;
When they said, "Does it buzz?"
He replied, "Yes, it does!"
"It's a regular brute of a Bee!"'

   By Edward Lear, from *The Nonsense Verse of Edward Lear* (1984), p28.

Limerick example 3

'There was an Old man who supposed
That the street door was partially closed;
But some very large rats
Ate his coats and his hats,
While that futile Old Gentleman dozed.'

> By Edward Lear, from The Penguin Book of Limericks. Compiled and Edited by E.O. Parrott (1983), p25.

Limerick example 4

'There was an Old Man who said: 'How
Shall I flee from that horrible cow?'
I will sit on this stile,
And continue to smile,
Which may soften the heart of that cow.'

> By Edward Lear, from *The Penguin Book of Limericks*, compiled and edited by E.O. Parrott (1983), p26.

Limerick example 5

'There was a Young Girl of Majorca,
Whose aunt was a very fast walker;
She walked seventy miles,
And leaped fifteen stiles,
Which astonished that Girl of Majorca.'

> By Edward Lear, from *The Penguin Book of Limericks*, compiled and edited by E.O. Parrott (1983), p27.

Limerick example 6

'There was an Old Man on whose nose
Most birds of the air would repose;
But they all flew away
At the closing of day,
Which relieved that Old Man and his nose.'

> By Edward Lear, from *The Penguin Book of Limericks*, compiled and edited by E.O. Parrott (1983), p27.

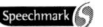

Limerick example 7

'There was an Old Man of Cape Horn,
Who wished he had never been born;
So he sat on a chair,
Till he died of despair,
That dolorous Man of Cape Horn.'

By Edward Lear, from *The Penguin Book of Limericks*, compiled and edited by E.O. Parrott (1983), p28.

Limerick example 8

'There was a Young Lady of Ryde
Whose shoelaces were seldom untied.
She purchased some clogs,
And some small spotted dogs,
And frequently walked about Ryde.'

By Edward Lear, from *The Penguin Book of Limericks*, compiled and edited by E.O. Parrott (1983), p28.

Limerick example 9

'There was a Young Lady of Norway,
Who casually sat in a doorway;
When the door squeezed her flat,
She exclaimed, "What of that?"
This courageous Young Lady of Norway.'

By Edward Lear, from *The Penguin Book of Limericks*, compiled and edited by E.O. Parrott (1983), p29.

Speechmark

Limerick example 10

'There's a Portuguese person named Howell,
Who lays on his lies with a trowel;
Should he give over lying,
T'will be when he's dying,
For living is lying with Howell.'

> By Dante Gabriel Rossetti, from *The Penguin Book of Limericks*, compiled and edited by E.O. Parrott (1983), p31.

Limerick example 11

'There was a painter named Scott,
Who seemed to have hair, but had not.
He seemed to have sense,
'Twas an equal pretence
On the part of the painter named Scott.'

> By Dante Gabriel Rossetti, from *The Penguin Book of Limericks*, compiled and edited by E.O. Parrott (1983), p31.

Limerick example 12

'There was an old man of the Cape,
Who made himself garments of crepe.
When asked: "Do they tear?"
He replied: "Here and there,
But they're perfectly splendid for shape." '

> By Robert Louis Stevenson, from *The Penguin Book of Limericks*, compiled and edited by E.O. Parrott (1983), p34.

Limerick example 13

'There was an Old Man who said "Hush!
I perceive a young bird in this bush!"
When they said, "Is it small?"
He replied, "Not at all!
It is four times as big as the bush!" '

> By Edward Lear, from *The Nonsense Verse of Edward Lear* (1984), p47.

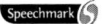

Limerick example 14

'There was an Old Man who said, "Well!
Will *nobody* answer this bell?
I have pulled day and night,
Till my hair has turned white,
But nobody answers this bell!"'

By Edward Lear, from *The Nonsense Verse of Edward Lear* (1984), p73.

Limerick example 15

'There was an Old Man of the coast,
Who placidly sat on a post;
But when it was cold
He relinquished his hold
And called for some hot buttered toast.'

By Edward Lear, from *The Nonsense Verse of Edward Lear* (1984), p71.

Limerick example 16

'There was a young lady of Whitby,
Who had the bad luck to be bit by
Two brown little things
Without any wings,
And now she's uncomfy to sit by.'

By Lewis Carroll, from *The Penguin Book of Limericks*, compiled and edited by E.O. Parrott (1983), p33.

Limerick example 17

His sister, called Lucy O' Finner,
Grew constantly thinner and thinner;
The reason was plain,
She slept out in the rain,
And was never allowed any dinner.'

By Lewis Carroll, from *The Penguin Book of Limericks,* compiled and edited by E.O. Parrott (1983), p33.

Limerick example 18

'There was a young lady of Riga,
Who smiled as she rode on a tiger:
They returned from the ride
With the lady inside,
And the smile on the face of the tiger.'

> By Cosmo Monkhouse, *from The Penguin Book of Limericks*, compiled and edited by E.O. Parrott (1983), p106.

Limerick example 19

'There was a Young Lady of Portugal
Whose ideas were excessively nautical;
She climbed up a tree
Just to look at the sea,
But declared she would never leave Portugal.'

> By Edward Lear, from *The Nonsense Verse of Edward Lear* (1984), p30.

Limerick example 20

'There was an Old Man on the Border,
Who lived in the utmost disorder;
He danced with the Cat,
And made tea in his Hat,
Which vexed all the folks on the Border.'

> By Edward Lear, from *The Nonsense Verse of Edward Lear* (1984), p37.

Limerick example 21

'There was an Old Person whose habits,
Induced him to feed upon rabbits;
When he'd eaten eighteen,
He turned perfectly green,
Upon which he relinquished those habits.'

> By Edward Lear from *The Nonsense Verse of Edward Lear* (1984), p42.

 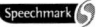

Limerick example 22

'There was an Old Man of Peru,
Who watched his wife making a stew;
But once by mistake,
In a stove she did bake
That unfortunate man of Peru.'

By Edward Lear, from *The Nonsense Verse of Edward Lear* (1984), p57.

Limerick example 23

'There was an Old Man, who when little
Fell casually into a Kettle;
But, growing too stout,
He could never get out,
So he passed all his life in that Kettle.'

By Edward Lear, from *The Nonsense Verse of Edward Lear* (1984), p77.

Limerick example 24

'There was an Old Man of New York,
Who murdered himself with a fork;
But nobody cried,
Though he very soon died,
For that silly Old Man of New York.'

By Edward Lear, from *The Nonsense Verse of Edward Lear* (1984), p123.

Limerick example 25

'There was a Young Lady whose chin,
Resembled the point of a pin;
So she had it made sharp,
And purchased a harp,
And played several tunes with her chin.'

By Edward Lear, from *The Nonsense Verse of Edward Lear* (1984), p205.

Teaching notes for Session 18

Encourage students to now make up their own limericks. They have heard quite a few and have chosen their favourites and given reasons for their choice. They can, if they wish, copy the theme of their favourite limerick, or start a completely new idea. Invite them to be as creative and flexible as they wish, using words and language in exciting, unique and eccentric ways. This is the time when they can pay less attention to grammar and using 'proper English' and really have some fun with their language. All they need to do is keep to the rhythmic structure of the limerick and adhere to the rhyming sequence and five-line limit. And then, they are completely free to play and go wild with words!

Students may like to work on their own, in pairs or in groups. Give them some time to make up their limericks, and once they have done this, get them to write them down and share them with the group members. They will also enjoy illustrating their limericks, so they become both poets and illustrators in this session!

Here are some guidelines which students will find helpful when constructing their limericks.

Tips on writing your own limerick

1   Choose a character and a name of a place.

2   Think of some words which rhyme with your place name. Remember that limericks are meant to be funny so your rhymes can be silly and you can even use nonsense words.

3   Find two rhyming words, which introduce your character and place, to end your first and second line of the limerick. For example: '**There was a crazy dude called Dane, who came from sunny old Spain**'.

4   Now, think of a main theme, problem or conflict that involves your character, and describe it in the next two rhyming lines. For example: '**He got into a big mess, while wearing a pink dress**'.

5   And finish the final and fifth line with some type of resolution or punch line which marks the ending, and which rhymes with the first two lines. For example: '**and from there on was always insane**!'

6   Remember the rhythmical sequence of the limerick:

> 'da da **DUM** da da **DUM** da da **DUM**
>
> da da **DUM** da da **DUM** da da **DUM**
>
> da da **DUM** da da **DUM**
>
> da da **DUM** da da **DUM**
>
> da da **DUM** da da **DUM** da da **DUM**'.

 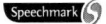

7   Your limerick must always adhere to the specific rhyme structure with the first, second and final lines rhyming and the middle third and fourth lines rhyming with each other. Remember the AABBA pattern.

8   Limericks often start with the first line identifying a character or a place or location.

9   Try and make your limerick funny, smart, clever or witty.

10 Use word play, double meanings and other literary devices that we have discussed previously.

11 Try ending your limerick with a surprise, cliffhanger or punch line. Surprise the listener!

12 And have fun writing them, telling them and listening to them!

Session 19

Names of students: _____

_____

Facilitator: _____ Date: _____

School: _____

Class: _____

Aims	Method/Activities	Materials
To revise and recap concepts from the previous sessions, with a focus on different ways of telling stories through **prose and poetry**.	Group discussion recapping the main ideas from the previous sessions. Revise the differences between prose and poetry and discuss the new terminology learned around poetry and the different literary devices that are used in both poetry and prose, but more so in poetry, to make the story more exciting and captivating. Emphasise for students that whatever form is used to tell a story, the main principles remain: the need for active listening by the listener, and the requirements for the story to be well structured with the appropriately sequenced main story elements making up the beginning, middle and end.	Flipchart or whiteboard, paper and pen. Story planner.
Explore with students their **favourite songs, and the stories that these tell, using the story planner to identify the different story elements.**	Discuss with students how songs are an excellent vehicle for storytelling and how many favourite and successful songwriters use this art form to share their hopes, feelings and dreams through story songs. Explore with students the main differences between prose, poetry and songs. Discuss how all three art forms tell stories and relay messages, and all use a variety of literary devices. Poetry and songs will use, by their very nature, a greater quantity and variety of these literacy devices. For example, they will find	Completed story planner from each student with details of favourite songs.

 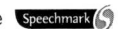

Aims	Method/Activities	Materials
	more examples of rhyme and alliteration in poetry than in prose. These literary devices are also evident frequently in songs. In addition to this, songs, like poems, have a definite rhythm to them. Songs, however, have an additional component in that their words and stories are set to music. Discuss with the group each student's favourite song and explore the reasons for their choice. Encourage students to consider why the specific song they have chosen touched them in such a powerful way. In what ways were they able to identify with the sentiments and messages expressed in the song? Students are to be encouraged to share the story that their chosen song tells, and use their prepared story planner to identify the main story components. Students are of course most welcome to sing their song choices! Discuss with students how the songwriters tell the story and what story techniques and literary devices they use to make their meaning more powerful and get their messages across to the listener. Encourage students to evaluate how successful these techniques are, and in what ways they are effective. Discuss with students how some songs aim to tell a story and may have a similar story structure to that of a more conventional story. These songs are called story songs.	
To **listen to and explore the meaning and stories of a variety of story songs.**	Introduce to students the story song, a song which tells a story using some or all of the story components discussed. The teaching notes include a range of examples of story songs which the facilitator reads to the students, many of which will be recognisable to them. The words of the suggested songs can be easily accessed	Flipchart or whiteboard, paper and pen. Story planner. Recommended titles of story songs in

Aims	Method/Activities	Materials
	through the internet or school library. The facilitator may choose not only to read the words of the songs to the students, but to play the songs as well. The facilitator may also like to bring the words and music of other story songs, not included in the programme, or use the words and themes of the songs brought in by students for their Mission to Achieve. Students take turns summarising the main themes or plots of the story songs, and identify the story components using the story planner. Students should be facilitated in identifying the setting of the story song, the main characters, time and place where the song takes place; the episodes of the story, the initial happening or event, the immediate response/s and actions and further reactions that take place. They are to discuss the main conflicts or problems faced by the characters, and explore how these problems are resolved, if they are resolved at all. Explore with students the outcome of the story song, the result and any meaning or message that the songwriter is trying to impart. Identify with students the literary devices that have been employed in the story song and discuss how effective these are. Encourage the group to discuss the role of the music in telling the story. Encourage students to consider in what ways the music adds power to the words and creates a certain ethos or mood which enhances the overall story. The group discuss which story songs are their most and least favourite and provide reasons for their choice. Encourage them to evaluate the story songs in the same way that they have been evaluating other stories and poems and their own stories. They might like to revisit the evaluative questions from the teaching notes for session 15 to help them with their evaluations.	teaching notes for session 19. The facilitator should bring to the session the words and/or music to all or some of the story songs. Evaluative questions from teaching notes for session 15.

 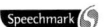

Aims	Method/Activities	Materials
	All of the chosen songs have their own meanings and messages that are being imparted to the listener. Encourage the students to listen carefully to the words of the songs and explore what the underlying meanings and messages are. Explore with students how these messages may relate to them and their lives. This discussion will lead well into the next activity where students are asked to tell their own stories around the message or meaning taken from their chosen song.	
To **construct and tell stories around the main theme** of one of their chosen story songs.	Students are asked to choose one story song from the story songs read to them in the previous activity, and identify the main theme, plot or message from the song. They are then to take this theme or message, and tell their own story around the same theme. However, their story should reflect their own life and experiences and should not be a reworking or repetition of the story from the story song. This is an opportunity for students to share something about their own life, a conflict or problem that they had to deal with, which has some similarity or resonance with the theme covered in their chosen song. Encourage students to choose any theme they wish from the story songs discussed in this session. The songs will have different meanings for each student, and students will interpret the songs in many different ways. Encourage them to find their own meaning and message from the song, which they can then weave into their own story about some episode or incident in their life. Below are some examples of themes and ideas from some of the story songs which can get students started. Some examples of themes and ideas from the songs are: **'The Windmills of Your Mind'** • The passing of time and of life	Story pencil or microphone. Story planner. Story template form 1. Story template form 2.

Aims	Method/Activities	Materials
	• Regrets	
	• Memories	
	• The circle of life	
	• Journey of life.	
	'Every Breath You Take'	
	• Death and loss	
	• Losing a loved one	
	• Missing a loved person	
	• Jealousy.	
	'Cats in the Cradle'	
	• Time is short and precious	
	• Doing what is important in life	
	• Prioritising and giving time to those you love	
	• You get out of life what you put into it	
	• People will treat you as you treat them.	
	'Leader of the Pack'	
	• First love	
	• Forbidden love	
	• Breaking up	
	• Loss and sorrow	
	• Loss at two levels: separation through break-up and final separation through death	
	• Grief and regret	
	• Guilt and feeling responsible.	
	'A Boy Named Sue'	
	• Living with some type of embarrassment	
	• Holding a long-term grudge	
	• Forgiving and forgetting	
	• Growing up	
	• Learning a lesson	
	• Changing a long-held view, belief or perspective.	

 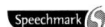

Aims	Method/Activities	Materials
	'At Seventeen' • Growing up • Growing pains • Loneliness • Not fitting in or being in the 'in' crowd • Dating and friendships. **'Starmaker'** • Longing, wishing, dreaming • Having aspirations • Settling down • Moving on • Making choices. **'The Gambler'** • Learning life lessons • Taking advice from someone more experienced • Knowing when you should keep pushing at something • And knowing when to walk away. **'Ben'** • The power of friendship • Friendship being blind • Acceptance • Belonging • Being different. **'Coat of Many Colours'** • Growing up in poverty • What it means to be truly rich or poor • Rich – much more than about money • Being loved and nurtured by parents • Being different at school • Being bullied • Being proud of your roots, where you come from.	

Aims	Method/Activities	Materials
	'Daniel' • Moving on • Loss of a loved one • Memories • Returning home • Longing for another place. **'Better Get to Livin'** • Living life • Forgiveness • Living each day • Life is short so make the best of it • Live a worthwhile life • The power to live the life you choose • The role of prayer and belief. **'Vincent (Starry Starry Night)'** • The power of visualisation • Freedom • Mental health and well-being • Life and death • Sorrow and loneliness • Unrequited love • The power of art and Vincent's paintings. **'Tears in Heaven'** • The power of love • Loss and bereavement • Life beyond what we know – heaven • Expression of one's feelings through song and other art forms. Students are to choose one of the themes or messages from the songs and make up their own story, their own personal narrative, to share with the group. They can choose any song and construct their own personal story around any of the themes or messages that they took from the song.	

 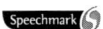

Aims	Method/Activities	Materials
	Remind students to make up well structured stories using the story planner to assist them in providing all the necessary story elements. Students may also like to use one of the story template forms to help them with their planning and sequencing. Encourage students to use a range of literary devices that have been discussed earlier to enhance their story, for example, hyperbole, repetition, simile. When telling their story, remind them to use the many different strategies that have been discussed to make the telling of the story more exciting and ensure the audience is captivated and engaged, for example, using direct speech and vocal variety. Ensure that when they are listening to the stories of their fellow group members, they show all the behaviours that have been identified for active listening.	
To **revise all the ideas, concepts and terminology of storytelling** covered through a word maze search activity.	Students take turns finding the words in the word maze included in the teaching notes. A list of words related to storytelling is provided and students are required to find each word in the word maze. All the words listed are in the word maze, except one! And students have to find all the words, and work out which is the one that is not in the maze. The words in the maze may be written in any direction: upwards or downwards, backwards or forwards as well as in a diagonal line. Please note that letters in the maze may be used twice for different words. Students need to show excellent observational skills to find all the words. They have lots of words to find, there are 59 of them in total! The students can complete this activity in smaller groups, and the group who manages to find the largest number of words in the maze is the winner. Alternatively students can complete the maze individually and compete with each member of the group.	Word maze in teaching notes for session 19.

Aims	Method/Activities	Materials
To sum up and revise contents of the session.	Get volunteers from the group to summarise the main content of the session. Ask other members of the group to help, adding in the parts that may have been omitted.	Flipchart or whiteboard, paper and pen.
Mission to Achieve: Students are asked to think about three of their favourite characters and episodes or events from books, movies or television.	Students are requested to choose three of their favourite characters from any book (for example, Lord Voldemort or Harry Potter from the *Harry Potter* book and film series), movie (perhaps James Bond himself!) or television series (for example, Freddie or Effy from *Skins* or the coach, Sue Sylvester in *Glee*), as well as three action events or episodes (for example, the Kung Fu tournament at the end of *The Karate Kid* movie or an episode from the television series *Dr Who*) and bring these six examples with them to the next session. They are to keep these a secret from the rest of the group, as they will be asked to act them out for the group in the next session, and for group members to see if they can guess which characters and events they are portraying.	

 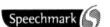

Evaluation of session/General comments

Teaching notes for Session 19

Examples of story songs

Here are some examples of famous favourite story songs. In preparation for this session, the facilitator will have chosen a selection of story songs from this list and accessed the words (and perhaps even the music) for each one. Read (and play) some of the songs to the students and encourage them to consider the following:

- The main story components using the story planner.

- The setting, time and place where the song is set.

- The main character or characters in the song.

- The main story theme or plot of the song.

- The initiating event or first thing that happens to start off the events of the story song.

- The immediate response/s of the character/s to this initial event.

- The subsequent actions taken by the character/s to resolve the story conflict or problem.

- The way the story song ends, the outcome, results and any messages or morals to be taken.

- The use of literary devices to enhance the storytelling.

- The role of the music and its impact and effect on the overall story and enjoyment of the song.

- Evaluation of all aspects of the story song and reasons for their comments.

- The relevance of the story and theme or message of the song for their own lives. Students will be asked, after listening to all the songs, to tell their own story around one of the themes or conflicts of the story songs they have just listened to, so they should be listening to them and thinking about whether they have experienced similar events, feelings, problems, etc.

Story song example 1

'The Windmills of Your Mind'

Words and music by Alan and Marilyn Bergman and Michel Legrand and written for the 1968 movie, *The Thomas Crown Affair*.

Story song example 2

'Every Breath You Take'

Words written by Sting and sung by The Police in 1983.

 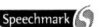

Story song example 3

'Cat's in the Cradle'

Written by Harry Sandy and Chapin in 1974 and performed by Cat Stevens.

Story song example 4

'Leader of the Pack'

Written by George Morton in 1964 and performed by The Shangri-Las.

Story song example 5

'A Boy Named Sue'

Written by Shel Silverstein and performed by Johnny Cash in 1969.

Story song example 6

'The Father of a Boy Named Sue'

Students may like to hear this follow-up song written by Shel Silvestein many years later in which he tells the old father's point of view.

Story song example 7

'At Seventeen'

Written and performed by Janis Ian in 1975.

'Story song example 8

'Starmaker'

Song written by Bruce Roberts and Carole Bayer Sager and performed by The Kids From Fame (Debbie Allen, Lee Curreri, Erica Gimpel, Carlo Imperato, Valerie Landsburg, PR Paul, Gene Anthony Ray and Lori Singer). It was released in September 1982.

Story song example 9

'The Gambler'

Written by Don Schlitz and performed by Kenny Rogers in 1978.

Story song example 10

'Ben'

Written by Walter Scharf and Don Black in 1972 and performed by Michael Jackson.

Story song example 11

'Coat of Many Colours'

Dolly Parton is reported to have written this famous song of hers in 1969 on the back of a dry cleaning receipt while on a bus tour! She recorded it in 1971.

Story song example 12

'Daniel'

Written by Elton John and Bernie Taupin and performed by Elton John. The song was released in 1973.

Story song example 13

'Better Get to Livin' '

Written and performed by Dolly Parton and released in 2007.

Story song example 14

'Vincent (Starry Starry Night)'

Written by Don McLean in 1971 in memory of the artist Vincent van Gogh.

Story song example 15

'Tears in Heaven'

A song written by Eric Clapton and Will Jennings about the pain Clapton felt following the death of his four-year-old son, Conor, who fell from a window of a New York apartment in 1991.

 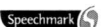

Teaching notes for Session 19

Word maze search

Can you find as many as possible of these words, related to storytelling which are listed below? The words can appear in any direction, they can be horizontal, vertical or diagonal, backwards or forwards. Some letters may also be used twice to make up different words. There is one small catch, though. One of the words, and only one, is not in the word maze. Can you identify which one that is?

1 Protagonist	22 Action	43 Soft
2 Setting	23 Autobiography	44 Horror
3 Listening	24 Narrative	45 Fable
4 End	25 Cliffhanger	46 Rhyme
5 Beginning	26 Fiction	47 Poem
6 Middle	27 Author	48 Loud
7 Result	28 Title	49 Body
8 Conflict	29 Time	50 Who
9 Adjective	30 Reaction	51 Plan
10 Limerick	31 Episode	52 Song
11 Onomatopoeia	32 Low	53 Rate
12 Moral	33 Outcome	54 When
13 Climax	34 Turntaking	55 Look
14 Character	35 Gesture	56 Voice
15 Plot	36 Pitch	57 Tell
16 Simile	37 Genre	58 Tale
17 Metaphor	38 Crime	59 Where
18 Hyperbole	39 Theme	60 Poet
19 Biography	40 High	
20 Place	41 Romance	
21 Illustrator	42 Mystery	

And remember, 59 words are in the maze, and one is not! Can you find the odd one out?

```
P  R  O  T  A  G  O  N  I  S  T  M  E  O  P  A
R  M  Y  S  T  E  R  Y  A  E  R  E  H  W  U  U
E  R  O  U  T  C  O  M  E  N  C  D  V  T  K  T
S  P  S  M  I  D  D  L  E  D  R  H  O  H  C  H
U  F  L  H  O  R  R  O  R  E  K  B  I  E  I  O
L  A  R  A  T  E  O  P  G  A  I  B  C  M  R  R
T  B  A  T  C  D  M  N  J  O  L  D  E  E  E  N
L  L  T  E  E  E  A  D  G  S  L  F  U  O  M  Q
A  E  E  L  T  H  B  R  Q  L  U  Y  I  O  I  C
R  W  A  L  F  T  A  E  S  I  S  I  M  I  L  E
O  R  D  F  R  P  H  V  F  S  T  W  N  A  L  P
M  N  I  P  H  S  I  I  F  T  R  S  O  N  G  I
E  L  E  Y  B  H  G  T  I  E  A  N  X  M  T  S
C  R  H  Y  M  E  H  A  C  N  T  Y  E  O  L  O
G  N  I  T  T  E  S  R  T  I  O  T  L  H  O  D
A  C  T  I  O  N  S  R  I  N  R  P  E  N  W  E
R  O  M  A  N  C  E  A  O  G  K  C  R  I  M  E
R  E  A  C  T  I  O  N  N  H  S  E  R  N  E  G
E  M  I  T  L  O  O  K  M  E  T  A  P  H  O  R
T  O  N  O  M  A  T  O  P  O  E  I  A  O  H  W
C  B  O  D  Y  X  T  U  R  N  T  A  K  I  N  G
A  D  G  U  A  A  T  H  Y  P  E  R  B  O  L  E
R  R  T  M  L  I  I  C  O  N  F  L  I  C  T  U
A  O  I  E  K  U  T  B  E  G  I  N  N  I  N  G
H  L  S  O  F  T  L  E  V  I  T  C  E  J  D  A
C  P  I  T  C  H  E  B  I  O  G  R  A  P  H  Y
```

Session 20

Names of students: _____

_____

Facilitator: _____ Date: _____

School: _____

Class: _____

Aims	Method/Activities	Materials
To revise and recap concepts from the previous sessions and draw together all the themes covered in the sessions.	Group discussion recapping the main ideas from the previous sessions. Encourage students to draw together the areas covered and identify the main elements to be aware of when telling a story. This is a good opportunity to review the whole programme and emphasise the most important aspects around storytelling. Get the students to help you do this as it provides you with an important picture of what aspects of the programme they have retained and what areas may still require some revision and expansion over the last two sessions and beyond.	Flipchart or whiteboard, paper and pen. Story planner.
Students act out their chosen favourite characters and episodes or events from books, movies or television series.	As part of their Mission to Achieve for the last session, students were asked to select three of their favourite characters from any book, movie or television series (for example, Neo from *The Matrix*, Lord Voldemort or Harry Potter from the *Harry Potter* series or even James Bond!), as well as three action events or episodes (for example, the Kung Fu tournament at the end of *The Karate Kid* movie, an incident from Hogwarts School of Witchcraft and Wizardry from a *Harry Potter* movie or the final scenes from *The Matrix*) and bring these six examples with them to this session. Students have the opportunity to take turns and	Story planner. Any props that students have and would like to use to role play their chosen characters and action events.

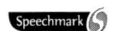

Aims	Method/Activities	Materials
	act out these examples for the rest of the group. So students will act out their favourite chosen character (for example, walk as they do, talk as they do) as well as act out their favourite chosen action or event in a movie, book or television series. The rest of the group have to guess the character or action or episode that the student is acting out. Students must try and act out their characters and action events as closely as possible to the 'real' characters and events to help with the guessing. The winner is the student who acts out the role plays so well, that group members guess them in the fastest time using the lowest number of guesses. Once the group have successfully guessed the character and/or event, they are to provide reasons why these were their favourites.	
To practise **story construction** incorporating all elements of the **story planner** and integrating all the information covered in the preceding sessions.	In this session, the focus is on practising the **storytelling skills** that have been covered previously and revisiting concepts that you feel are less understood by the students. This is the opportunity to revise skills and concepts that have been covered previously. The students are presented with seven different objects and have to choose four. The suggested objects all provide much interest and allow for many different storytelling options and interpretations. However the facilitator may like to bring in other objects, or even get the students to choose their own objects. What is important in this task is that students get an opportunity to construct a story and share it with the group, practising the many skills they have gained. Students are required to construct a well structured and coherent story using all four objects. Students are encouraged to work on their stories in pairs or smaller groups using the story planner to ensure that their story contains	Flipchart or whiteboard, paper and pen. Story planner. Story template form 1. Story template form 2. Students may find it useful to have the story F1 race track, the story football match or the story athletics race track available to assist them with this activity. Story pencil or microphone.

Aims	Method/Activities	Materials
	all the required story elements. Encourage the students to recall what they need to include, to make their stories more interesting. They should try use a range of the literary devices that have been discussed previously. The objects need to be integrated seamlessly into the story plot. This will be a challenge as it is a difficult task. Students need to think about how each object will contribute to the overall story plot and how each object will be introduced in the story and add to the overall meaning. Encourage students to take time to PLAN and discuss with other group members. They may like to use a pen and paper to record their ideas. Students should also be encouraged to plan their stories using the story template forms to assist them in the sequencing of ideas. After a period of preparation time, students take turns (using the story pencil or microphone) to share their story with the rest of the group. Encourage those listening to actively listen to each student using the positive active listening behaviours that have been identified in session 2. Encourage the storytellers to use greater variety in their vocal delivery, discussed in session 16, for example, different loudness and pitch levels, as well as to use facial expression and body language. The group evaluate whether the students have managed to integrate all four objects into an interesting and exciting story. They are also encouraged to evaluate whether the story has all the required elements from the story planner, is exciting, uses a variety of literary devices, has a logical sequence and order and	Story objects: including: **plaster, train ticket, part of a map (torn part), lock and key, whistle, money, battery.** You may also have brought in other interesting objects to use. Students to choose four of the above objects around which they are to base their stories. Students to draw on all the information that has been used in previous sessions and this information should be available to them in the form of photocopies. These should include strategies for active listening, strategies to make a story more interesting, ways of varying vocal delivery, etc. Students will use both the story planner and the story templates, where appropriate, to help structure their stories.

 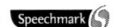

Aims	Method/Activities	Materials
	has captured the attention of the listeners. The students should be encouraged to ask questions about each story which will assist them in their evaluation of the stories produced. Suggested questions are included in the teaching notes for session 15. Each story is rated using a 1–10 rating scale and the person or group with the highest score is the story king or queen of this activity.	Evaluative questions in teaching notes for session 15.
To practise constructing different **types of stories or story genres**.	In this activity, students give each other three objects. They therefore do not choose the objects themselves. They can be the same objects used in the activity above, or the students can choose any three objects that are around them. They are then required to construct different types of stories. Students take turns (using the story pencil or microphone) to make up and share the following types of stories using the three objects given to them by their fellow group members: • Romantic story • Adventure story • Mystery story • Science fiction story • Horror story • Narrative poem. Encourage students to use the story planner and the story template forms to assist them with their story construction. Reinforce the importance of building a story using the main story elements they have learned about from the story planner, and structuring their story following a logical sequence of events. Students are to be encouraged to make their stories as unique and captivating as possible, using a story climax, cliffhanger, exciting plot, detailed character, time and place descriptions, use of descriptive words and various literary devices to enhance their storytelling.	Story planner. Story template forms 1 and 2. Story pencil or microphone. Objects as above.

Aims	Method/Activities	Materials
	Discuss with the group some of the main differences between the different story genres (types) given above. What plot would they need to devise for a romantic story that would be different for a horror story or a mystery? Where would a climax be most appropriate – in a romance or in a mystery story? Encourage students to consider the need to build up the suspense and even to have a cliffhanger for a horror story. Get them to discuss how this would be different from a romantic story, and how this would then differ from a mystery. Group discussion to observe how the objects are used differently depending on the type of story being told. Stories are again evaluated by the group and rated. Once again, a story king or queen is chosen.	
To construct a **narrative around a historical figure** that they have learned about in class.	In this task, students have the opportunity to choose a famous historical figure that they have learned about in class. It could be a famous historical character from any of their lessons, for example, history or English. Students should not tell the rest of the group who they are but each student will have the opportunity to tell a story about this historical figure. They are to provide as much of a detailed character description of the historical figure as possible, and provide details of the time and place when and where the character lived. Their story should contain the main or one of the most important episodes in that historical figure's life, as well as information on how it was resolved and ended. For example, students may choose Queen Victoria, Oliver Cromwell, Abraham Lincoln or Napoleon as their historical figure. The student is to construct and share this story with the rest of the group. They should be reminded that the story needs to be well	Story planner. Story template form 1. Story template form 2. Story pencil or microphone.

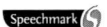

Aims	Method/Activities	Materials
	structured with all the main story elements from the story planner. They should not divulge to the group which historical figure they are talking about, but should provide enough clues in their story that members of the group are able to successfully guess the historical figure under discussion.	
To sum up and revise contents of the session.	Get volunteers from the group to summarise the main content of the session. Ask other members of the group to help, adding in the parts that may have been omitted.	Flipchart or whiteboard, paper and pen.
Mission to Achieve: To **choose a book** they would like to begin to read after completion of the programme. To **revisit and complete their learning profiles** and evaluate what they have learned.	For the final session, students are asked to think about a book that they would now like to begin reading. It can be any book, a book that they have wanted to read for a long time but haven't, a book which was covered and discussed in the programme, a book from school, or a new book that they have only just discovered. They are asked to bring the name of the book to the final session. Students are also asked to revisit the learning profiles that they completed at the beginning of the programme. They are given a new learning profile to take home and complete for next session, thinking about what they have learned from the programme and whether they have met their targets. They are also to consider what areas they still wish to explore further.	Learning profiles completed by each student in the first session. Facilitator to distribute these profiles to students.

Evaluation of session/General comments

 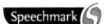

MY LEARNING PROFILE

Name: _____

Date: _____

Class: _____

1   In this programme, I have learned all about…

```



```

2   After having taken part in this storytelling/narrative programme, I can now see different ways that speaking, listening and storytelling are important in my life. These include…

```



```

3   The best part about participating in this narrative programme was…

4   The worst part about participating in this narrative programme was…

5   The three main areas that I have got better at in speaking, listening and storytelling are:

-

-

-

 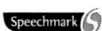

6   I know that I have got better in these areas because…

7   The three areas which are sometimes still difficult for me around speaking, listening and storytelling are:

-
-
-

8   I know that these are still difficult for me because…

9   Some of the things I learned to do in this programme, to help me with these difficult areas include…

10 The three main targets that I wanted to work and improve on by being involved in this programme were:

-

-

-

11 I have achieved the following targets which I chose at the start of the programme.

 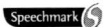

12 I know I have achieved these targets because…

13 I have not achieved the following targets which I identified for myself at the start of the programme…

14 The reason I have not achieved them is because…

15 The areas that I still want to improve on in speaking, listening and storytelling are…

16 I am going to work on them by…

17 The three ways that I am going to use what I have learned from this programme in school are:

-
-
-

18 The three ways that I am going to use what I have learned in this programme at home are:

-

-

-

19 The three ways that I am going to use what I have learned in this programme when spending time with my friends are:

-

-

-

I have worked very hard on this programme and am proud of everything I have achieved.

⭐ **WELL DONE** ⭐

Name: _____

Signature: _____

Signature and comments of facilitator: _____

_____

_____

Session 21

Names of students: _____

_____

Facilitator: _____ Date: _____

School: _____

Class: _____

Aims	Method/Activities	Materials
To revise and recap on the main aims and content of the storytelling programme. Explore with students whether there are any specific aspects that are more difficult for them that they would like to revisit and revise.	Group discussion recapping the main targets and ideas from the previous sessions. Encourage students to summarise the main aims and content of the entire programme. The facilitator writes the ideas on a flipchart or whiteboard and adds important concepts that are omitted. It is important to allow the students to summarise the contents of the programme as this enables you to observe what has been learned and what requires further expansion and explanation. Encourage students to highlight specific areas of which they are unsure and revisit those specific areas. Ask students what they would like to focus on in this final session and allow for flexibility to ensure these areas or ideas are covered.	Flipchart or whiteboard, paper and pen. Story planner. All teaching notes from previous sessions.
To discuss the Mission to Achieve from the previous session discussing the **choice of book/s** chosen by students as their next reading material for pleasure.	Each student to give details about the **book** they have chosen which they will begin reading. This is a book that they will read for pleasure and can be any book of their choice. The students are to share their choice with the group and provide reasons for their decision. Other students may give their own opinions of the book if they have already read it. Encourage an open and free discussion. Students to identify what kind of book they have chosen, i.e. a fictional or non-fictional story, a romance, horror or thriller.	Story pencil. Flipchart or whiteboard, paper and pen. Book choices from students, and reasons for their choices.

 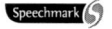

Aims	Method/Activities	Materials
To construct **personal narratives** for a favourite star and/or personality.	In this task, students have the opportunity to choose a favourite star and act as that star. This could be a famous pop star, an actor or actress, a singer, dancer, footballer, athlete, model, etc. Students should not tell the rest of the group who they are but each student will have the opportunity to share a personal narrative about the star, telling the story as if they are the star in question. For example, if one student chooses to be David Beckham, they would perhaps tell the story about leaving Real Madrid and Spain and moving to LA Galaxy in America with his family. The story could also contain the juicy gossip about why England did so poorly in the World Cup, and how David was kicked out of the England team. The student is to share a personal experience of the star that they are pretending to be, ensuring that their story consists of all the story components from the story planner. The group then have to try and guess who the star is from the personal narrative given.	Story planner. Story template form 1. Story template form 2. Story pencil or microphone.
To **revise main concepts, content areas** and strategies covered.	**Group quiz:** The facilitator asks the group questions about the content covered in the programme. This includes questions about the story planner and the elements that make up the planner, techniques for active listening, different types of stories, techniques for making a story more exciting, etc. The quiz should cover all content areas of the programme. Each student to adopt a special identifying sound as their 'buzzer' and the first student to know the answer to the question makes their specific sound and is called upon to answer the question. There is an eventual winner to the game who has answered the most questions correctly.	All materials used previously should be available as photocopies so that students can use them if they are unable to answer the questions asked. Flipchart or whiteboard, paper and pen.

Aims	Method/Activities	Materials
	The facilitator is to prepare and ask the questions. These should include a range of questions covering the content of the sessions. Refer to teaching notes for session 21 for suggested questions. If appropriate, students can also be given the opportunity to ask each member one or two questions about what they have learned. This further involves the students actively in the session. It is important to ensure that corrective feedback is given throughout the quiz. Do not accept incorrect answers but provide positive and constructive feedback.	Suggested questions for end of programme quiz in teaching notes.
To share with group members their **learning profiles** and feed back to the group on their current and future targets.	Provide opportunities for students to complete and share their learning profiles. Students will have begun this process as part of their Mission to Achieve from the last session. They are invited to think about what they have learned from the programme, whether they have met their targets, how they will use their new skills in school and at home, and what their future areas for development are. Group discussion around the areas of the learning profiles. Below are some specific areas to target for discussion that make up parts of the learning profiles.	Individual learning profiles of students. Flipchart or whiteboard, paper and pen.
To revisit the reasons for learning about stories and generate reasons from the students. For students to identify three specific ways that they will use the storytelling skills in their home, school and social settings.	Discuss with the students the **importance of stories and storytelling** and why they feel learning about stories is important to them. Get students to explore specifically how this knowledge will help them. Each student to identify three specific ways that they will use the new understanding of telling stories in school, home and other social settings. Students to use their completed learning profiles to support them during this discussion.	Flipchart or whiteboard, paper and pen. Individual student learning profiles.

 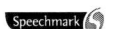

Aims	Method/Activities	Materials
To share three specific **skills** that they have learned from the sessions.	Students are to share **three specific skills or strategies** that they have learned from the storytelling programme. Explore with the students how they feel they have improved as storytellers. Encourage them to be specific about skills and knowledge learned. Students will find it helpful to answer these questions using their completed learning profiles. This is an opportunity to ensure that each group member feels empowered by the sessions and is able to explicitly identify the new skills they have learned which they can use at home and at school. This enhanced confidence will then hopefully be transferred to other learning contexts.	Flipchart or whiteboard, paper and pen. Completed individual learning profiles.
For students to provide two examples of how the other **group members have improved in storytelling**.	Group discussion: students to take turns in telling every group member how they have improved in areas of storytelling over the duration of the programme. This is to encourage positive reinforcement and acknowledgement by others. At this stage the group will have established themselves as a cohesive unit and will have worked together on storytelling for some time. They are therefore in an excellent position to comment on improvements made by their fellow group members – improvements and progress that sometimes students miss in their own performance. The facilitator should provide support and guidance during this process and ensure every member is given two positive comments.	Flipchart or whiteboard, paper and pen.
To share with group members the areas for future focus, attention and development, using	Students have the opportunity to discuss with the group the areas that continue to present some difficulties and challenges for them, and their plans to work on these areas in the future after the end of the programme.	Flipchart or whiteboard, paper and pen.

Aims	Method/Activities	Materials
their learning profiles.	Students should be encouraged not only to identify the areas they wish to focus on in the future, but also to identify how they will do this, and the support structures that they will draw upon to help them continue to work at enhancing their language and storytelling skills. The facilitator will support this discussion and provide ideas on how the students can extend their learning and what the most appropriate support structures will be after completion of the programme.	Completed individual learning profiles.
Mission to Achieve – future plans: Students to begin reading their chosen book, and to follow up on all the areas they wanted to explore further with regards to storytelling.	Students to be encouraged to see this programme as simply the start of their journey into learning and loving language, storytelling and communication. Encourage them to begin reading their chosen book, and to share their feelings and thoughts about the book with their peers. Remind them that the story planner and other story templates can be used effectively when they are telling or writing stories both in school and at home, and are secret weapons when doing homework! Encourage students to take home their narrative folders and revisit the themes and ideas from the programme. They should revisit their learning profile and follow up the themes and areas that they identified as needing further development. If appropriate, it may be possible to arrange a revision session for the group, or identify for the students someone at school they can go to if they have any further questions around storytelling. Students should not feel that this is the end of the road or that they do not have any follow-up support. If appropriate, problem solve with students ways of taking the programme further and using the principles in their school and home settings.	Students to keep their narrative folders.

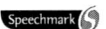

Evaluation of session/General comments

Teaching notes for Session 21

End of programme quiz

Conduct a fun quiz which explores the students' understanding of the contents of the entire programme. Play 'first on the buzzer' game where students adopt a specific sound which they make as soon as they have the answer to the specific questions. The winner is the person who answers the most questions. Please ensure that answers are discussed and corrective feedback is provided. It is important for students to get feedback so that they know the correct answers.

Here is a list of suggested questions for the quiz. You will want to add others. Also allow students to ask questions. Ensure that the questions cover the content of the programme:

- Define a fictional story

- Define a personal story

- What is the difference between an autobiography and a biography?

- Is an autobiography fiction or non-fiction?

- Give three examples of non-fiction

- Give three examples of fiction

- Name five different types of stories or story genres

- What are the three main elements of a story?

- What elements make up the beginning of a story?

- What elements make up the middle of a story?

- What elements make up the end of a story?

- Give five examples of possible settings for a story

- What is the climax of a story?

- What do we use to pause in written language?

- What is the story plot?

 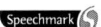

- Provide an example of alliteration

- What does the moral refer to?

- Name five behaviours which show that you are listening actively

- Name five ways of making the beginning of a story more interesting

- Where do you usually find the moral of the story?

- Name five ways of making the end of a story more interesting

- What is the title of a story?

- What is a narrative poem?

- What is a metaphor? Can you give an example?

- Give an example of a simile

- Name three authors that you know

- Name three poems that you know

- What should you think about when making up a title for your story?

- What do we call the person who writes a story?

- Give two similarities and two differences between prose and poetry

- What is a headline?

- What do we call someone who writes poems?

- What is the structure and rhyme sequence of a limerick?

- Give three examples of story poems

- What is alliteration?

- What does the illustrator do?

- Name five things you can do with your voice to make the telling of your story more exciting

- What is a good way of beginning a story?

- Give an example of hyperbole

- Name three ways of capturing an audience's attention

- What does figurative language or double meaning refer to?

- What is personification? Can you provide an example?

- Name three ways you can use your body language to make a story more exciting

- How can you make a written story look more exciting?

- Name three poets that you know

- What is onomatopoeia? Can you provide an example?

 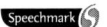

References

Applebee AN (1978) *The Child's Concept of Story: Ages Two To Seventeen*, University of Chicago Press, Chicago.

Beitchman JH, Wilson B, Johnson CJ, Atkinson L, Young A, Adlaf E, Escobar M and Douglas L (2001) 'Fourteen-year follow-up of speech/language-impaired and control children: psychiatric outcome', *Journal of the American Academy of Child and Adolescent Psychiatry*, 40, pp75–82.

Bercow J (2008) The Bercow Report: *A Review of Services for Children and Young People (0–19) With Speech, Language and Communication Needs*, DCSF, Nottingham.

Bishop DVM and Adams C (1990) 'A prospective study of the relationship between specific language impairment, phonological disorders and reading retardation', *Journal of Child Psychology and Psychiatry*, 31, pp1027–50.

Bishop DVM and Edmundson A (1987) 'Language impaired four-year-olds: distinguishing transient from persistent impairment', *Journal of Speech and Hearing Disorders*, 52, pp156–73.

Botting N and Conti-Ramsden G (2000) 'Social and behavioural difficulties in children with language impairment', *Child Language Teaching and Therapy*, 16, pp105–20.

Cirrin F and Gillam R (2008) 'Language intervention practices for school-age children with spoken language disorders: a systematic review', *Language, Speech, and Hearing Services in Schools*, 39, S110–S37.

Clegg J, Hollis C, Mawhood L and Rutter M (2005) 'Developmental language disorders a follow-up in later adult life. Cognitive, language and psychosocial outcomes', *Journal of Child Psychology and Psychiatry*, 46 (2), pp128–49.

Conti-Ramsden G, Durkin K, Simkin Z and Knox E (2009) 'Specific language impairment and school outcomes I: Identifying and explaining variability at the end of compulsory education', *International Journal of Language and Communication Disorders*, 44 (1), pp15–35.

Department for Education and Schools (2006) *National Statistics. First Release Special Educational Needs In England*, DfES, London.

Dockrell J and Lindsay D (2001) 'Children with specific speech and language difficulties – the teachers' perspective', *Oxford Review of Education*, 27 (3), pp369–92.

Durkin K and Conti-Ramsden G (2007) Language, social behavior, and the quality of friendships in adolescents with and without a history of specific language impairment', *Child Development*, 78 (5), pp1441–57.

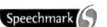

Durkin KZ, Simkin Z, Knox E and Conti-Ramsden G (2009) 'Specific language impairment and school outcomes II: educational context, student satisfaction and post-compulsory progress', *International Journal of Language and Communication Disorders*, 44 (1), pp36–55.

Fazio B, Naremore R and Connell P (1996) 'Tracking children from poverty at risk for specific language impairment: a 3-year longitudinal study', *Journal of Speech and Hearing Research*, 39, pp 611–24.

Gillam R, Loeb D, Hoffman L, Bohman T, Champlin, C, Thibodeau L, Widen J, Brandel J and Friel-Patti S (2008) 'The efficacy of fast forWord language intervention in school-age children with language impairment: a randomized controlled trial', *Journal of Speech, Language and Hearing Research*, 51, pp97–119.

Joffe VL (2006) 'Enhancing language and communication in language-impaired secondary school-aged children', Ginsborg J and Clegg J (eds), *Language and Social Disadvantage*, Wiley, London.

Joffe, VL (2008) 'Minding the gap in research and practice in developmental language disorders'. Joffe VL, Cruice M and Chiat S (eds), *Language Disorders in Children and Adults: New Issues in Research and Practice*, Wiley-Blackwell, Chichester.

Joffe VL, Cruice M and Chiat S (2008) 'Introduction: language disorders in children and adults: current themes, issues and connections', Joffe VL Cruice M and Chiat S (eds), *Language Disorders in Children and Adults: New Issues in Research and Practice*, Wiley-Blackwell, Chichester.

Johnson CJ, Beitchman JH and Brownlie EB (2010) 'Twenty-year follow-up of children with and without speech-language impairments: family, educational, occupational, and quality of life outcomes', *American Journal of Speech Language Pathology*, 19, pp51–65.

Law J, Lindsay G, Peacey N, Gascoigne M, Soloff N, Radford J and Band S (2000) *Provision for Children with Speech And Language Needs In England And Wales: Facilitating Communication Between Education and Health Services*, DfEE/DoH, London, research report 239.

Liles B (1993) 'Narrative discourse in children with language disorders and children with normal language: a critical review of the literature', *Journal of Speech and Hearing Research*, 36, pp868–82.

Liles BZ, Duffy RJ, Merritt DD and Purcell SL (1995) 'Measurement of narrative discourse ability in children with language disorders', *Journal of Speech and Hearing Research*, 38, pp415–25.

Lindsay G and Dockrell J (2000) 'The behaviour and self-esteem of children with specific speech and language difficulties', *British Journal of Educational Psychology*, 70, pp583–601.

Lindsay G, Dockrell J and Mackie C (2008a) 'Vulnerability to bullying and impaired social relationships in children with specific speech and language difficulties', *European Journal of Special Needs Education*, 23, pp1–16.

Lindsay G, Desforges M, Dockrell J, Law J, Peacey N and Beecham J (2008b) *Effective and Efficient Use of Resources in Services For Children and Young People with Speech, Language and Communication Needs*, DCSF, Nottingham, DCSF-RW053.

Meek M (1991) *On Being Literate*, Bodley Head, London.

Mello R (2001) 'The power of storytelling: how oral narrative influences children's relationships in classrooms', *International Journal of Education and the Arts* 2 (1), online, www.ijea.org (accessed June 2010).

Merritt DD and Liles BZ (1987) 'Story grammar ability in children with and without language disorder: story generation, story retelling and story comprehension', *Journal of Speech and Hearing Research*, 30, pp539–52.

Naremore R, Densmore A and Harman D (1995) *Language Intervention with School-Aged Children: Conversation, Narrative and Text*, Singular Publishing Group, San Diego.

Nippold M (1998) *Later Language Development. The School-Age and Adolescent Years*, Pro-Ed, Austin, Texas.

Nippold M (2004) 'Research on later language development: international perspectives' Berman RA (ed), *Language Development Across Childhood and Adolescence*, John Benjamins Publishing Company, Amsterdam.

Nippold M (2007) *Later Language Development. School-age Children, Adolescents, and Young Adults*, Pro-Ed, Austin, Texas.

Nippold M (2010a) *Language Sampling with Adolescents*, Plural Publishing, San Diego.

Nippold M (2010b) 'It's NOT too late to help adolescents succeed in school', *Language Speech and Hearing Services in Schools*, 41, pp137–8.

Peterson C (1990) 'The who, when and where of early narratives', *Journal of Child Language*, 17, pp433–55.

Sievers R (2005) 'Time to plug a shocking gap in service provision', *Bulletin: The Official Magazine of The Royal College of Speech and Language Therapists*, 643, p22.

Snow PC and Powell MB (2004) 'Developmental language disorders and adolescent risk: a public-health advocacy role for speech pathologists?' *Advances in Speech Language Pathology*, 6 (4), pp221–9.

Snowling MJ, Adams JW, Bishop DVM and Stothard SE (2001) 'Educational attainments of school leavers with a preschool history of speech-language impairments', *International Journal of Language and Communication Disorders*, 36 (2), pp173–83.

 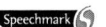

Snowling MJ, Bishop DVM, Stothard SE, Chipchase B and Kaplan C (2006) 'Psychosocial outcomes at 15 years of children with a preschool history of speech-language impairment', *Journal of Child Psychology and Psychiatry*, 47 (8), pp759–65.

Stein N and Glenn C (1979) 'An analysis of story comprehension in elementary school children', Freedle R (ed), *New Directions in Discourse Processing*, Erlbaum, Hillsdale, NJ.

Stothard S, Snowling M, Bishop D, Chipchase B and Kaplan C (1998) 'Language-impaired preschoolers: a follow-up into adolescence', *Journal of Speech, Language and Hearing Research*, 41, pp407–18.

Tomblin JB, Records N, Buckwalter P, Zhang X, Smith E and O'Brien M (1997) 'Prevalence of specific language impairment in kindergarten children', *Journal of Speech, Language and Hearing Research*, 40 (6), pp1245–69.

Van der Lely, HJK (1997) 'Narrative discourse in grammatical specific language impaired children: a modular language deficit?', *Journal of Child Language*, 24, pp221–56.

Wadman RK, Durkin K and Conti-Ramsden G (2008) 'Self-esteem, shyness and sociability in adolescents with specific language impairment (SLI)', *Journal of Speech Language and Hearing Research,* 51 (4), 938–52.

Wadman RK, Durkin K and Conti-Ramsden G (2011) 'Close relationships in adolescents with and without a history of specific language impairment', *Language Speech and Hearing Services in Schools*, 42, pp41–51.

Wells G (1986) *The Meaning Makers: Children Learning Language and Using Language to Learn*, Heinemann, Portsmouth.

References to stories

Books

Alcott LM (2003) *Little Women*, Chrysalis Classics, London.

Attenborough D (1984) *The Living Planet: A Portrait of the Earth*, Collins, London.

Attenborough D (1995) *The Private Life of Plants: A Natural History of Plant Behaviour*, BBC Books, London.

Attenborough D (1998) *The Life of Birds*, BBC Books, London.

Austen J (2003) *Pride and Prejudice*, Penguin Books Ltd, London.

Bach R (1973) *Jonathan Livingston Seagull: A Story*, Pan Books, London.

Banks LR (1999) *An Indian in the Cupboard*, Collins, London.

Beckham D (2004) *David Beckham: My Side – The Autobiography*, Harper Collins Willow, London.

Beckham T (2006) *David Beckham: My Son*, Pan Books, London.

Blume J (1980) *Are you there, G-D? It's Me, Margaret*, Pan Books, London.

Blume J (2001) *Blubber*, Macmillan, London.

Blyton E (1991) *Five go to Smuggler's Top,* Hodder and Stoughton, London.

Boyne J (2007) *The Boy in the Striped Pyjamas*, Black Swan Books, Random, London.

Brontë E (2006) *Wuthering Heights*, Penguin Classics, London.

Burnett FH (2002) *The Secret Garden*, Kingfisher Publications, London.

Burnett FH (2009) *A Little Princess*, Hodder Children's Books, London.

Carnegie D (2003) *How to Win Friends and Influence People*, Vermilion, London.

Carroll L (1946) *Alice's Adventures in Wonderland*, Puffin Books, London.

Carroll L (1994) *Through the Looking-Glass*, Puffin Books, London.

Cartland B (1976) *The Proud Princess*, Corgi Books, London.

Christie A (1959) *Murder on the Orient Express*, Fontana, London.

Cartland B (2009) *A Castle of Dreams*, Cartland Promotions, Great Britain.

Christie A (1959) *Murder on the Orient Express*, Fontana, London.

Christie A (1960) *Death on the Nile*, Fontana, London.

Christie A (1993) *The Murder of Roger Ackroyd*, Harper Collins, London.

Christie A (2001) *Cards on the Table*, Harper Collins, London.

 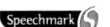

Cole C (2010) *Through My Eyes*, Bantam Press, London.

Collins T (2005) *Tony Blair*, Lerner Publications, Minneapolis.

Dahl R (2008) *Charlie and the Chocolate Factory*, Puffin Books, London.

Dahl R (2008) *James and the Giant Peach*, Puffin Books, London.

Dahl R (2008) *Matilda*, Puffin Books, London.

Dahl R (2008) *The Twits*, Puffin Books, London.

Dahl R (2008) *The Witches*, Puffin Books, London.

Defoe D (1981) *Robinson Crusoe*, Penguin Books, London.

Dickens C (1979) '*A Christmas Carol*, Cedric Chivers Ltd, Bath.

Dickens C (2000) *A Tale of Two Cities*, Penguin Books, London.

Dickens C (2003) *Hard Times*, Penguin Books, London.

Dickens C (2008) *The Haunted House*, Oneworld Classics Ltd, Surrey.

Doyle AC (1993) *The Case-Book of Sherlock Holmes*, Oxford University Press, Oxford.

Doyle AC (2006) *The Hound of the Baskervilles*, Headline Review, London.

Doyle AC (2007) *A Study in Scarlet*, Penguin Books, London.

Echols J (2007) *The Boys Next Door*, Simon Pulse Publication, New York.

Eliot G (2008) *Adam Bede*, Penguin Classics, London.

Fitzgerald FS (2006) *The Great Gatsby*, Penguin Books, London.

Fothergill A & Attenborough D (2007) *Planet Earth: As You've Never Seen It Before*, BBC Books, London.

Frank A (2008) *The Diary of A Young Girl*, Penguin Books, London.

Golding W (1958) *Lord of the Flies*, Faber, London.

Grafton S (1995) *K is for Killer*, Pan, London.

Hanson JR (2005) *First Man: The Life of Neil Armstrong*, Simon Schuster UK Ltd, London.

Hardy T (1998) *Tess of the d'Urbervilles*, Penguin, London.

Hemingway E (1978) *The Old Man and the Sea*, Heinemann, London.

Irving W (2007) *A History of the Life and Voyages of Christopher Columbus, Volume 2*, Kessinger Publishing LLC, MT.

Keller H (1990) *The Story of My Life*, Bantam Classics, New York.

King S (1975) *Carrie*, New English Library, London.

King S (1977) *The Shining*, Doubleday, New York.

Lalor B (1998) *Ireland: Blue Guide*, A&C Black Publishers Limited, London.

Lawson N (2007) *Nigella Express: Good Food Fast*, Chatto and Windus, London.

Lee H (1991) *To Kill a Mockingbird*, Minerva, London.

Lewis CS (1980) *The Lion, the Witch and the Wardrobe*, Collins, London.

Lindgren A (2002) *Pippi Longstocking*, Oxford University Press, Oxford.

London J (1989) *White Fang*, Tor Books, New York.

Lubrich O (ed) (2010) *Travels in the Reich, 1933–1945, Foriegn Authors Report from Germany*, The University of Chicago Press, Chicago.

McCall Smith A (2003) *The No. 1 Ladies' Detective Agency*, Abacus, London.

McKenna P (2006) *Instant Confidence: The Power to go for Anything you Want!* Bantam, London.

McKenna P (2007) *I Can Make You Rich*, Bantam, London.

Mandela N (1994) *Long Walk to Freedom: The Autobiography of Nelson Mandela*, Little, Brown and Company, London.

Marks G (2006) *Snatched*, Usborne Publishing, London.

Meyer S (2005) *Twilight*, Little, Brown and Company, New York.

Montgomery LM (1994) *Anne of Green Gables*, Puffin Books, London.

Morpurgo M (2007) *Born to Run*, Harper Collins, London.

Morton A (1997) *Diana: Her True Story*, Michael O'Mara Books Ltd, London.

Morton A (2003) *Posh and Becks*, Michael O'Mara Books Ltd, London.

Nesbit E (1991) *The Railway Children*, Oxford University Press, Oxford.

Orwell G (2003) *Animal Farm*, Penguin Books, London.

Oxford Atlas of the World: Seventeenth Edition (2010) Oxford University Press, New York.

Paxman J (2010) *The Victorians*, Random House Group Limited, London.

Pike A (2010) *Spells*, Harper Collins, London.

Price K (2005) *Being Jordan: My Autobiography*, Blake Publishing, London.

Ramsay G (2001) *Gordon Ramsay's Just Desserts*, Quadrille Publishing Ltd, London.

Rowling JK (1999) *Harry Potter and the Chamber of Secrets*, Bloomsbury, London.

Rowling JK (2000) *Harry Potter and the Goblet of Fire*, Bloomsbury, London.

Sachar L (2000) *Holes,* Bloomsbury Publishing, London.

Sanderson G (2009) *Cheryl Cole: Her Story – an Unauthorized Biography*, Michael O'Mara Books Ltd, London.

Sewell A (2001) *Black Beauty*, Kingfisher Publications, London.

Shakespeare W (1980) *Hamlet, Penguin, London*

 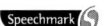

Shakespeare W (2004) *Romeo and Juliet,* Bantam Books, New York.

Stephens P (2004) *Tony Blair: The Making of a World Leader,* Viking, New York.

Stevenson RL (1996) *The Strange Case of Dr Jekyll and Mr Hyde*, Puffin Classics, London.

Stevenson RL (2008) *Treasure Island*, One World Classics, London.

Stevenson RL (2009) *Kidnapped*, Puffin Books, London.

Stoker B (1993) *Dracula*, Wordsworth Editions Limited, Hertfordshire.

Tolkien JRR (1978) *Lord of the Rings*, Unwin Paperbacks, London.

Twain M (2008) *Adventures of Huckleberry Finn*, Puffin Classics, London.

Weir A (2007) *The Six Wives of Henry VIII*, Vintage Books, London.

Wilde O (1989) *Salome*, Faber, London.

Wilde O (1995) *The Importance of Being Earnest*, Penguin Books, London.

Wilson J (1999) *Buried Alive*, Corgi Yearling Books, Random House, London.

Wilson J (2008) *Kiss*, Corgi, London.

Wilson J (2006) *The Story of Tracey Beaker*, Yearling Books, London.

Zindel P (1978) *My Darling, My Hamburger*, Fontana, London.

Poems

Belloc H (2000) 'Matilda who told lies, and was burned to death', *The Nation's Favourite Poems of Childhood*, BBC Worldwide Limited, London.

Causley C (1999) '*I saw a jolly hunter*', Rhys-Jones G (ed), *The Nation's Favourite Twentieth Century Poems,* BBC Worldwide Limited, London.

Day Lewis C (2000) 'Walking away. For Sean', *The Nation's Favourite Poems of Childhood*, BBC Worldwide Limited, London.

De La Mare W (1996) 'The listeners', *The Nation's Favourite Poems of Childhood*, BBC Worldwide Limited, London.

Duffy CA (2000) 'Chocs', *The Nation's Favourite Poems of Childhood*, BBC Worldwide Limited, London.

Frost R (1996) 'The road not taken', *The Nation's Favourite Poems*, BBC Worldwide Limited, London.

Hardy T (1996) 'The darkling thrush', *The Nation's Favourite Poems*, BBC Worldwide Limited, London.

Joseph J (1996) 'Warning', *The Nation's Favourite Poems*, BBC Worldwide Limited, London.

Lear E (1996) 'The owl and the pussy-cat', *The Nation's Favourite Poems of Childhood*, BBC Worldwide Limited, London.

Milligan S (1968) 'On the Ning Nang Nong', *Silly Verse for Kids*, Penguin Books, London.

Noyes A (1996) 'The highwayman', *The Nation's Favourite Poems of Childhood*, BBC Worldwide Limited, London.

Owen W (1996) 'Dulce et decorum est', *The Nation's Favourite Poems*, BBC Worldwide Limited, London.

Patten B (2000) 'Gust becos I could not spel', *The Nation's Favourite Poems of Childhood*, BBC Worldwide Limited, London.

Silverstein S (2001) 'Kidnapped!!!', Sweeney M (ed), *The New Faber Book of Children's Poems*, Faber & Faber, London.

Smith S (1996) 'Not waving but drowning', *The Nation's Favourite Poems*, BBC Worldwide Limited, London.

Wordsworth W (1996) 'Daffodils', *The Nation's Favourite Poems*, BBC Worldwide Limited, London.

Limericks

Carroll L (1983) Parrott EO (ed), *The Penguin Book of Limericks*, Penguin Books, London.

Lear E (1983) Parrott EO (ed), T*he Penguin Book of Limericks*, Penguin Books, London.

Lear E (1984) *The Nonsense Verse of Edward Lear,* Penguin Books, London.

Marquis D (1983) Parrott EO (ed), *The Penguin Book of Limericks*, Penguin Books, London.

Monkhouse C (1983) Parrott EO (ed), *The Penguin Book of Limericks*, Penguin Books, London.

Rossetti GR (1983) Parrott EO (ed), *The Penguin Book of Limericks*, Penguin Books: London.

Stevenson RL (1983) Parrott EO (ed), *The Penguin Book of Limericks*, Penguin Books, London.

 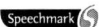

Appendix 1

Narrative checklist

NAME: _____ DATE: _____

SEX: _____ SCHOOL: _____

TESTER: _____ D.O.B: _____

'I am going to ask you some questions about telling stories. Tell me as much as you can for each question. When answering, think about all the stories you may have heard, read, watched on television or told'.

1 Tell me in your own words what a story is.

> Response

2 Can you give me four examples of famous stories that you have heard or read? So, for example, you could say *Little Red Riding Hood* or *Black Beauty*.

1

2

3

4

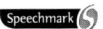

3 What different types of stories are there, for instance, a detective story?

Response

4 Can you name as many different parts that make up a story?

Response

5 Can you tell me a good way to begin a story?

Response

6 Can you tell me a really good way to end a story?

Response

7 Can you tell me three different ways that you can make a story more exciting?

1

2

3

8 Can you give me an example of how to get someone's attention when you are telling them a story?

Response

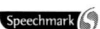

9 What does the 'climax' of a story mean?

Response

10 What are some of the important things that you should do when listening to someone tell a story?

Response

11 Can you name any tour literary devices that you can find in stories?

Response

1

2

3

4

12 Can you explain what a cliffhanger means?

Response

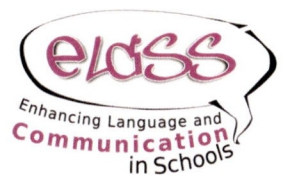

An overview of the Enhancing Language and Communication in Secondary Schools (ELCISS) research programme

The narrative intervention programme was originally part of a research project funded by the Nuffield Foundation. The research programme was entitled: 'Enhancing language and communication in secondary school students (ELCISS) with language and communication impairments through two intervention programmes: narrative and vocabulary enrichment.' The aims of the research programme were to:

- Describe the nature and type of language and communication difficulties in secondary school age students.

- Investigate and compare the effectiveness of two language intervention programmes (narrative and vocabulary enrichment), delivered by teaching assistants, on the language and communication of a group of year 8 and year 9 (12–13 years) secondary school students identified as having language and communication difficulties.

- Train teaching and support staff on speech, language and communication difficulties, and on using language strategies to enhance language and communication in the classroom, and hence build capacity within the existing schools.

Preliminary results of the ELCISS Research Programme

The focus of the ELCISS programme was two-pronged: delivery of language intervention support (storytelling and vocabulary enrichment) by teaching assistants to secondary school students with significant SLCN, as well as a structured whole school training programme on speech, language and communication to raise awareness, knowledge and skills in this area across mainstream schools. Preliminary results of the research suggest substantial positive outcomes for the students, teaching assistants who delivered the training and schools who participated in the knowledge transfer workshops.

Initial data analysis indicates significant differential improvement by the students in areas of language targeted by the interventions. This means that students who participated in the **narrative intervention** performed better on measures of **narrative** than the control group, who received no training, at post intervention, a finding not evident with the students in the vocabulary group. As a result of this intervention, students told more interesting stories using more story components. They also showed improved knowledge around what it entails to tell a 'good story'.

Conversely, the same pattern was observed with vocabulary knowledge in the group of students

 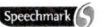

receiving the **vocabulary enrichment intervention**. These students scored higher at post intervention on measures of **vocabulary** than students in the control group who did not receive any intervention.

Therefore, students attending the narrative training scored more highly on narrative measures compared with a control group at post intervention, and students receiving the vocabulary intervention scored better on vocabulary measures compared with the control group. These findings therefore suggest that the interventions were effective at enhancing the language and communication of secondary school students with speech, language and communication difficulties. It is important to note that these improvements were specific to the group receiving the targeted intervention. This evidence is encouraging and shows the positive impact of both the narrative and vocabulary intervention programmes in enhancing narrative and vocabulary ability respectively in a group of secondary school students with SLCN.

What has been said about the ELCISS research programme?

Feedback about the ELCISS programme and specifically the two interventions has been extremely positive, and provides further evidence for the benefits of the ELCISS intervention programmes from the perspectives of the students, teaching staff, teaching assistants and representatives from the local education authorities of the participating boroughs. Some examples of this feedback are presented below:

The children

The children reported benefits in the areas of **language ability** ('I really liked the storytelling best, it helps me with my talking and I hope we are going to do it again' and 'It helped me to bring out my language properly and I enjoyed it too'); and **self-esteem** and **social skills** ('I felt confident and started socialising more', 'Didn't have to **worry** about getting something wrong', 'Working in a team' and 'Helping me understand people'). Other comments from the students participating in the programme include:

'I enjoyed the project and learned a lot. I used to feel nervous but now I can express myself much more' (Student G)

'I thought it was good because it taught me to concentrate and listen more' (Student D)

'…I liked when we learned what autobiography and fiction and non-fiction is. I know how to put a story in order. I've learned a lot of new words: autobiography, biography, fiction, non-fiction' (Student Sh)

'I really learned a lot about the stories and I improved on how to describe characters and the beginning and end of a story' (Student M)

'I liked the story making also when we had to read the story. I also liked the card games because we had to make up stories using cards' (Student L)

'[It was] fun because we told our stories that happened to us' (Student BM)

'I liked the games and it helped me to work things better and it's a shame it's finished now' (Student J)

'It was fun and I would tell anyone who got the chance to do it. I would like to do it again' (Student KA)

'It was really good and now I am able to understand more and have more confidence when I am talking to people' (Student S)

'It helped me to bring out my language properly and I enjoyed it too' (Student KE)

'I really enjoyed it and the activities were fun. I would like to do it again' (Student P)

'I found some of it quite hard but it was fun too and you learn stuff' (Student Th)

'It was quite good and I liked the puzzle bits. I think it has helped my English too' (Student R)

'I thought it was fun to do and Miss was really helpful. I wish I could carry on with it' (Student N)

'I really enjoyed all the activities and games and doing work just by myself. In class the teachers are busy and they don't give you enough attention and I don't always understand what I have to do.' (Student T)

'I liked it because it is a fun way of learning' (Student JA)

'Didn't have to worry about getting something wrong. No pressure' (Student JG)

 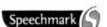

'I liked beening [being] in a group and Talking about stuff' (Student MK)

'I liked making storys because it was fun and making a story on the spot' (Student CL)

'It was fun. We learned a lot of things that are useful' (Student JB)

'I learned how to write better stories. Good words. Discriptive [descriptive] words' (Student Ha)

'It was fun. I learned a lot of things! Some of my English levels have gone up… You meet new people. It has help[ed] me with English and how to cope with over [other] people' (Student Ge)

'I liked meeting and knowing [finding] out more about the people I see around the school. I also liked working in a team. Also showing how myself and others are simu[i]lar' (Student KP)

The teachers

'Over the last three years the school has been involved in the "Enhancing Language and Communication in Secondary Schools" project. The 22 students identified to participate in this initiative have made outstanding progress in their literacy skills which has impacted on their attainment across all curriculum areas. Progress has been measured in terms of NC (National Curriculum) Levels attained at the end of the Key Stage. The TA trained to deliver the Speech and Language interventions has benefited in terms of her ability to impact on the learning of students in addition to progressing in her own professional development. She has now gained HLTA (higher level teaching assistant) status. The school now wishes to increase capacity and sustainability in order to ensure that all learners benefit from the Speech and Language strategies through improved "Quality First Teaching". The benefits of ELCISS are such that the school wishes to embed the Speech, Communication and Language strategies within the teaching culture of the classroom.'

Michelle, Assistant Head Teacher and SENCO (Special Educational Needs Coordinator)

'Each student has absolutely loved being part of the project and they often come and ask when it is their turn again. "Being noticed" has already been a major strength of the success of this project. The children realise this and are all very appreciative of what has been done so far for them. They were unanimous in their response to the ELCISS project and could not stop praising the positive impact the project has had on their learning experience at school. They all felt that it had helped them gain confidence, enabling them to approach their learning in a much more positive manner. The strategies taught in the small groups as part of the intervention were useful and easily applied in all their lessons. All these students have looked forward to each session and thoroughly enjoyed participating. The parents have fully supported this project and we have received excellent feedback from all of them. They are enormously grateful that their children have been identified and chosen to participate in such a positive and successful intervention programme. They have all commented on the confidence their children have gained and the enjoyment they have experienced throughout each session. Most parents stated that their children's views towards school have been transformed as a result of this intervention programme. As a school we too have noticed what an amazing transformation the ELCISS project has made to our students.'

   (Anita, Deputy SENCO)

The following quotes are from SENCOs at the secondary schools involved in the ELCISS programme and were collected anonymously by the local education authorities.

'The ELCISS programme has highlighted the importance of this area of need. We have been able to develop a focused LSA (Learning Support Assistant) lead and we have a well thought through intervention. It has been a very useful framework to train LSAs in small group intervention work.'

   (SENCO A)

'We plan on continuing to use this as an intervention group. Students' understanding will affect their ability to access the curriculum and academic performance.'

   (SENCO B)

'Groups enjoyed it very much and felt a sense of achievement and…the impact it has had (on) the LSA's in the school and their confidence to deliver specific programmes.'

   (SENCO C)

'The materials are a very valuable resource.'

   (SENCO D)

'ELCISS has raised an awareness of problems that students with language and communication difficulties face. ELCISS offers the opportunity to test strategies that might help those students. Selected students have had the chance to receive language therapy sessions in small groups, using many picture prompts and other visual material.'

   (SENCO E)

 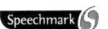

'Lesson plans and materials can be used in future across the school. Also it is possibly beneficial for work with EAL (English as an additional language) students.'

(SENCO F)

'Overall it has contributed to strengthening the students' self-confidence and has given strategies to become a more independent learner.'

(SENCO G)

'The material is very good with detailed lesson plans and a clear structure. What has been previously learnt is reinforced throughout the programme. Word maps/story planner etc are particularly useful and pictures help to engage the students and allow for enjoyable activities and caters for different learning styles.'

(SENCO H)

The teaching assistants

The teaching assistants reported feeling more confident helping other children in the classroom, after conducting the intervention sessions, as well as more confident working with the teachers. Our data from the training with teaching assistants shows the limited understanding they had around the areas of speech, language and communication, even with regards to basic definitions of language and communication. The training has resulted in a significant increased awareness of speech, language and communication and in methods and strategies to support students with SLCN in the classroom.

Feedback from the participating TAs included:

'The training has given me the knowledge and understanding to effectively support students with language and communication impairments. It has also given me greater insight into understanding the difficulties students encompass in all aspects of their everyday lives. I have been able to give students the strategies they need to make learning more accessible to them and to make learning fun. The students involved have benefited greatly from being part of the programme and being part of a small group learning new skills. Some have gained more confidence in social situations and are happier in class because of this. Others have gained academically as well. This can be seen in their achievements on the progress tracker for their year group. They are also finding it easier to access parts of the curriculum that previously they struggled with. Furthermore, the training has aided greatly my personal development. It will enable me to not only pass my skills onto the students but to share them with the staff as well. By sharing my knowledge and skills with other teachers I will be making them aware of communication and language impairment. This will greatly influence the teaching given by them. I will also be able to continue to use the resources in the packs as a teaching aid for communication and language impaired children.'

(Sharon, TA)

'I am a Specialist Teaching Assistant…and I work with students in Years seven to eleven. I have been interested in language and communication difficulties in children for a long while and have been on several courses involving the subject. Whilst they were informative none of them ever provided me with strategies or skills to support these children in a more positive way. When I was given the opportunity by the City University team to take part in the ELCISS study I was delighted.

The students taking part really enjoyed their time in our sessions and they knew they were learning as well. They loved being part of a small group where they were able to "express themselves" as one student told me. They knew that if they said something wrong they would not be laughed at. They got the chance to discuss and to evaluate what we were doing. These are the children that are great at fading into the background so as not to be noticed and asked to contribute. It really became apparent to me how much the children's language and communication skills had improved when we had some visitors to meet and talk to them. Not only has this project helped the children taking part I feel it has helped all the children I support in lessons.'

(Pat, TA)

'It [ELCISS] has been a turning point in my career, the fantastic training given to all participating TA's has given me an in-depth understanding of the needs of students with Speech, Language and Communication Needs (SLCN), and up to now, there has been a lack of relevant programmes and strategies available for secondary school students to help them overcome these difficulties.

I have witnessed the impact this therapy has had on these students. In addition to enhancing language and vocabulary skills; ELCISS has helped with the broader, sometimes immeasurable aspects of education such as debating, problem solving, accepting their own and others' differences through effective communication. It has shown that the most disengaged students, that are all too typically seen on the wrong side of the classroom door, have not only been offered, but have embraced the opportunity to access learning through communication, verbal participation, effective visual resources and the use of all the senses, to name but a few strategies. The well researched, curriculum based lesson plans and teaching notes within the ELCISS packs ensure this. It is evident, through whole school activities that the students have responded well to the sessions. The most negative of learners, at first convinced that they did not need to be there, did in fact, engage, enjoy and indeed learn.

I was excited about the project at my first involvement but now that I have been part of delivering the ELCISS sessions and have seen students' progress, ELCISS has exceeded even my expectations. I feel both grateful and proud to be involved in this wonderful project.'

(Tracey, TA)

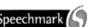

'I think the students will make a lot more progress in all of their subjects with the strategies that are provided in the groups…I have taken great pleasure in being involved with this course. I have learnt a great deal myself, as much as the students.'

(Jane D, TA)

'The material was explained/delivered in a fun, motivational way. The project appears comprehensive and covers what will enhance the students' learning.'

(Jean, TA)

'The story telling I think to me was the most valuable, a child can express so much through storytelling.'

(Jayne, TA)

'The sessions were full of useful and practical schemes – the students were constantly motivated and keen. This programme covered so much that is relevant to mainstream English and school life.'

(Jean R, TA)

'Thank you for allowing me to take part in something that I feel the students have gained so much benefit from.'

(Nicola, TA)

School/local education authorities

'The impact of ELCISS has been far reaching with large numbers of TAs trained to deliver SLT programmes. There will be a huge knock on effect for us as the confidence of our TAs has increased to such an extent that we will be able to develop their skills of delivery even further and ass their knowledge and experience onto other members of staff. It has raised the profile of S CNs in schools not only with the TAs but also with whole school staff, which will have an effect on th perception of SLCNs as a whole school issue. The opportunity for further work would be wel omed by all our secondary schools as they found it to be such a worthwhile programme to be invol d in.'

(Sen r SEN Advisor, LEA)

'I am writi g to extend my thanks to you and your team following the success of the Enhancing Language nd Communication in Secondary Schools project…It is evident that the dissemination of skills and knowledge through the project has gone from strength to strength. Staff in secondary schools are demonstrating greater knowledge, awareness and understanding of SLCN issues and the implications for pupils in their classrooms. It is evident that the success of the project has been far reaching because schools are requesting whole school training…This also includes a training request from the special school that has pupils with social, emotional and behavioural difficulties which demonstrates a developing understanding of [the] impact of language and communication on pupil behaviour. Language and communication are essential skills for young people to possess for their health, well-being and participation in society. Participating in the project with you and your team has been fundamental to the LA [Local Authority] engaging in the debate about effective provision for SLCN that has led us to think creatively about developing our existing workforce. Furthermore…we have also recognised an unmet need for secondary aged pupils who are experiencing difficulties with speech, language and communication. We would be extremely keen to continue with the programme…with all our secondary schools. We feel that developing the skills of staff to provide effective quality first teaching and communication friendly schools will enable effective identification and provision for those students who require targeted interventions.'

  (Annita, SEN manager, LEA)

'The Local Authority has been involved in the above, very innovative, project…Feedback from the schools, parents and young people has been extremely encouraging. Parents have seen positive progress. Staff have reported that the materials are of high quality and have enabled them to be effective in supporting individual pupils through developing their skills and understanding of speech, language and communication needs. The Local Authority has valued the project because of its high engagement of schools and the positive progress of children and young people with communication needs. We would like to continue and extend the project.'

  (Ann, Group manager inclusion, LEA)

"Enhancing Language and Communication in Secondary Schools" has been a valuable project with high quality training and materials. It has had a positive impact in raising the profile of speech, language and communication skills in secondary school for children and young people whose needs have long been neglected or unidentified. Without this programme these children and young people are unlikely to achieve the outcomes of the "Every Child Matters" agenda. It has had a noticeable impact on staff skill, knowledge and confidence both at the individual and whole school level. Pupils have responded positively to the materials and are using the strategies and skills taught in the wider context. Parents report positive progress in communication and confidence. The Local Authority Education Inclusion Team has welcomed the support that this project has provided. It has highlighted the speech, language and communication needs of pupils previously identified as having behavioural or literacy difficulties. It has created an interest that will accelerate the process of change and begin to address the communication needs of secondary age pupils, enhancing their life opportunities.'

  (Karen, Coordinator Speech and Language Needs, LEA)

 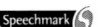